BASIC NUTRITION AND
DIET THERAPY

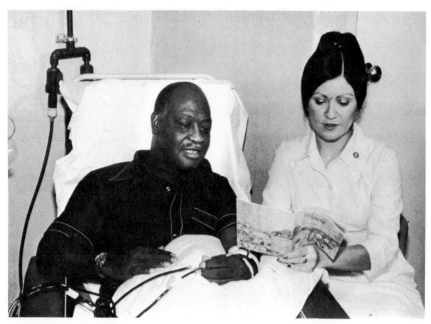

Veterans Administration Medical Center, Washington, D.C.

FOURTH EDITION

BASIC NUTRITION
AND
DIET THERAPY

CORINNE H. ROBINSON

M.S., D.Sc. (Hon.), R.D.

Professor of Nutrition Emeritus.
Formerly, Head, Department of Nutrition
and Food, Drexel University, Philadelphia

MACMILLAN PUBLISHING CO., INC.

NEW YORK

COLLIER MACMILLAN PUBLISHERS

LONDON

MACMILLAN PUBLISHING CO., INC.
866 Third Avenue, New York, New York 10022

COLLIER MACMILLAN CANADA, LTD.

Figures 5–1, 8–2, 9–2, 9–3, 11–1, 12–2, 12–3, 12–4, and 12–5 herein are reproduced from C. H. Robinson and M. R. Lawler, *Normal and Therapeutic Nutrition,* 15th ed. (New York: Macmillan Publishing Co., Inc., 1977).

Library of Congress Cataloging in Publication Data

Robinson, Corinne Hogden.
  Basic nutrition and diet therapy.

  Includes bibliographies and index.
  1. Diet therapy. 2. Nutrition. I. Title.
[DNLM: 1. Diet therapy. 2. Nutrition. WB400.3 R658b]
RM216.R652 1980   613.2   79–14678
ISBN 0–02–402450–3

Printing: 1 2 3 4 5 6 7 8   Year: 0 1 2 3 4 5 6

PREFACE TO THE FOURTH EDITION

The aim of the fourth edition of this textbook is to present the fundamental principles and practices that are essential in nutritional care to maintain health, to prevent illness, and to provide support and therapy during illness. It is intended especially for students of practical and vocational nursing, associate-degree nursing, dietetic technology, and other health-related fields. The book is also useful for the layman who desires a basic understanding of nutrition so that he can make appropriate choices for himself and his family.

The American public today has an unprecedented interest in nutrition and in the food supply. Technical and professional health personnel must be able to provide factual information, and to recognize areas that remain controversial. Throughout this book some of the major concerns of the public have been addressed, such as the controversies regarding sugar and fat and their effect on health; the role of fiber; the advantages and problems associated with vegetarianism; vitamin supplementation and megadoses; the uses of additives; and food labeling and regulation of the food supply.

The 1979 Recommended Dietary Allowances are included in Chapter 4 and in each of the chapters pertaining to the nutrients. Clinical problems associated with imbalanced nutrient intake have been highlighted in each of the chapters of Unit II, "The Nutrients."

The Dietary Goals developed by the Senate Select Committee on Nutrition and Human Needs in 1977 have been adopted by many Americans and criticized by others. They are presented along with other dietary guidelines in Chapter 4. Their application to food selection is discussed in chapters pertaining to fats (Chapter 6), carbohydrates (Chapter 7), energy metabolism (Chapter 8), and meal planning (Chapter 13).

Two new chapters appear in Unit IV, "Diet Therapy." Chapter 19, "Nutrition Education and Dietary Counseling," presents a discussion of ways the technical health worker as well as professional health personnel can contribute substantially to nutrition education of the layman. Chapter 31, "Nutrition and Diet in Cancer," describes the importance of nutrition for the wellbeing of the patient, some problems associated with food intake, and some suggestions for alleviating these problems.

The 1976 Exchange Lists for Meal Planning are presented in Table A-2 and are used in the calculation of modified diets (Chapters 21, 22, and 23). Other recent developments in diet therapy have been included: behavioral modification in weight control; dietary modifications for the types of hyperlipidemias; high-fiber diet; and meeting nutritional needs in surgical conditions.

The Appendix includes two new tables: Table A-6, "Some Examples of Drug and Food/Nutrient Interactions," and Table A-7, "Proprietary Formulas for Oral and Tube Feedings."

The users of the earlier editions of this book—students and faculty alike—have contributed valuable suggestions that are incorporated into the current edition. They are sincerely appreciated. Materials and photographs have been supplied through the generosity of private and public agencies and personal acquaintances. For new illustrations in this edition the author is especially grateful to Dr. Susan Calvert, Director, Nutrition Services, Ross Laboratories; Mr. Alvin S. Goodman, Director, Publications Division, Bureau of Public Education, Commonwealth of Pennsylvania; Ms. Marilyn R. Lawler, University of Minnesota and Metropolitan Hospital, Minneapolis; Ms. Evelyn Davis McCormick, Nutritionist-Manager, Gerber Products Company; and Ms. Edna S. Strand, Director, Dietetic Service, Veterans Administration, Washington, D.C.

Dr. Glenn A. Robinson, my son, has given useful suggestions, and has been enthusiastic and supportive throughout the course of the preparation of this edition.

For the first three editions of this book it has been a privilege to have the guidance of Miss Joan C. Zulch, Executive Editor, Medical Books Department of Macmillan. She has given unstintingly of her professional skills and time, and her ideas have led to innovations with each edition. I especially treasure a friendship with Miss Zulch that has grown with the years.

Mr. John J. Beck, Macmillan Publishing Company, has assumed the role of editor beginning with this edition. His suggestions and cooperation are sincerely appreciated.

Corinne H. Robinson

CONTENTS

APPENDIXES

APPENDIX A

TABLE

APPENDIX B

BASIC NUTRITION AND DIET THERAPY

INTRODUCTION TO FOOD AND NUTRITION— INDIVIDUAL AND COMMUNITY GOALS

1

FOOD, NUTRITION, AND HEALTH

POPULAR INTEREST IN FOOD

People of all ages and all socioeconomic groups are keenly interested in food, and concerned about its wholesomeness, nutritive qualities, and cost. These interests have an almost unlimited range. More and more people are again preparing food "from scratch" in the belief that these foods are better for them. Gourmet foods and cooking schools appeal to some who are affluent. Health professionals are especially concerned about ways to feed families adequately in these days of inflation. Those on limited income seek to stretch their food dollar. Many people are involved in legislation that promotes nutrition programs for vulnerable groups.

The environmental movement has changed the way many people think about food. Are chemical fertilizers as good as manures and plant composts for producing nutritious foods? What are the benefits and risks of using pesticides? What is the best use of land and water resources to produce food? Can we justify such great use of animal protein foods in the western world when most of the world's people have too little food? Can vegetarian diets be planned to meet nutritional needs?

Some people are also worried about the effects of food processing. What are the nutritive values of canned, frozen, dehydrated, refined, and fortified foods? Are vitamin-mineral supplements needed? Why are so many additives used in food processing? How can we be sure these additives are safe?

Food habits are constantly changing. "Fast foods," "junk foods," "snack foods," "convenience foods"—what are their nutritive values? Many nutritionists and physicians believe we are consuming too many calories, too much fat,

3

too much cholesterol, too much sugar, too much salt, and too little fiber. What is the evidence that these excesses are related to many chronic diseases? What are some ways by which nutritional balance can be achieved?

Perhaps you can think of other questions that you have about the foods you eat, and about nutrition. To find the answers to so many questions is indeed a challenge. Your study of nutrition will give you the background for answering many questions. You will also find that there remain many unanswered questions; that there are several answers to some questions; and that you must keep an open mind for new information as it becomes available from nutrition and food scientists.

THE MANY SIDES OF FOOD

From birth to death food is a dominant factor in our lives. In a single year, on a three-meal-a-day basis, most of us eat well over 1000 meals. We know that the food we eat is necessary for our very being—we know it provides the energy for the quiet breathing at night and the full activity of the day—we know too that it builds, maintains, and regulates muscles and bones, nerves and brain, eyes, hair, and all our physical being.

But food does much more than nourish, for most of us enjoy eating. Food makes us feel secure and happy; we use food as a link in our friendships, as an expression of pleasure during our holidays, and as a symbol of our religious life.

Food is the world's biggest business. A large part of the world's work is concerned with the growing, processing, and preparation of food. We spend an important amount of our income for food. In the United States and in other highly developed countries there is food in abundance and variety.

Most of the world's people spend the greater part of their working days and most of their income for food. In some countries of the world three fourths or more of the working population is directly concerned with growing food; yet it seldom manages to grow quite enough. Tonight millions of the world's people will go to bed more or less hungry. Is it any surprise that these people are discontented, diseased, and die an early death?

From this brief introduction you can see that good nutrition depends upon the understanding, knowledge, and cooperation of many people. Good nutrition alone cannot guarantee good health, but without good nutrition health cannot be at its best.

SOME DEFINITIONS

Before we can begin the study of nutrition, some definitions need to be made.

Food is that which nourishes the body. No two foods are alike in their ability to nourish, because no two foods contain identical amounts of nutrients.

Nutrients are those 50 or more chemical substances in food that are needed by the body. They are divided into six classes: proteins and amino acids; fats and fatty acids; carbohydrates; mineral elements; vitamins; and water.

Nutrition refers to the processes in the body for making use of food. It includes eating the correct kinds and amounts of foods for the body's needs; digestion of foods so that the body can use the nutrients; absorption of the nutrients into the bloodstream; use of the individual nutrients by the cells in the body for the production of energy, the maintenance and growth of cells, tissues, and organs; and elimination of wastes.

Nutritional care is the application of the art and science of nutrition to the feeding of people. It deals with the assessment of nutritional status; the planning of meals according to physiologic and psychologic needs at any stage in the life cycle; the implementation of the plan through the preparation and service of meals; the education that is necessary so that individuals may apply the principles of nutrition to their daily needs; and the continuous evaluation so that changes can be made as situations require. Nutritional care is personalized for each individual, but the concepts of nutritional care also involve everyone in a group situation.

GOOD AND POOR NUTRITION

Nutritional status is the condition of health as it is related to the use of food by the body. It is evident in some very obvious ways we can all see, such as changes in weight. However, an accurate measure of nutritional status can be made only by the expert examination that a physician can give and through a variety of blood and urine tests. Some contrasts in good and poor nutrition are listed in Table 1–1. You should remember that other reasons for poor health might be lack of sleep, poor sanitation, poor housing, and so on.

NUTRITION AS A SCIENCE

Throughout all of history man has written about food and its effects on the body. Ancient Egyptian writings on tablets of stone record the use of food for the treatment of numerous diseases. In the Old Testament of the Bible we can learn much about the foods available to the Jewish people, the religious symbolism of food, and the laws governing the use of food. Hippocrates, the famous Greek physician who lived several hundred years before Christ, wrote of the proper foods for treating disease. He observed, "Persons who are naturally very fat are apt to die earlier than those who are slender." [1] The thinking of Hippocrates, Galen, and other philosophers governed the whole practice of medicine down through the Middle Ages.

---

[1] G. Lusk, *Nutrition* (New York: Paul B. Hoeber, Inc., 1933), p. 8.

TABLE 1-1 SOME CONTRASTS IN NUTRITION

Good Nutrition	Poor Nutrition
Normal weight for height, body frame, and age	Overweight; underweight; failure to grow; sudden loss of weight
Erect posture; arms and legs straight; abdomen in; chest up; chin in	Poor posture: chest forward; rounded shoulders, protruding abdomen
Firm, strong muscles; moderate padding of fat	Thin, flabby muscles, lack of padding of fat, or excessive fat
Firm, clear skin with good color; healthy, pink mucous membranes	Dry, scaly, pale skin; pale mucous membranes
Well-formed jaw and even teeth	Poorly formed jaw with teeth poorly aligned
Soft, glossy hair	Dull, dry hair
Clear, bright eyes, not unduly sensitive to light	Dull eyes, sensitive to light; burning, itching; circles and puffiness under eyes
Good appetite and digestion	Poor appetite; complaints of indigestion; diarrhea; constipation
Abundance of energy and endurance	Listlessness, fatigue, and lack of endurance
Resistance to disease	Many infections; longer convalescence from disease
Ability to concentrate	Short attention span
Cooperative, interested, agreeable, cheerful	Irritable, apathetic, worried, depressed

People have learned through the ages that some foods were more nourishing than others, and that some plants were, in fact, poisonous and could not be eaten. Along with this experience a great deal of superstition about foods also arose. Some of these false notions are believed even today by many people.

The science of nutrition developed only after the groundwork had been laid for the sciences of chemistry and physiology, and had its beginnings in the late eighteenth century—just about the time of the American Revolution. Most of the understanding of the functions of the nutrients in the body, the nutritive values of foods, the body's requirements for nutrients, and the role of nutrition in health and disease belongs to the last 60 or 70 years. It must be emphasized that nutrition is indeed one of the youngest of sciences, and that much still remains to be learned.

Scientists learn about nutrition through laboratory studies on experimental animals, using rats, mice, guinea pigs, hamsters, chickens, dogs, cattle, and even microorganisms. Many studies have likewise been conducted on healthy human volunteers, since not all of the results obtained on animals can be applied directly to humans.

Studies conducted on animals and on humans usually measure certain physical changes; for example, growth in height and weight, skin condition, and many other conditions that the researcher can note. The amount of nutrients in the food intake and the amount of specific substances excreted in the urine and feces are measured in balance experiments. Thus, if the intake and excretions are equal, the subject is said to be in *balance,* or in *equilibrium.* Many constituents may also be measured in the blood and tissues, for changes in diet will, sooner or later, bring about changes in the level of certain substances in the blood. The techniques of the physician, biologist, physiologist, chemist, and nutritionist are required in nutrition research.

To summarize, when you study nutrition, you will become aware that this is a well-organized science with a tremendous body of knowledge. There is no room for the food faddist or the quack who tries to substitute oratory, unrealistic promises, and emotional appeal for sound knowledge and wise applications to the healthful feeding of people.

TEAMWORK IN NUTRITION

As a nurse you are part of the health team that cares for the sick. (See Fig. 1–1.) The most important member of the team is the patient. Indeed, the patient is the sole reason for the team's existence. Health professionals must always remember that they must work *with* the patient, and permit him to share in decisions as far as he is able. Many professional people work with the physician: nurses, dietitians, dietetic technicians, social workers, pharmacists, physical therapists, occupational therapists, laboratory technicians, and others.

Teamwork in nutritional care means that the physician prescribes the diet; the dietitian supervises the planning of menus and the purchase and preparation of food for all patients; the nurse helps the patients at mealtime and records

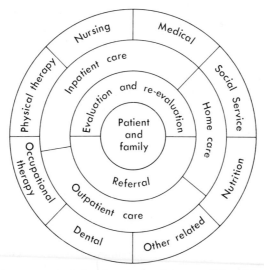

FIGURE 1–1 The concentric circles of comprehensive care radiate out from the patient and his family. *(Miss Geraldine Piper and* Journal of the American Dietetic Association, *Chicago.)*

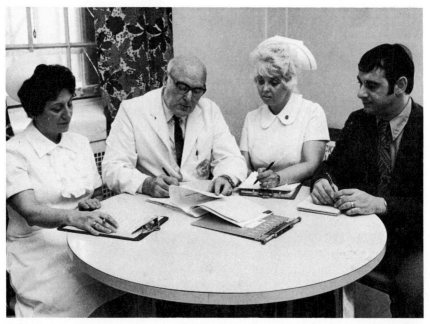

FIGURE 1-2 The nurse, physician, dietitian, and social worker discuss the patient's progress and make plans for his continuing care. (*Veterans Administration Hospital, Coatesville, Pennsylvania. Photo by J. A. Josephs.*)

the acceptance of the meal. The nurse and dietitian work with the patient on menu selection, food acceptance, and dietary counseling. From time to time the nurse and dietitian may consult with the physician concerning any nutritional problems presented by the patient. (See Fig. 1–2.)

YOUR RESPONSIBILITY IN NUTRITION

First of all, you have a responsibility to *yourself.* You will personally benefit from good nutrition, for you will look and feel better; you will be better able to meet the demands of your profession; and you will set an example for others.

You have a responsibility to your *family.* Perhaps this lies in planning and preparing better meals for the family, in helping a child to develop good food habits, or in guiding an elderly person in making adjustments in his diet according to a doctor's prescription. Perhaps this is a responsibility you will assume more fully at some later time.

You have a responsibility as a *nurse* or *other health worker.* Nutrition is an essential part of the total care of a patient. You will need an appreciation of what food means to the patient, how illness changes his feelings about food, and how to help him with his day-to-day meals. See Chapter 18 for specific details on the nutritional care of patients.

You have a responsibility as a *citizen*. Because you are a health worker, many people look to you for an example and for advice. You will need to know how to answer simple questions. But you will also need to know when to refer people to physicians if questions concerning diagnosis and treatment are asked. You can give your support to the school lunch program and other activities that improve the nutrition of people. You can take a positive stand for any action by the community government aimed toward better nutrition.

GOALS FOR NUTRITION STUDY

If you accept seriously the responsibilities outlined, you will find the following goals to be helpful in the study of nutrition:

Understanding and appreciation of:
    the relation of food and nutrition to health, happiness, efficiency, and long life for
        yourself as well as for others
    the meanings of food to people—religious, cultural, social, psychologic, and economic;
        respect for individual differences
    the importance of having the right attitude toward food
    the opportunities to help people in the selection of a good diet
    the difficulties involved in changing food habits
    the importance of nutrition to the recovery of the patient
    the need for teamwork in the improvement of nutrition of people
    your responsibility for the nutritional care of patients
Knowledge concerning:
    basic principles of nutrition
        functions of the nutrients
        requirements for nutrients by various age groups
        foods as sources of nutrients
    cultural food patterns
    techniques for development of good food habits
    principles for modifying diets for disease conditions
    reliable sources of information on nutrition

Behavioral outcomes.   Having achieved the understanding, appreciation, and knowledge outlined above, the student should expect to be able to act in the following ways:

    Selects own diet for good nutrition
    Uses tables of food composition to learn values of foods
    Interprets labeling and advertising of food products
    Makes adjustments in meal plans for cultural, psychologic, and economic factors
    Helps patients use a selective menu
    Helps patients at mealtime
    Encourages and reassures patient; explains importance of diet
    Observes food intake of patients and reports to nursing supervisor or dietitian

Answers simple questions posed by patient; or refers questions to the dietitian
Works with the supervising nurse, dietitian, and physician
Makes use of community resources in helping the patient to care for himself
Uses nutrition knowledge to help well people improve their diets.

REVIEW QUESTIONS AND PROBLEMS

1. Define nutrient, nutrition, nutritional status, nutritional care.

2. List some signs of good nutrition.

3. In addition to poor diet what factors might be responsible for poor health?

4. Look for advertisements on food in magazines and newspapers. Discuss the good features of the advertisements. What are some of the bad features?

5. Start a file for articles on food and nutrition from current newspapers and magazines. From time to time compare the content of these articles with what you learn in your study of nutrition.

6. Examine the list of goals for nutrition. As you proceed in the study of nutrition, evaluate yourself against these goals. Are there other aims you should include?

NUTRITION IN THE COMMUNITY

Nutrition in the United States

The patterns of American diet have resulted from a bountiful and varied food supply and from the cultural impact of many nationality backgrounds. The creativity of the food technologist, the skill of the food engineer, and the speed of transportation from east to west and from north to south have all contributed to the variety of readily available foods.

CHANGING PATTERNS OF LIVING

Dietitians and nurses must take changes in the patterns of living into account when they try to help people toward better food habits. Most Americans today have more money, more education, more leisure, and more opportunity to travel both here and abroad. Women make up about 40 per cent of the work force; some of these are second wage earners in the family, and many others are the sole wage earners. With so many women working, the purchase of food and the meal preparation are often shared with other family members. There is much greater reliance upon convenience foods. Children have lunches at school and sometimes breakfasts as well, and working members of the family eat in restaurants or at quick-lunch counters or carry their own lunches. Business and social obligations and the school activities of children often interfere with families having dinner together. People are eating much more frequently, partly because of the many attractive snacks that are available. Numerous new foods are introduced in the markets each year. Since there is a limit to the amount

11

of food a person can eat, each new food that is adopted replaces another. Is the new food a good replacement or not? Obviously, the food patterns of individuals as well as families differ widely and must be taken into account when counseling is provided.

NUTRITIONAL PROBLEMS

Nutritional problems may arise from dietary deficiencies or excesses. (See Fig. 2–1.) For example, obesity is the result of excessive caloric intake. Dental decay is more complex and may result from an excess of sugar as well as a deficiency of fluoride and other factors.

Nutritional problems in the United States are identified by surveys of population groups. The National Nutrition Survey by the Nutrition Program of the Public Health Service was carried out in 1967 on people living in low-income areas in ten states. Another survey, the Health and Nutrition Examination Survey (HANES) was carried out in the early 1970s and was representative of the national population.

Among the important problems identified by the surveys was the high incidence of obesity, dental caries, and iron-deficiency anemia. Growth retardation

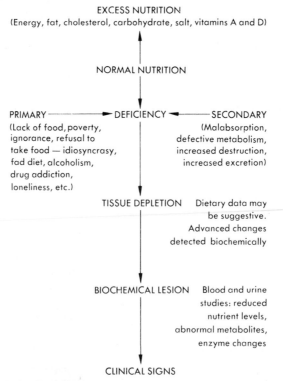

FIGURE 2–1 The levels of nutrition *(From C. H. Robinson, Fundamentals of Normal Nutrition, 3rd ed., New York: Macmillan Publishing Co., Inc., 1978.)*

was present in some young children. Low serum levels of vitamin A were observed in preschool children. Low serum ascorbic acid levels occurred in about one of every eight persons; one person in every 25 had scorbutic gums. Occasionally pediatricians see infants who have symptoms of protein-calorie malnutrition, scurvy, or rickets. Usually such occurrences are the results of ignorance concerning the child's nutritional needs or child neglect.

Dietary excesses of calories, fat, cholesterol, sugar, salt, together with a lack of fiber have been associated with a high prevalence of heart disease, hypertension, cancer, various gastrointestinal disorders, diabetes mellitus, and others in the United States. In each of these conditions factors other than diet also are contributing to risk. Further discussion on these factors will be presented in other chapters in this text. At this point it is important to emphasize that more research is needed to prove the claims that are being made.

FAULTY FOOD HABITS

Every ten years the U.S. Department of Agriculture conducts a survey of family food consumption. The most recent survey was carried out in 1977–78, but an analysis of the results is not yet available. Nonetheless, the nutrition surveys cited together with the 1965 family food consumption survey are good indicators of faulty food habits that exist in many of today's families.

The quality of the American diet is directly related to income. People at the lowest income level had poor diets four times as often as those at the highest income level. (See Fig. 2–2.) But the fact that some people at higher income levels also had poor diets indicates that adequate nutrition education has not reached as many people as it should.

Insufficient money, ignorance of the essential foods for an adequate diet, poor facilities for preparing food, and lack of skills must share the blame for the malnutrition seen in this country. The following points need to be recognized in setting up programs for improved nutrition.

1. Infants, preschool children, adolescent girls, and pregnant women are the most vulnerable to the effects of poor food habits.

2. Milk, deep green and yellow vegetables, and citrus fruits require greater emphasis in dietary planning. The trend among Americans today seems to be away from milk as a beverage, substituting coffee, tea, soft drinks, and fruitades.

3. The use of convenience foods has greatly increased and no doubt will continue to do so. Homemakers need much more assistance in making the best choices for the money they can spend because the products are so numerous.

4. Snacks are too often made up of foods high in starches, sugars, and fats but providing little by way of other nutrients. These snacks may lead to excessive weight gain, they may replace nutritionally essential foods, or they may destroy the appetite for meals. Teenagers especially need to learn to control the quality and the amounts of snack foods they consume.

5. Breakfast is often skipped. Lack of time, uninteresting foods, and poor appetite are usually given as reasons. It is hard to make up in the rest of the day for the nutrients that a good breakfast can provide.

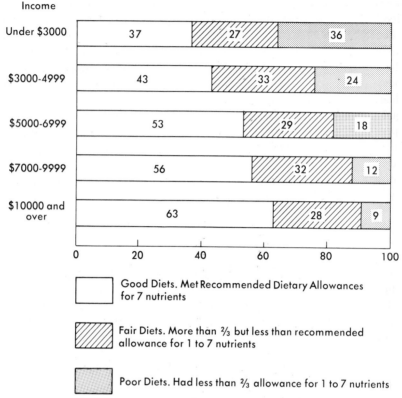

Income

Under $3000	37	27	36
$3000-4999	43	33	24
$5000-6999	53	29	18
$7000-9999	56	32	12
$10000 and over	63	28	9

☐ Good Diets. Met Recommended Dietary Allowances for 7 nutrients

▨ Fair Diets. More than ⅔ but less than recommended allowance for 1 to 7 nutrients

▨ Poor Diets. Had less than ⅔ allowance for 1 to 7 nutrients

FIGURE 2–2 As income goes down, the percentage of people having a good diet also goes down. Lack of income is not the sole reason for inadequate diets, however. Note that only 63 per cent of people at the highest income level had good diets. *(Data from family dietary survey, 1965; Agricultural Research Service, U.S. Department of Agriculture, Washington, D.C.)*

6. Lunch is likely to be skimpy, or may consist of high-calorie foods low in nutrients.
7. Too many meals are eaten in a hurry with little enjoyment of them.

Nutritional improvement means public concern for the poor. It means much greater emphasis on nutrition education for people of all ages. Elementary and secondary schools must strengthen their classroom programs in nutrition; school feeding programs need to be expanded; and all segments of the population must be reached through wider use of mass media such as television, radio, and newspapers and magazines.

FOOD MISINFORMATION AND FADDISM

A *fad* is a style or custom that many people are interested in for a short time. Just as dress fashions come and go, so food fads come and go. *Nutritional quackery* pertains to false claims made for the health virtues or curative properties of foods.

People often adopt a dietary regimen, or subscribe to claims for specific foods or supplements because someone has told them about the particular virtues, or because they have read about these claims in articles or advertisements. When they have had little or no education in nutrition, they are unable to evaluate whether the claims are justified. Thus, they often fall prey to faddism or quackery. Some dietary fads are harmless. Others create an economic hardship for people of limited income because the foods or supplements may be expensive. Still others are nutritionally inadequate and could lead to serious nutritional deficiencies. Sometimes the harm from a fad comes about because a person substitutes self-therapy for the advice of a physician. By such action he might delay effective treatment until it is too late.

IDENTIFYING THE FOOD QUACK

It is not always easy to determine who is a food quack. Such a person can be very persuasive. He appeals to the emotions and makes extravagant claims for his product: youth, beauty, glamour, long life, cure of disease. He is out to sell something, whether it be a book, an appliance, or a food product. Many of his products are sold door to door, often with "money back" guarantees of cure for some disease in a matter of weeks or months. The product is usually more expensive than similar products sold in food markets.

The food quack frequently accuses the medical profession of not giving the full facts to the public, or he claims to be persecuted by scientists or governmental agencies. He quotes from the scientific literature and sounds very learned. Yet, a careful search of his sources will often show that he has lifted ideas out of books and journals and is placing his own interpretation upon them.

You should become suspicious if someone talks about specific foods or supplements as "wonder foods," "miracle foods," "health foods," "natural foods," "organic foods," or a "secret formula." Claims are sometimes made for special virtues of foods such as yogurt, raw sugar, honey, sea salt, stone-ground flour, vegetable juices, wheat germ oil, vitamin E supplements, lecithin, and so on.

No single food possesses unique qualities for health. Rather, good nutrition is served by any combination of foods that will provide the necessary nutrients. The Food and Drug Administration considers a food to be misbranded if it is called a "health" food. (See also Chapter 17).

RELIABLE SOURCES OF INFORMATION

The best defense against food misinformation and faddism is through sound nutrition education at all levels—in the elementary and secondary schools, to consumers by mass media, and through health agencies in the community.

Among the individuals who work in a community who can be especially helpful in supplying sound information are the following:

Nutritionists working in city, county, or state offices of health
Dietitians in hospitals, health agencies, food industries, school food services, nutrition programs for children, the elderly
Nutritionists in county and state cooperative extension services
Professors of nutrition in colleges and universities

Nutrition, a World Concern

INTERNATIONAL NUTRITION PROBLEMS

The central problem in nutrition today is that millions of people in underdeveloped countries of the world do not have enough to eat. Yet, each day approximately 200,000 persons are added to the world's population, and they, too, must somehow be fed. Asia contains one third of the earth's land surface, but it must feed two thirds of the world's people. Thus, supplying more food to keep up with the increase in population as well as trying to improve the state of nutrition is truly a staggering problem.

Infants and young children suffer most from the lack of food. The death rate among infants in many countries is appallingly high. Of infants who survive the first year, many will die before the age of five. The infants and children fail to grow, they are quite susceptible to infection, and many of them die of protein-calorie malnutrition known as *kwashiorkor*. Even though these severely malnourished children live, their mental development may have been permanently retarded.

Other deficiency diseases are still quite prevalent in many parts of the world. Anemias caused by lack of iron and of the B-complex vitamins are frequent. Goiter is widespread in areas where there is a lack of iodine. Beriberi occurs because of lack of thiamin; pellagra from lack of niacin; xerophthalmia and blindness from lack of vitamin A; and rickets from lack of vitamin D. As you study nutrition, the characteristics of some of these diseases will become more familiar.

INTERNATIONAL ORGANIZATIONS

The *Agency for International Development* (AID) of the U.S. Department of State and numerous charitable organizations are pledged to providing aid in many ways: direct food supplies; technical assistance in the development of agriculture and industry; education of youth; education of homemakers in food preparation, child care, and sanitation; and many other ways. Several organizations of the United Nations illustrate the humanitarian efforts of the great international body. (See Fig. 2–3.)

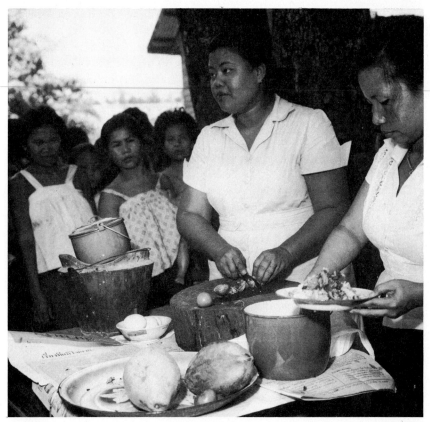

FIGURE 2–3   A nurse in Thailand gives a cooking demonstration using local foods. *(UNICEF.)*

The *Food and Agriculture Organization* (FAO) aims especially to improve the growth, distribution, and storage of food. To carry out its aims it might be involved in such widely different activities as irrigation for crops; development of varieties of grain that will grow in a given climate; sponsoring home economics programs to show people how to prepare their foods and to better feed their families; and setting up a food processing plant.

The *World Health Organization* (WHO) aims to eliminate diseases of all kinds, including those that relate to nutrition. It works closely with FAO. Diseases such as malaria and others keep millions from working. When people are treated for these diseases they are able to work and produce food for themselves and their families. WHO works closely with communities to improve the sanitation through insect control, water supplies, housing, and waste disposal.

The *United Nations Children's Fund* (UNICEF) is concerned with all aspects of the health and welfare of children everywhere. Some of its activities include the distribution of nonfat dry milk; immunization of children; provision of tools and seeds for gardening programs; school materials; development of safe water supplies; and many others.

The *United Nations Education, Scientific, and Cultural Organization* (UNESCO) aims to eliminate illiteracy and thus to help people through education to use science and to understand cultural forces for the improvement of their lives.

REVIEW QUESTIONS AND PROBLEMS

1. Prepare a list of false ideas about foods that you have heard. What is your basis for saying that each is false?

2. What are some ways by which you can identify a quack?

3. What nutritional problems do you know of in your community?

4. List some food habits of people you know that could be improved. What are some ways you would use to try to help them?

5. Find five examples of materials prepared by food manufacturers that are useful in obtaining a better diet.

6. What organizations in your community include nutrition as part of their work?

7. Prepare a report for your class on a state, national, or international organization that has the major goal of promoting good nutrition.

REFERENCES

Calderbank, D. A.: "Facing the Food Crisis," *Nurs. Times,* 71:366–67, 1975.

"Dietary Goals: A Statement by the American Dietetic Association," *J. Am. Dietet. A.,* 71:227–28, 1977.

Harrison, G. G., *et al.:* "Food Waste Behavior in an Urban Population," *J. Nutr. Educ.,* 7:13–16, 1975.

"Highlights from the Ten-State Nutrition Survey," *Nutr. Today,* 7:4–11, July 1972.

Latham, M. C., and Stephenson, L. S.: "U.S. Dietary Goals," *J. Nutr. Educ.,* 9:152–54, 1977.

Mayer, J.: "The Fad Diet Bust," *Family Health,* 10:42–43, July 1978.

Stare, F. J., *et al.:* " 'Health' Foods: Definitions and Nutrient Values," *J. Nutr. Educ.,* 4:94–97, 1972.

Winckler, I.: "Nutrition Today. Moderation in All Things," *Nurs. Times,* 72:1917–19, 1976.

3

NUTRIENTS AND BODY COMPOSITION | FUNCTIONS OF FOOD | CONTROLS FOR DIGESTIVE ACTIVITY | ROLE OF DIGESTIVE ORGANS | DIGESTIBILITY OF FOOD | ABSORPTION | METABOLISM

THE NUTRIENTS AND THEIR UTILIZATION

NUTRIENTS AND BODY COMPOSITION

Whatever you eat turns into you. It is quite reasonable to suppose that there is a relationship between the substances present in the body and the kinds of nutrients present in food. Also it is quite reasonable to suppose that the body can be properly built and maintained only if the correct materials are available.

The cell is the unit of body structure. Cells in different body tissues carry out specific kinds of functions; thus liver, bone, muscle, and blood cells differ from each other. Likewise, the kinds and amounts of nutrients that make up cells vary from one type of cell to another. At least 50 nutrients are required by the cells of the body.

Four chemical elements account for 96 per cent of the body weight. They are carbon, hydrogen, oxygen, and nitrogen. Water is by far the most abundant compound in the body; it accounts for about two thirds of the body weight. Protein represents roughly one fifth of the body weight, and fat constitutes one fifth, more or less, of the body weight. The proportions of these major body constituents will vary widely from individual to individual. Obviously, a lean person will have a much lower proportion of fat than an overweight person. A baby has a higher proportion of body water than an adult.

Carbohydrate, so important in the diet for its energy value, actually is present only in limited amounts in body tissues. About 300–350 gm occurs in the adult body in the forms of liver and muscle glycogen and the blood sugar.

Mineral matter accounts for about 4 per cent of the body weight, but a

19

wide variety of mineral elements is needed for the structure of the tissues. The total store of vitamins in the body would add up to only a few grams.

FUNTIONS OF FOOD

Some nutrients function in three categories, whereas others are restricted to one or two classes of functions.

Nutrients that furnish energy: carbohydrates, fats, proteins
Nutrients that build and maintain body tissues: water, proteins, fats, carbohydrates, mineral elements
Nutrients that regulate body functions: water, mineral elements, vitamins, proteins, fats, carbohydrates

CONTROLS FOR DIGESTIVE ACTIVITY

Digestion includes the mechanical and chemical processes by which foods are broken down to their nutrients so that they may be absorbed into the circulation. Mechanical and chemical changes take place simultaneously on the carbohydrates, fats, and proteins in foods. The autonomic nervous system continuously controls the motor and secretory activity of the intestinal tract.

The mechanical processes include the chewing of food, the churning actions in the stomach, and the muscular contractions of the intestinal tract. The rhythmic contractions, known as *peristalsis*, break up food into smaller and smaller particles, mix them intimately with the digestive juices, and continually move the food mass along the intestinal tract. (See Fig. 3–1.)

The chemical reactions in digestion involve the addition of water to the protein, fat, and carbohydrate molecules and their splitting up into nutrients that the tissues can use. This process is known as *hydrolysis*. The final end products of digestion are

Carbohydrates to the simple sugars—glucose, fructose, galactose
Fats to fatty acids and glycerol
Proteins to amino acids

Water, mucin, hydrochloric acid, enzymes, and hormones are interrelated in the orderly processes of digestion.

Water. The digestive juices supply an abundance of water at all points of the intestinal tract. Water holds the foods in suspension during movement throughout the tract, facilitates the peristaltic movements, and brings food particles into intimate contact with the enzymes.

Mucin. The glands of the intestinal tract secrete mucin, a polysaccharide that gives the slippery consistency to mucus. The walls of the stomach are protected from irritation and erosion by acid because of the coating of mucus.

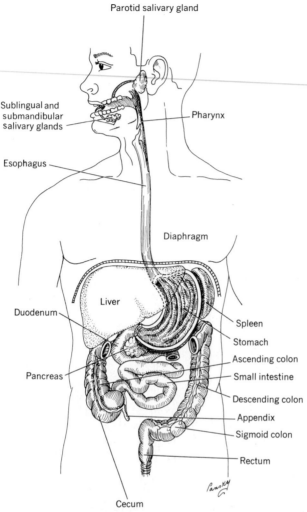

Parotid salivary gland

Sublingual and submandibular salivary glands

Pharynx

Esophagus

Diaphragm

Liver

Duodenum

Spleen

Stomach

Ascending colon

Small intestine

Pancreas

Descending colon

Appendix

Sigmoid colon

Rectum

Cecum

FIGURE 3–1 The digestive tract. *(From Ben Pansky:* Dynamic Anatomy and Physiology. *New York: Macmillan Publishing Co., Inc., 1974, p. 412.)*

Foods move more readily along the tract because of the lubricating effect of mucus.

Enzymes. The chemical reactions require helpers called *enzymes.* Sometimes enzymes are called living catalysts. A catalyst is any substance that hastens a chemical reaction but does not itself become a part of the compounds that are formed.

Enzymes are composed of specific proteins. They are named for the substance upon which they act; for example, *protease* is an enzyme that digests protein, and *oxidase* is involved in the addition of oxygen. Each enzyme is highly individ-

TABLE 3-1   SUMMARY OF CHEMICAL REACTIONS IN DIGESTION

Site of Activity	Enzyme	Substrate	Products of Enzyme Activity
Mouth	Salivary amylase (ptyalin)	Cooked starch	Dextrins, maltose
Stomach	Protease (pepsin)	Proteins	Proteoses, peptones, polypeptides
	Rennin	Milk casein	Calcium caseinate
	Lipase	Emulsified fats	Fatty acids, glycerol
Small intestine	Pancreatic juice		
	Protease (trypsin)	Proteins	Proteoses, peptones, polypeptides, some amino acids
	Lipase (steapsin)	Fats	Di- and monoglycerides, fatty acids, glycerol
	Amylase (amylopsin)	Starch	Maltose
	Intestinal juice		
	Peptidases (erepsin)	Peptones, poly-peptides	Amino acids
	Sucrase	Sucrose	Glucose, fructose
	Maltase	Maltose	Glucose (2 molecules)
	Lactase	Lactose	Glucose, galactose

ual in its action. An enzyme that digests fat will not digest starch. Some enzymes act only in an acid medium, such as pepsin in the stomach, whereas others act only in an alkaline medium, such as trypsin in the small intestine. See Table 3–1 for a summary of enzyme activity.

Hormones are chemical messengers that control the mechanical and chemical processes of digestion. They are produced at a given site in the presence of a specific stimulant such as acid chyme, polypetides, or fat. See Table 3–2 for summary of hormones involved in digestive processes.

ROLE OF DIGESTIVE ORGANS

Digestion in the mouth.   The digestion of food begins in the mouth with the chewing of food and its mixing with saliva. Chewing is important because it increases the surface area of the food particles for later digestive action. Saliva contains *amylase,* a starch-splitting enzyme, but food remains in the mouth for such a short time that only a small amount of starch can be broken down to dextrins and maltose.

Digestion in the stomach.   Food passes from the esophagus into the stomach by relaxation of the cardiac sphincter. Following the entrance of food

TABLE 3–2   HORMONES THAT REGULATE DIGESTIVE ACTIVITY

Hormone	Where Produced	Stimulus to Secretion	Activity
Gastrin	Pylorus; duodenum	Proteins, caffeine, spices, alcohol	Stimulates flow of gastric juice
Enterogastrone	Duodenum	Acid chyme; fats	Inhibits acid secretion; reduces motility
Cholecystokinin	Duodenum	Fats	Contracts gallbladder; bile flows into duodenum
Secretin	Duodenum	Polypeptides; acid chyme	Pancreas secretes thin, enzyme-poor juice into duodenum
Pancreozymin	Duodenum; jejunum	Polypeptides; acid chyme	Pancreas secretes thick, enzyme-rich juice into duodenum
Enterocrinin	Upper small intestine	Chyme	Intestinal juices secreted by intestinal glands

into the stomach the sphincter closes, thus preventing the regurgitation of food. The stomach serves as a temporary storehouse for food, brings about partial digestion of protein, and prepares food for further digestion in the small intestine. The food is continually churned and mixed with gastric juice until it reaches a liquid consistency known as *chyme*. Rhythmic contractions move the chyme toward the pylorus where small portions are gradually released through the pyloric sphincter into the duodenum.

Gastric juice contains hydrochloric acid, pepsin, rennin, mucin, and other substances. Hydrochloric acid has several important functions: (1) it swells the proteins so as to make them more easily attacked by the enzymes; (2) it provides the acid medium necessary for the action of pepsin; (3) it increases the solubility of calcium and iron salts so that they are more readily absorbed; and (4) it reduces the activity of harmful bacteria that may have been present in the food.

Pepsin, a protease, splits proteins into smaller molecules called proteoses and polypeptides. Very little digestion of carbohydrates and fats occurs in the stomach. In the upper (cardiac) portion of the stomach the salivary amylase continues to act upon starch to change it to dextrins and maltose. As soon as the food mass is mixed with hydrochloric acid this action ceases. Lipase in the stomach has some effect on emulsified fats as in milk, cream, butter, and egg yolk, but most of the hydrolysis of fats takes place in the small intestine.

Digestion in the small intestine. Most of the digestive activity takes place in the small intestine, which includes the duodenum, the jejunum, and the ileum. Bile, manufactured by the liver and stored in the gall bladder, is essential for fat digestion. As soon as fats enter the duodenum the secretion of a hormone, *cholecystokinin*, is stimulated. Cholecystokinin causes the gallbladder to contract and to release bile into the duodenum. Bile emulsifies the fats, that is, breaks them down into tiny globules so that the fat-splitting enzymes have greater contact with the fat molecules. Bile, being highly alkaline, neutralizes the acid chyme and provides the alkaline reaction necessary for the action of the intestinal enzymes.

As soon as acid chyme enters the duodenum, two hormones, *secretin* and *pancreozymin* are produced. They are carried by the bloodstream to the pancreas where they stimulate the secretion of pancreatic juice. The pancreas also pours its secretions into the duodenum. Pancreatic amylase splits starch to maltose; a protease, *trypsin*, breaks down proteins and polypeptides to much smaller molecules; and lipase, *steapsin*, completes the digestion of fats to fatty acids and glycerol.

A hormone, *enterocrinin*, stimulates the flow of intestinal juice from glands in the walls of the small intestine. The intestinal juice contains protein and sugar-splitting enzymes. Lactase splits lactose to the simple sugars glucose and galactose; maltase acts on the maltose molecule to yield glucose; and sucrase brings about the hydrolysis of sucrose to glucose and fructose. A group of enzymes known as *peptidases* completes the breakdown of proteins and polypeptides to amino acids.

Function of the large intestine. The large intestine includes the cecum, colon, rectum, and anal canal. Digestion and the absorption of nutrients have been essentially completed by the time the food mass reaches the large intestine, but much water and digestive juices are reabsorbed so that the intestinal contents gradually take on a solid consistency. The feces contain the fibers of food, small amounts of undigested food, bile salts, cholesterol, mucus, bacteria, and broken-down cellular wastes.

DIGESTIBILITY OF FOOD

By digestibility is meant the completeness of digestion and also the ease or speed of digestion. The efficiency of digestion is remarkably high. Based upon the typical American diet, 98 per cent of the carbohydrate, 95 per cent of the fat, and 92 per cent of the protein in the food eaten is digested and absorbed.

Fibers and seeds are not digested. Therefore, a diet made up of many fruits, vegetables, and whole-grain products could have a digestibility of carbohydrate of only 85 per cent. The completeness of digestion is greatly reduced in some disorders of the gastrointestinal tract such as severe diarrhea. In some hereditary diseases such as celiac disease, cystic fibrosis of the pancreas, and lactose intolerance, the enzymes for the digestion of fats and carbohydrates may be missing, so that much fat or starch is eliminated in the feces.

The speed of digestion varies widely according to the size of the meal and the composition of the diet and also depends upon certain psychologic factors. As little as 9 hours or as much as 48 hours may elapse from the time food is eaten until the wastes are eliminated. Small meals will remain in the stomach for a far shorter time than will large meals. Foods that are poorly chewed are likely to require a longer time for digestion.

Foods are sometimes said to "stick to the ribs." In other words, they stay in the stomach longer, so that they delay hunger contractions and are therefore more satisfying. They are said to have high *satiety* value. A breakfast of juice and dry toast, being chiefly carbohydrate, has little satiety value. But a breakfast of juice, toast, eggs, and bacon also contains proteins and fats. Because the digestion takes somewhat longer in the stomach, this meal would be more satisfying. An excessive amount of fat, especially in the form of fried foods, slows up digestion so much that discomfort sometimes results.

Extractives in meat increase the flow of digestive juices. A cup of broth or bouillon is sometimes used at the beginning of a meal to stimulate the appetite and to increase the digestive action. The secretion of digestive juices is also increased by the pleasant sight, smell, and taste of food. On the other hand, the secretion is likely to be decreased when foods are unattractively served or when the surroundings are unpleasant. An individual who is excessively tired or who is under emotional stress such as fear, grief, or anger often experiences digestive upsets or may be unable to take food.

ABSORPTION

Absorption is the process whereby the nutrients released from food by digestion are transferred from the intestinal lumen into the blood and lymph circulation. The intestinal wall is lined with 4 to 5 million tiny fingerlike projections called *villi*. (See Fig. 3–2.) Each villus is a complex organ with a surface layer of epithelium over a layer of connective tissue (lamina propria) that is supplied with capillaries and lacteals. On the surface of each villus are 500 to 600 *microvilli*, also known as the *brush border*. Thus, the villi and microvilli give an immense surface area through which nutrients can be absorbed—an area comparable to the size of a third of a football field!

The nutrients are carried across the epithelial cell walls by several complex processes. Small particles such as glucose and some minerals can move from an area of greater concentration to one of lesser concentration by *passive diffusion;* this accounts for only a small part of absorption. Some nutrients must be attached to a *carrier* before they can be ferried across the cell membrane. One of the most complex examples of a nutrient attached to a carrier is vitamin B_{12}. This vitamin must be attached to a factor produced in the stomach known

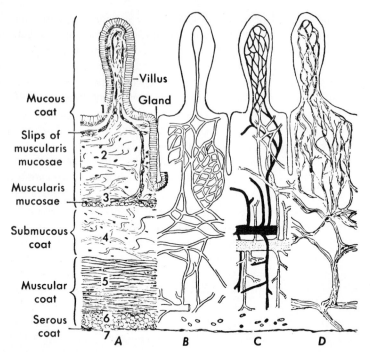

Mucous coat

Slips of muscularis mucosae

Muscularis mucosae

Submucous coat

Muscular coat

Serous coat

Villus

Gland

FIGURE 3–2 Diagram of a cross section of small intestine. *A* shows coats of intestinal wall and tissues of coats: *(1)* columnar epithelium, *(2)* areolar connective tissue, *(3)* muscularis mucosae, *(4)* areolar connmective tissue, *(5)* circular layer of smooth muscle, *(6)* longitudinal layer of smooth muscle, *(7)* areolar connective tissue and endothelium. *B* shows arrangement of central lacteal, lymph nodes, and lymph tubes. *C* shows blood supply; arteries and capillaries *black,* veins *stippled. D* shows nerve fibers, the submucous plexus lying in the submucosa, the myenteric plexus lying between the circular and longitudinal layers of the muscular coat. *(From M. A. Miller, and L. C. Leavell,* Kimber-Gray-Stackpole's Anatomy and Physiology, *16th ed., New York: Macmillan Publishing Co., Inc., 1972).*

as *intrinsic factor,* but it is not absorbed until it reaches the ileum. Most of the nutrients must be "pumped" across the cell wall by *active transport.* This requires energy which is supplied by glucose in the cell.

From the lamina propria the fatty acids, some molecules of fat, and fat-soluble vitamins enter the lacteals and enter into the lymph circulation. Glucose, amino acids, mineral salts, and water-soluble vitamins enter into the blood capillaries and are carried by the portal circulation to the liver.

METABOLISM

Metabolism is an inclusive term that describes all the changes that take place in the body. *Anabolism* is a more specific term that is used to indicate the building up of complex substances from simpler substances. Building new bone, or hemoglobin, or muscle tissue would be examples of anabolism. *Catabolism,* by contrast, refers to the breaking down of complex substances into simpler substances. The breakdown of glucose or fatty acids to yield energy is an example of catabolism.

The terms "dynamic equilibrium" and "homeostasis" are sometimes used to indicate that the processes of anabolism and of catabolism are continuously taking place and that the one is equal to the other. In growing children, during pregnancy, and during recovery from illness the processes of anabolism are greater than those of catabolism. On the other hand, excessive catabolism takes place with high fever, during acute illness, following surgery, fractures, and burns, or when certain hormones are produced in excessive amounts by the body.

The innumerable reactions in metabolism require the activity of enzymes. Many of these enzymes require another substance called a *coenzyme* in addition to the protein. One of the important functions of vitamins and certain mineral elements is to act as coenzymes.

Hormones maintain a system of checks and balances on metabolism. To name just a few: thyroxine, produced by the thyroid gland, regulates energy metabolism; insulin, produced in the pancreas, controls the level of the blood sugar; an adrenal hormone controls the amount of sodium retained or excreted.

In addition to (1) ingestion, (2) digestion, and (3) absorption, metabolism includes these categories.

4. Transportation of the nutrients to the cells where they are needed and of the wastes to the organs of excretion is the function of the blood circulation.

5. Respiration. In the lungs oxygen is taken into the blood so that the nutrients may be combined with oxygen (oxidized). Through the lungs carbon dioxide is given off as a waste.

6. Utilization. Within every cell are found hundreds of enzymes that bring about the appropriate functions in terms of energy, building or maintenance, and regulation. In a complex series of steps glucose combines with oxygen to release the energy for the body's work. Fats, likewise, are oxidized for energy. Carbohydrates and fats are also stored as potential energy in the form of adipose tissue. Amino acids are used to build new cells, to form hormones, or enzymes, or as a source of energy. Mineral elements enter into the structure of the cell or into any one of many regulatory activities. An important aspect of the study in the chapters to follow will be concerned with more detail of the functions of the nutrients.

7. Excretion of wastes is accomplished by the kidney, which removes nitrogenous wastes, water, mineral salts, and excess water-soluble vitamins; by the bowel, which eliminates indigestible fiber, bile pigments, cholesterol and other products of metabolism, and bacterial wastes; by the skin, through which water, mineral salts, and some nitrogenous wastes are removed; and by the lungs, which remove carbon dioxide and water.

REVIEW QUESTIONS AND PROBLEMS

1. Name the three functions of food in the body. What functions are performed by fats, by carbohydrates, by mineral elements, by proteins, by vitamins?

2. Define metabolism, anabolism, catabolism, enzyme, hormone.

3. Name three enzymes in the digestion of foods, and tell what they do.

4. What percentage of food eaten is digested under normal circumstances?

5. What products result from the complete digestion of proteins, fats, carbohydrates?

6. List five factors that may determine the speed with which a meal is digested.

7. What relation exists between the oxygen you breathe in and the food you eat?

8. How could you explain the fact that your output of urine may be less on a very warm day when you are exercising vigorously?

9. What kinds of waste products are excreted in the urine? Refer to a table of constituents in the urine.

REFERENCES

Pansky, B.: *Dynamic Anatomy and Physiology.* New York: Macmillan Publishing Co., Inc., 1975, chap. 12.

Robinson, C. H., and Lawler, M. R.: *Normal and Therapeutic Nutrition,* 15th ed., New York: Macmillan Publishing Co., Inc., 1977, chap. 2.

GUIDES FOR NUTRITIONAL PLANNING

Do you weigh what you should? Are you getting enough protein? Is a small glass of tomato juice a good substitute for a small glass of orange juice? How much milk should you drink each day? Are you eating too much fat or sugar?

Almost everything we do is according to some design. We use recipes for cooking, patterns for sewing, and rules for behavior. Likewise, we have certain guides to answer questions such as the above and to help us in the maintenance of good nutrition and health. Let us examine more closely some of the guides that can be especially useful.

STANDARDS OF BODY WEIGHT

Probably no aspect of one's health is more often discussed than one's weight. Some people are trying to take off weight, others are trying to put on weight, and still others are fortunate in weighing just what they should. How do you measure up according to the standards of height and weight?

During the teen years boys and girls reach their full height, but in the early twenties they continue to mature somewhat in their body frame and muscle development. The adult is at the peak of his physical development between 20 and 30 years of age. Many people, however, continue to gain somewhat throughout life, so that the average weights for men and women at 35, 45, and 55 years are steadily increased.

Medical and insurance authorities have shown that it is not desirable for men and women to continue to gain throughout their lives. Height and weight tables are, therefore, set up on the basis of weight at age 25 to 30 years. (See

29

Table A-3, p. 351.) One should aim to keep the desirable weight for one's height and body frame at age 25 years for the rest of one's life.

In using this table, some differences are allowed for body frame. Some people with small bones—small wrists, narrow shoulders, and narrow hips—would be classified as "low." Other people of a generally stocky build—large wrists, broad shoulders, wide hips—would have a desirable weight range between "median" and "high." You should note that the heights indicated in this table are without shoes and that the weights are without clothing.

At best, height-weight tables are only an approximate guide to body fatness. Many athletes could be considered overweight by these standards, but the excess weight results from well-developed muscles, and not fat. On the other hand, some inactive people appear to be of normal weight but have little muscular development and much body fat. Many physicians use the thickness of fat layers under the skin as an estimate of fatness. They use the skin-fold pinch test, or obtain a more precise measurement by using a caliper.

If your weight is less than 10 per cent over or under the desirable weight for your body frame, your weight is about what it should be. If you are between 10 and 20 per cent overweight, you should correct the situation before it gets more severe. If you weigh more than 20 per cent over or under your desirable weight, it would be a good idea to consult your physician about bringing your weight more nearly in line.

USING METRIC MEASURES

Scientists and health workers have long used metric measures: micrograms, milligrams, grams, kilograms; milliliters, liters; millimeters, centimeters, meters; degrees Celsius. Gradually, in the United States, the metric system of measures is replacing the English measures. Children are becoming familiar with these measures in school, but older persons will find the transition to be a little more difficult.

To use the metric system you will need to learn what relationships exist between it and our present system. For example, if you now weigh 120 pounds, what is your weight in kilograms? If you buy 5 pounds of potatoes, how many kilograms would you buy? Some conversion factors are shown in Table A-5. In this text weights and measures are expressed in metric terms, with the present system of measures placed in parenthesis. The following relationships are important to remember:

1 kilogram (kg) = 1000 grams
1 gram (gm) = 1000 milligrams
1 milligram (mg) = 1000 micrograms (mcg or μg)
1 liter = 1000 milliliters (ml); this is used for fluid measures

RECOMMENDED DAILY DIETARY ALLOWANCES

The Food and Nutrition Board of the National Research Council is the recognized authority for setting standards of nutrition in the United States. This board has set up a table of Recommended Daily Dietary Allowances, which is revised about every five years to include new research as it becomes available. (See Table 4–1.)

If you examine this table carefully, you will find recommendations listed for infants, preschool and school children, older boys and girls, men and women of varying ages, and for pregnancy and lactation. Thus the table is intended to be used as a guide for the entire healthy population.

For each age an individual of given size has been used as a standard. For example, the "reference woman" is 163 cm (64 in.) tall and weighs 55 kg (120 lb) and is assumed to be normally active and to live in a temperate climate. Using this guide, one can estimate what allowances might be suitable for a woman who is larger or smaller, who is younger or older, who lives in a warmer or colder climate, or who is more or less active.

For each age category specific allowances are listed for protein, minerals, and vitamins. The body requires other nutrients that are not listed, but the average well-planned diet will furnish sufficient amounts of these.

The correct interpretation of this table is important. Each person differs from all other individuals in his exact nutritional requirements. There is no practical way to determine which persons use nutrients more or less efficiently than the average. To ensure that these differences are taken into account, the recommended allowances provide a "margin of safety."

An individual who fails to get the full allowances in his diet is not necessarily poorly nourished, since he may be one of those persons whose needs are lower. Nutritional status can be determined only by a thorough physical examination, laboratory tests, and a dietary history. Your goal in dietary planning for yourself and others should be toward obtaining the full allowances each day. If you were catching a plane at a particular time, you would surely allow a little extra time to get to the airport in the event of a traffic tie-up. Why not allow yourself the margin of safety in your nutrition by meeting fully the recommended allowances each day?

TABLES OF FOOD COMPOSITION

In order to use the table of recommended allowances you need to know the nutritive values of the foods you eat. Table A-1, Appendix A, lists numerous foods and the values for many of the nutrients recommended in the table of allowances. The nutritive values are averages of many samples of food analyzed in laboratories. Many factors determine the nutritive values of the foods we eat: the conditions of growing; the handling from farm to market to consumer; the care given to food in the home; and the manner in which food is cooked.

TABLE 4-1 FOOD AND NUTRITION BOARD, NATIONAL ACADEMY OF SCIENCES–NATIONAL RESEARCH COUNCIL

Recommended Daily Dietary Allowances,[1] Revised 1979

Designed for the maintenance of good nutrition of practically all healthy people in the U.S.A.

	Age (years)	Weight (kg)	Weight (lbs)	Height (cm)	Height (in)	Protein (g)	Fat-Soluble Vitamins Vitamin A (μg R.E.)[2]	Vitamin D (μg)[3]	Vitamin E (mg α T.E.)[4]	Water-Soluble Vitamins Vitamin C (mg)	Thiamin (mg)	Riboflavin (mg)	Niacin (mg N.E.)[5]	Vitamin B6 (mg)	Folacin (μg)[6]	Vitamin B12 (μg)	Minerals Calcium (mg)	Phosphorus (mg)	Magnesium (mg)	Iron (mg)	Zinc (mg)	Iodine (μg)
Infants	0.0–0.5	6	13	60	24	kg × 2.2	420	10	3	35	0.3	0.4	6	0.3	30	0.5	360	240	50	10	3	40
	0.5–1.0	9	20	71	28	kg × 2.0	400	10	4	35	0.5	0.6	8	0.6	45	1.5	540	360	70	15	5	50
Children	1–3	13	29	90	35	23	400	10	5	45	0.7	0.8	9	0.9	100	2.0	800	800	150	15	10	70
	4–6	20	44	112	44	30	500	10	6	45	0.9	1.0	11	1.3	200	2.5	800	800	200	10	10	90
	7–10	28	62	132	52	34	700	10	7	45	1.2	1.4	16	1.6	300	3.0	800	800	250	10	10	120
Males	11–14	45	99	157	62	45	1000	10	8	50	1.4	1.6	18	1.8	400	3.0	1200	1200	350	18	15	150
	15–18	66	145	176	69	56	1000	10	10	60	1.4	1.7	18	2.0	400	3.0	1200	1200	400	18	15	150
	19–22	70	154	177	70	56	1000	7.5	10	60	1.5	1.7	19	2.2	400	3.0	800	800	350	10	15	150
	23–50	70	154	178	70	56	1000	5	10	60	1.4	1.6	18	2.2	400	3.0	800	800	350	10	15	150
	51+	70	154	178	70	56	1000	5	10	60	1.2	1.4	16	2.2	400	3.0	800	800	350	10	15	150
Females	11–14	46	101	157	62	46	800	10	8	50	1.1	1.3	15	1.8	400	3.0	1200	1200	300	18	15	150
	15–18	55	120	163	64	46	800	10	8	60	1.1	1.3	14	2.0	400	3.0	1200	1200	300	18	15	150
	19–22	55	120	163	64	44	800	7.5	8	60	1.1	1.3	14	2.0	400	3.0	800	800	300	18	15	150
	23–50	55	120	163	64	44	800	5	8	60	1.0	1.2	13	2.0	400	3.0	800	800	300	18	15	150
	51+	55	120	163	64	44	800	5	8	60	1.0	1.2	13	2.0	400	3.0	800	800	300	10	15	150
Pregnant						+30	+200	+5	+2	+20	+0.4	+0.3	+2	+0.6	+400	+1.0	+400	+400	+150	8	+5	+25
Lactating						+20	+400	+5	+3	+40	+0.5	+0.5	+5	+0.5	+100	+1.0	+400	+400	+150	8	+10	+50

[1] The allowances are intended to provide for individual variations among most normal persons as they live in the United States under usual environmental stresses. Diets should be based on a variety of common foods in order to provide other nutrients for which human requirements have been less well defined. See text for detailed discussion of allowances and of nutrients not tabulated. See Table 8–2 (p. 72) for suggested average energy intakes.

[2] Retinol equivalents. 1 Retinol equivalent = 1 μg retinol or 6 μg β-carotene. See text for calculation of vitamin A activity of diets as retinol equivalents.

[3] As cholecalciferol. 10 μg cholecalciferol = 400 I.U. vitamin D.

[4] α tocopherol equivalents. 1 mg d-α-tocopherol = 1 α T.E.

[5] 1 NE (niacin equivalent) is equal to 1 mg of niacin or 60 mg of dietary tryptophan.

[6] The folacin allowances refer to dietary sources as determined by Lactobacillus casei assay after treatment with enzymes ("conjugases") to make polyglutamyl forms of the vitamin available to the test organism.

[7] The RDA for vitamin B12 in infants is based on average concentration of the vitamin in human milk. The allowances after weaning are based on energy intake (as recommended by the American Academy of Pediatrics) and consideration of other factors such as intestinal absorption.

[8] The increased requirement during pregnancy cannot be met by the iron content of habitual American diets nor by the existing iron stores of many women; therefore the use of 30–60 mg of supplemental iron is recommended. Iron needs during lactation are not substantially different from those of nonpregnant women, but continued supplementation of the mother for 2–3 months after parturition is advisable in order to replenish stores depleted by pregnancy.

Reproduced from: Recommended Dietary Allowances, Ninth Edition (1979) with the permission of the National Academy of Sciences, Washington, D.C.

The study of the individual nutrients in the chapters that follow will point out some of the effects of food preparation.

Generally speaking, the values listed in Table A-1 are for household measures of food. Some measures are greater than the usual serving portions—for example, a cupful of vegetables. Note that the foods in this table are grouped by classes such as Milk, Cream, Cheese; Meat, Poultry, Fish; Vegetables; and so on. This arrangement makes it easy to compare the nutritive value of one food in a group with another food in that same group.

Suppose you were going to calculate the nutritive value of your own diet for one day. You would need to list each meal in terms of the kinds and amounts of every food, not forgetting the sugar, butter, jelly, coffee, cream, and other incidentals. You should also record the kinds and amounts of every food that you eat between meals. For example, your breakfast might have included juice, toast, cereal, milk, and coffee. In order to look up the nutritive value you would need to have an exact record such as the following:

Grapefruit juice	1 small glass (120 gm)
Cornflakes	1 cup (28 gm)
Milk, whole	½ cup (120 gm)
Sugar on cereal	1 teaspoon (5 gm)
Raisin toast	1½ slices (38 gm)
Butter	2 pats (10 gm)
Cream for coffee	2 tablespoons (30 gm)

When your day's record is complete, it is a good idea to add up the daily total for all foods that are the same, such as milk, butter, sugar. You may wish to calculate the value of your diet for all nutrients listed in the table; or you might look up the values for only one nutrient at the time. As you study each of the chapters on the nutrients it is a good idea to calculate your own intake of that nutrient. In this way you begin to know the good and poor sources of the nutrients and you also learn how to improve your own diet.

When you have calculated the value of your diet, compare the totals with the recommended allowances for a person of your age. Does your diet add up to the allowances? There is no harm in being a little bit over, but if you are under the allowances, you should look for ways to improve your diet. For the correct calorie intake, your weight is your best guide: if you weigh too much, you are consuming too many calories; if you weigh too little, you are not eating enough to keep your weight at the desirable level.

FOUR FOOD GROUPS

If you have calculated the nutritive value of a diet for one day, you would agree that this is somewhat time consuming. Fortunately, some short cuts have been developed. The Four Food Groups is a useful guide when properly used. * (See Fig. 4–1.)

* *A Daily Food Guide.* U.S. Department of Agriculture, Washington, D.C.

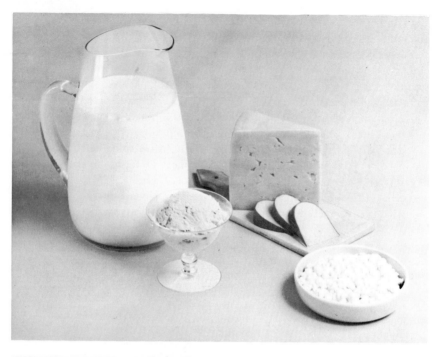

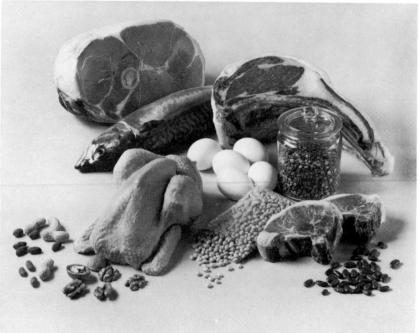

FIGURE 4–1   A Daily Food Guide: the Four Food Groups *(National Dairy Council, Chicago.)*

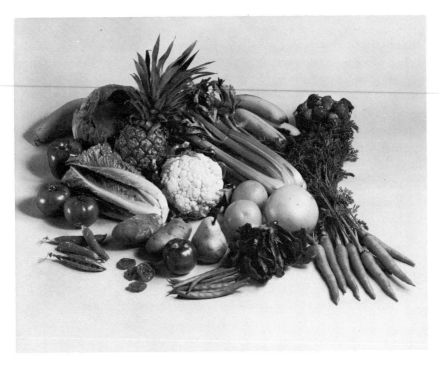

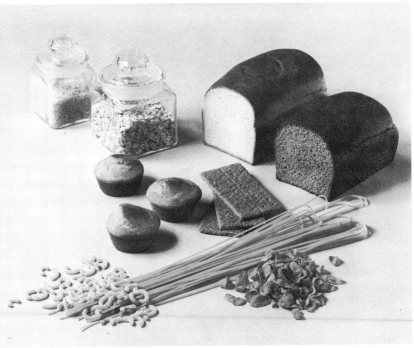

Milk group
  2 cups for adults
  2 to 3 cups for children under 9 years
  3 to 4 cups for children 9 to 12 years
  3 to 4 cups for teenagers
  3 cups or more for pregnant women
  4 cups or more for lactating women

Meat group
  2 servings. Count as one serving:
    2 to 3 ounces lean, cooked beef, veal, pork, lamb, poultry, fish—without bone
    2 eggs
    1 cup cooked dry beans, dry peas, lentils
    4 tablespoons peanut butter

Vegetable-fruit group
  4 or more servings per day, including:
    1 serving of citrus fruit, or other fruit or vegetable as a good source of vitamin C, or 2 servings of a fair source
    1 serving, at least every other day, of a dark green or deep yellow vegetable for vitamin A
    2 or more servings of other vegetables and fruits, including potatoes

Bread-cereals group
  4 or more servings daily (whole grain, enriched, or restored). Count as one serving:
    1 slice bread
    1 ounce ready-to-eat cereal
    ½ to ¾ cup cooked cereal, corn meal, grits, macaroni, noodles, rice, or spaghetti

Each of the food groups includes a variety of foods that contribute important nutrients. No single food group furnishes all needed nutrients. Nor are all foods in each group equally valuable for their nutrients. Therefore, in menu planning from day to day choices should be made from a wide variety of foods that belong to these groups. The chapters that follow in Unit II will identify the nutritive contributions of foods in each group.

The Four Food Groups have been criticized for a number of reasons. (1) They are only an approximate measure of the nutritive quality of the diet. They do not guarantee that the recommended allowances will be met for all nutrients; for example, iron for women. (2) It is difficult to use the groupings when food mixtures or many new foods in the market are used. For example, into which group or groups would you place lasagna or pizza? (3) Substantial modifications would be required if the Dietary Goals are to be implemented. (See p. 38.)

A BASIC DIET

The nutritive values for a basic diet pattern are shown in Table 4–2. This pattern includes the minimum amounts of foods listed for adults from each

Table 4-2 NUTRITIVE VALUE OF A BASIC DIET PATTERN FOR THE ADULT IN HEALTH *

Food	Measure	Weight gm	Energy kcal	Protein gm	Fat gm	Carbo-hydrate gm	Minerals		Vitamins				
							Ca mg	Fe mg	A I.U.	Thia-mine mg	Ribo-flavin mg	Niacin mg	Ascorbic Acid mg
Milk	2 cups	488	320	18	18	24	576	0.2	700	0.14	0.82	0.4	4
Meat Group													
Egg	1	50	80	6	6	tr	27	1.1	590	0.05	0.15	tr	0
Meat, fish, poultry (lean cooked) †	4 ounces	120	240	33	10	0	17	3.6	35	0.32	0.26	7.4	0
Vegetable-Fruit Group													
Leafy green or deep yellow	¼ to ⅓ cup ‡	50	15	1	tr	3	14	0.5	3700	0.03	0.04	0.3	14
Other vegetable	¼ to ⅓ cup §	50	15	1	tr	3	10	0.4	240	0.03	0.03	0.3	7
Potato	1 medium	122	80	2	tr	18	7	0.6	tr	0.11	0.04	1.4	20
Citrus fruit ‖	1 serving	100	40	1	tr	10	10	0.2	160	0.07	0.02	0.3	40
Other fruit #	1 serving	100	60	1	tr	16	12	0.5	600	0.04	0.04	0.4	9
Bread-Cereal Group													
Cereal, enriched or whole grain **	¾ cup	30 (dry)	105	3	tr	22	10	0.8	0	0.12	0.04	0.8	0
Bread, enriched or whole grain	3 slices	75	210	6	3	39	63	1.8	tr	0.18	0.15	1.8	tr
			1165	72	37	135	746	9.7	6025	1.09	1.59	13.1 ††	94
Recommended Dietary Allowances													
Woman (over 23 years)			2000	44			800	18	4000	1.0	1.2	13	60
Man (over 23 years)			2700	56			800	10	5000	1.4	1.6	18	60

* Values for foods in the meat, vegetable-fruit, and bread-cereal groups are weighted on the basis of the approximate consumption in the United States.
† Calculations based upon an average weekly intake for meat of 11 ounces beef, 7½ ounces pork, 6½ ounces poultry, 1½ ounces lamb and veal, and 1½ ounces fish.
‡ Dark green leafy and deep yellow vegetables include carrots, green peppers, broccoli, spinach, endive, escarole, and kale. It is assumed that an average serving of ½ cup is eaten at least every other day.
§ Other vegetables include tomatoes, lettuce, cabbage, snap beans, lima beans, celery, peas, onions, corn, cucumbers, beets, and cauliflower. It is assumed that an average serving of ½ cup is eaten at least every other day.
‖ Citrus fruit includes fresh, canned, and frozen oranges, orange juice, grapefruit, and grapefruit juice.
Other fruit includes apples, peaches, pears, apricots, grapes, plums, prunes, berries, and bananas.
** Cereals include corn flakes, wheat flakes, macaroni, oatmeal, shredded wheat, and enriched rice.
†† The protein in this diet contains about 720 mg trytophan, equivalent to 12 mg niacin; thus, the niacin equivalent of this diet is 25 mg.

of the Four Food Groups. The nutritive values have been calculated on the basis of food consumption in the United States. From this calculation you can see that a young woman who chooses a variety of foods from the Four Food Groups would meet the recommended allowances for all nutrients except iron and calories. Additional foods from the Four Food Groups or desserts, fats, and sweets will easily bring the calories to the level to maintain desirable weight. Sufficient iron remains a special problem, which will be discussed further in Chapter 9.

DIETARY GOALS

A third guide has received prominent attention in recent years. The Senate Select Committee on Nutrition and Human Needs in 1977 issued a list of dietary goals to recommend to people in the United States. These goals were based on the fact that many research reports have related excessive calories, too much fat, too much cholesterol, too much sugar, and too little fiber to increased risk of obesity, heart disease, cancer, various disorders of the digestive tract, diabetes mellitus, and others. Many nutritionists and physicians have accepted these findings and strongly support the Dietary Goals. Others state that proof of these relationships is lacking.

The Dietary Goals can be used with appropriate modifications of the Four Food Groups. Since the intake of fats and sugars is reduced, the choices of foods for daily menus must come from increasing amounts of fruits, vegetables, breads, and cereals. Thus, the nutritive value of the diet may actually be improved. If these goals are practiced over a lifetime, they should, in fact, improve the nutritional quality of the diet. They might have a preventive effect against the disease problems mentioned, but there is no guarantee that this is so.

The second edition of the Dietary Goals was published in late 1977.

Goals

1. To avoid overweight, consume only as much energy (calories) as is expended; if overweight, decrease energy intake and increase energy expenditure.
2. Increase the consumption of complex carbohydrates and "naturally occurring" sugars from about 28 per cent of energy intake to about 48 per cent of energy intake.
3. Reduce the consumption of refined and processed sugars to account for about 10 per cent of total energy intake.
4. Reduce overall fat consumption from approximately 40 per cent to about 30 per cent of energy intake.
5. Reduce saturated fat consumption to account for about 10 per cent of total energy intake; and balance that with polyunsaturated and monounsaturated fats, which should account for about 10 per cent of energy intake each.
6. Reduce cholesterol consumption to about 300 mg a day.
7. Limit the intake of sodium by reducing the intake of salt to about 5 gm a day.

The Goals suggest the following changes in food selection and preparation:

1. Increase consumption of fruits and vegetables and whole grains.

2. Decrease consumption of refined and other processed sugars and foods high in such sugars.

3. Decrease consumption of foods high in total fat, and partially replace saturated fats, whether obtained from animal or vegetable sources, with polyunsaturated fats.

4. Decrease consumption of animal fat, and choose smaller portions of lean meats, poultry and fish which will reduce saturated fat intake.

5. Except for young children, substitute low-fat and nonfat milk for whole milk, and low-fat dairy products for high-fat dairy products.

6. Decrease consumption of butterfat, eggs, and other high cholesterol sources. Some consideration should be given to easing the cholesterol goal for premenopausal women, young children, and the elderly in order to obtain the nutritional benefits of eggs in the diet.

7. Decrease consumption of salt and foods high in salt content.

REVIEW QUESTIONS AND PROBLEMS

1. What is your present weight in pounds? in kilograms? what is your present height in inches? in centimeters? (See Table A-5, p. 354.)

2. Compare your present weight with your desirable weight. Calculate the percentage overweight or underweight. How do you compare in size with the reference person of your age?

3. Keep a record of the foods you eat for one day. Check this against the recommended amounts from the Four Food Groups. Which foods should you add to your diet? Why?

4. Using Table A-1 (p. 322), list six foods that are specially rich in protein. How much of these foods would you be likely to eat in one meal?

5. Compare the ascorbic acid values for ½ cup grapefruit juice, 1 raw medium peach, 1 raw plum, 1 baked sweet potato, and ½ cup cooked spinach.

6. List the calorie values for 1 slice enriched bread, 1 tomato, 1 oz. sweetened milk chocolate, 1 teaspoon sugar, 1 teaspoon butter, 1 cup buttermilk, and 1 pork chop.

7. Write a menu for one day including only the minimum amounts of foods recommended for adults in the Four Food Groups. What foods would you ordinarily add to this menu pattern?

8. From Table A-1 determine whether these statements are correct.
   a. A 4-oz glass of apricot nectar is not a good substitute for 4 oz of orange juice.
   b. Green peas and broccoli are about equal in value for vitamin A and ascorbic acid.

9. List the changes you would need to make in the Four Food Groups if you were also adopting the Dietary Goals.

REFERENCES

Caly, J. C.: "Assessing Adults' Nutrition," *Am. J. Nurs.*, 77: 1605–1609, 1977.

Cullen, R. W., *et al.:* "Sodium, Hypertension, and the U.S. Dietary Goals," *J. Nutr. Educ.*, 10:59–60, 1978.

"Dietary Goals: A Statement by the American Dietetic Association," *J. Am. Dietet. A.*, 71:227–28, 1977.

Food and Nutrition Board: *Recommended Dietary Allowances*, 9th ed. National Academy of Sciences—National Research Council, Washington, D.C., 1979.

King, J. C., *et al.:* "Evaluation and Modification of the Basic Four Food Guide," *J. Nutr. Educ.*, 10:27–29, 1978.

Mayer, J.: "Food for a Healthy Heart," *Family Health*, 8:38–40, November 1976.

Sorenson, A. W., *et al.:* "An Index of Nutritional Quality for a Balanced Diet," *J. Am. Dietet. A.*, 68:236–42, 1976.

THE NUTRIENTS

5

NATURE AND PROPERTIES | QUALITY OF FOOD PROTEINS | SOURCES |
FUNCTIONS | PROTEIN ALLOWANCES | CLINICAL PROBLEMS | SOME FALLACIES
AND FACTS

PROTEINS AND AMINO ACIDS

The abundant food supply in the United States provides its people with a protein intake far in excess of requirements. Even most poor people consume protein at levels above the recommended allowances. Protein deficiency is less likely to occur in the United States than is deficiency of any other nutrient.

NATURE AND PROPERTIES

Like carbohydrates and fats, proteins contain carbon, hydrogen, and oxygen. In addition, proteins contain about 16 per cent nitrogen. Sulfur, phosphorus, iron, and sometimes other elements such as iodine are found in small amounts. Proteins are built from 20 or so simpler building stones called *amino acids.* Just as the 26 letters of the alphabet can be combined in an amazing number of words, so the different amino acids can be joined to give an almost infinite variety of proteins. For example, the proteins found in bones, or teeth, or fingernails are quite different from those in hair, or muscle, or liver. The proteins in egg are different from those in milk, or wheat, or rice, and so on.

The amount of protein present in a food or in a tissue can be determined in the laboratory by an analysis for the nitrogen content. Each gram of nitrogen found in a food sample is equal to 6.25 gm protein.

Proteins coagulate when they are exposed to heat or to acid. Thus egg white and meat coagulate when they are cooked; if too high heat is used, or if the food is cooked too long, the protein becomes dried out and tough. Perhaps at some time you have added a little vinegar to milk when you did not have the sour milk called for in a recipe. The milk thickens or curdles with the addition of the acid; in other words, the milk protein has been *coagulated.*

43

QUALITY OF FOOD PROTEINS

The body can manufacture some of the amino acids required by the tissues, but it is unable to make others. Those amino acids that cannot be manufactured by the body must be present in the protein of the diet, and are called *essential amino acids*. It is a good idea to be able to recognize the names of these essential amino acids when you see them. They are

histidine (infants and children; possibly adults)	phenylalanine
isoleucine	threonine
leucine	tryptophan
lysine	valine
methionine	

Biologic value. The foods we eat supply the amino acids that the cells require for synthesis of proteins. Not all foods are of equal quality in meeting the cellular needs. Each cell must have a sufficient supply of all the amino acids it needs in order to build a new protein. All of these amino acids must be present at the same time; if one or more are missing, the protein cannot be synthesized and the rest of the amino acids will be more or less wasted. Suppose there were half the needed amount of one of the amino acids: then the cell can build only half as much protein.

If a food furnishes amino acids in the proportions and amounts needed by the body cells for tissue replacement and growth, it is said to furnish protein of *high biologic value;* the protein is often referred to as *complete*. Eggs, milk, cheese, meat, fish, and poultry are examples of foods high in biologic value.

Foods that lack adequate amounts of one or more essential amino acids are of *poor biologic value* or *incomplete*. These include the proteins found in cereals, legumes, nuts, and vegetables.

Complementarity. Fortunately, the same amino acids are not missing from all plant foods. When one food provides the amino acids that are missing in another is it said to *complement* (to make complete) the second food. For example, neither corn nor dry beans, when eaten at separate times, provide the amino acids needed by the tissues. But if they are eaten at the same meal, as Mexicans often do, the two foods will supply sufficient amounts of the amino acids for protein synthesis to take place in the cells. Thus, cheese complements the protein in macaroni; milk makes up for some amino acids missing in the breakfast cereal; and black-eyed peas and corn bread, eaten together, complement each other in their amino acids.

Protein efficiency ratio. One of the methods used to measure the quality of a protein is to determine its *protein efficiency ratio* (PER). You may occasionally see reference to this ratio on a food label. To determine the PER a single protein to be tested is fed in an adequate diet to very young rats for a four-week period. The PER is the weight gain of the rats divided by the amount of protein eaten. For example, suppose the rats gained 5 grams for each 2 grams of protein fed, then the PER would be 2.5. Such a ratio is typical of milk, eggs, meat, poultry, and fish. If cereals alone, or legumes alone, were fed the ratio would be much lower. If cereal, such as wheat, were fed with a legume, such as beans, the PER would be nearly that of milk, meat, or egg protein.

SOURCES

When the word "protein" is mentioned most people immediately think of meat. Mistakenly, they also think that diets cannot be adequate in protein if they do not include meat. In the United States foods of high biologic value—meat, poultry, fish, eggs, milk, and cheese—provide just over three fifths of the protein in the average diet. The approximate amount of protein contributed by typical foods of the Four Food Groups is shown in Table 5–1 and Fig. 5–1.

TABLE 5–1 AVERAGE PROTEIN COMPOSITION OF SOME FOODS

Food	Serving	Protein gm	Protein Quality
Milk group			
Milk, whole, skim, buttermilk	1 cup	9	Complete
Cheese, American, process	1 oz	7	Complete
Cheese, cottage	¼ cup	8	Complete
Cheese, cream	2 tablespoons	2	Complete
Ice cream	⅛ qt	3	Complete
Meat group			
Meat, fish, poultry	3 oz, fatty	15–20	Complete
	3 oz, lean	20–25	Complete
Egg	1 whole	6	Complete
Dried beans or peas	½ cup cooked	7–8	Incomplete
Peanut butter	1 tablespoon	4	Incomplete
Vegetable-fruit group			
Fruit juice	½ cup	Trace	
Fruits	1 serving	Trace–1	Incomplete
Vegetables	½ cup	1–3	Incomplete
Bread-cereal group			
Breakfast cereals	½ cup cooked	2–3	Incomplete
	¾ cup dry	2–3	Incomplete
Bread	1 slice	2	Incomplete
Macaroni, noodles, rice, spaghetti	½ cup cooked	2	Incomplete

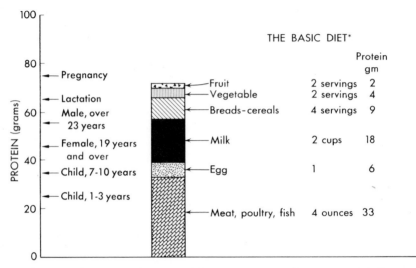

FIGURE 5-1 The Four Food Groups of the Basic Diet meet the recommended allowances for protein for all categories except the pregnant woman. See Table 4–2 (p. 37) for complete calculation.

Legumes (navy beans, pinto beans, chick peas, soybeans, split peas, peanuts) are rich in protein, as are also nuts of many kinds. Presently legumes do not form an important part of the American diet, but their potential uses are great; they are widely used in some parts of the world.

Food technologists have developed procedures to extract the protein from plant foods such as soybeans, cottonseed, wheat, and others. The extracted protein is spun into fibers which are almost pure protein. The fibers can be formulated into *textured vegetable protein* foods that simulate chicken, beef, ham, bacon, sausage, tuna, and others in terms of appearance, texture, and flavor. Because of these similarities to the animal foods they are also referred to as *analogs*. Since these products are intended as a replacement for meat, it is important that they provide the same variety and quantity of nutrients as contained in meat. These products are widely used to replace meat in the diets of vegetarians.

Breads and cereals contain about 2 to 3 gm protein per serving. However, the amount of bread and cereal eaten may be sufficiently great to provide an important proportion of the total protein requirement. For example, a boy of 16 who eats eight slices of bread in a day is thus obtaining 16 to 20 gm protein from this source alone.

The average serving of vegetables contributes 1 to 3 gm protein, and fruits are even lower in protein content. This food group accounts for only a small part of the protein in typical American diets.

FUNCTIONS

Proteins are digested to amino acids (see Chapter 3) which are absorbed through the walls of the small intestine into the portal blood circulation for delivery to the liver and the tissues of the body. The cells of each tissue and organ remove the kinds and amounts of amino acids required for a given function.

Structural role. Proteins are essential components of the cells of all living things—plants, animals, and even microorganisms. Every tissue and fluid in the body except bile and urine contains some protein. The human body consists of about 18 to 20 per cent protein. Muscles account for most of this protein. It is not always realized that the framework of the skeleton into which minerals are deposited also consists of protein.

The need for protein continues throughout life since there is a constant need for new cells to replace those that have broken down. For example, the red blood cells have a life span of about 60 to 120 days, while cells of the intestinal mucosa are renewed every few days. When cells are broken down, there must be equal numbers of new ones to take their places.

Throughout the period of pregnancy, and in infancy, childhood, and adolescence, protein is continuously required for the building of the marvelous variety of new tissues as well as for replacement to take care of wear and tear.

Regulatory functions. Most of the regulatory materials of the body, including enzymes and hormones, are protein in nature. For example, the digestion of food requires certain enzymes that are constructed from amino acids. Thyroxine, a hormone that regulates energy metabolism, and insulin, which regulates the blood sugar level, contain specific kinds and amounts of amino acids. The red coloring matter of the blood, *hemoglobin,* is an iron-containing protein that carries oxygen to the tissues. Other proteins in the blood regulate osmotic pressure and water balance. The body's defense against disease is brought about by antibodies that are composed of protein.

Energy. Proteins furnish 4 kcal per gram. If the diet contains more protein than is needed, the nitrogen will be removed from the excess amino acids by the liver. The nitrogen is excreted in the form of urea by the kidney. The remainder of the amino acid molecule is then used as an immediate source of energy, or it may be stored in the form of fat. If the diet does not contain sufficient calories from carbohydrate and fat, the protein will be used for energy rather than for building or replacing tissues.

PROTEIN ALLOWANCES

The protein need of the adult is based on body size. The recommended allowance is 0.8 gm per kilogram body weight. This amounts to 56 gm for the 70-kg man and 44 gm for the 55-kg woman. (See Table 4–1, p. 32.) Hard work and exercise do not increase the protein requirement. On the other hand, advancing age does not decrease the requirement.

Under certain conditions the adult can maintain nitrogen balance with a protein intake as low as 25 to 40 gm. The quality of the protein in these circumstances must be excellent, and sufficient calories must be provided by carbohydrate and fat so that protein is not used for energy. Such reduction of protein intake becomes imperative when the food supply is very limited, and also when the kidneys are failing. (See Chapter 27.)

When new tissues are being built, the amount of protein eaten must be greater than the amount used for tissue wear and tear. Persons who are building new tissues are said to be in *positive nitrogen balance.* Infants, because of their rapid growth, are allowed 2.2 gm protein per kilogram (1.0 gm per pound) for the first 6 months, and then 2.0 gm per kilogram for the remainder of the first year. The recommended allowance for children 7 to 10 years is 36 gm, which is about three fourths of the woman's allowance. Teenage boys and girls should include 44 to 54 gm daily, depending upon age and body size.

The pregnant woman should include an additional 30 gm protein. To supply the nursing infant with sufficient protein, the lactating woman needs to include 20 gm protein above her normal needs.

In planning diets it is generally recommended that each meal contain some complete protein foods or foods that complement each other so that all of the amino acids will be available to the tissues at the same time.

CLINICAL PROBLEMS

Protein deficiency is not common in the United States. Under certain circumstances an individual might be in *negative nitrogen balance.* This means that his body is breaking down protein tissues faster than they are being replaced. Thus the excretions contain more nitrogen than is being supplied by the diet. Just as overdrawing a bank account is not a good thing, so the excess removal of nitrogen from the tissue is also harmful. When negative nitrogen balance exists, the individual is less able to resist infections, he may withstand the stress of injury or surgery poorly, and his general health will deteriorate.

Negative nitrogen balance can exist when an individual does not eat enough protein-containing foods, or eats protein foods of poor quality, or obtains insufficient calories. Some persons use crash diets for reducing and thus have a very low protein intake. Many elderly persons are unable to chew well, or don't like milk, or believe they don't need protein foods such as meat or eggs. Injury, infections, and surgery increase the protein need but patients in these situations often have a poor appetite. Nurses and dietitians should be particularly alert to the possibility of protein malnutrition in patients with poor appetites. They should take steps to improve food intake before serious problems arise.

Protein-calorie malnutrition. Two forms of protein-calorie malnutrition (PCM), *kwashiorkor* and *marasmus,* are seen in infants and young children in

Africa, Central and Latin America, and parts of the Orient. Although rare in the United States, these conditions are sometimes seen in conditions of severe poverty, or as a result of parental ignorance regarding infant feeding, or in child neglect.

Kwashiorkor usually appears after the child is weaned from the mother's breast. Usually the infant obtains enough calories, but the high-carbohydrate foods do not supply enough protein. The infants fail to grow, the appetite is poor, the skin and hair change in texture and color, diarrhea follows, the tissues hold water (edema), and death sometimes follows if there is no treatment. (See Fig. 5-2.)

Marasmus occurs in infants who are weaned very early and who are fed diets that are low in calories as well as protein. These infants are emaciated

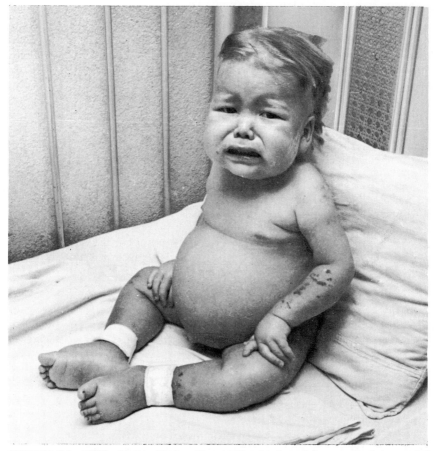

FIGURE 5-2 Child with kwashiorkor. Note swollen hands and feet, patchy hair, mottled skin, and uncomfortable appearance. (UNICEF. Photo by Nagata.)

in appearance. Because the severe malnutrition has occurred very early in life, the brain cells have had less opportunity to develop. If the infant survives, there is the possibility of mental retardation taking place.

Protein-calorie malnutrition can be prevented or treated with inexpensive sources of protein-rich foods. Dry milk supplied through UNICEF to many infants and children has been highly effective. Many countries have developed protein-rich foods by combining locally available plant foods. *Incaparina*, the best known of these, is a food powder that can be mixed with water for child feeding. It is made from corn, cottonseed, sorghum, and mineral-vitamin supplements. Soybean protein, peanut protein, and others have been used in various mixtures.

SOME FALLACIES AND FACTS

1. *Fallacy*. Athletes need more protein than nonathletes.

Fact. The protein requirement of the adult depends on the body size and not on the amount of exercise.

2. *Fallacy*. Older people need less protein than young adults.

Fact. The need for replacing the protein of tissues continues throughout life. Older people need the same amount of protein as the young adult of the same body size.

3. *Fallacy*. Gelatin is an excellent source of protein.

Fact. Dry gelatin is about 90 per cent protein, but the average gelatin dessert would furnish about 2 gm protein. Gelatin lacks some of the essential amino acids; as a sole source of protein it cannot maintain life or support growth.

4. *Fallacy*. Protein foods should not be eaten in the same meal as starches.

Fact. There is no reason to separate protein foods and starches. In fact, many common foods contain both protein and carbohydrate. The digestive tract efficiently digests protein, carbohydrate, and fat components of the diet at the same time. Each meal should contain one fourth to one third of the day's protein so that the amino acids will be most efficiently used for tissue synthesis.

REVIEW QUESTIONS AND PROBLEMS

1. Define amino acid, essential amino acid, complete protein, complementary protein, biologic value, nitrogen balance, antibody, phenylalanine.

2. How do proteins differ from fats and carbohydrates?

3. Keep a record of the food you eat for one day. Using the approximate values on p. 45, estimate the amount of protein in your diet. What foods provided you with complete protein?

4. What happens if you eat more protein than your tissues need for maintenance?

5. How does the protein need of a ten-year-old boy compare with your need?

6. How could you improve these meals for protein?

I	II
Large fruit salad	Baked beans
Roll with butter	Brown bread with butter
Cucumber-water cress sandwich	Sliced tomato salad
Iced tea	Jello with whipped cream

7. Name three substances in the body that are of a protein nature and that regulate body functions. Tell what each does.

8. What is kwashiorkor? How may it be prevented?

9. A 75-year-old woman refuses to drink milk or to eat meat because she thinks these foods are not good for her. How would you respond to this situation?

REFERENCES

Breeling, J. L.: "Marketing Protein for the World's Poor," *Today's Health*, **47**:42, February 1969.

Council on Foods and Nutrition: "Zen Macrobiotic Diets," *J.A.M.A.*, **218**:397, 1971.

Mayer, J.: "Textured Vegetable Proteins," *Family Health*, 8:40, September 1976.

Robinson, C. H.: *Normal and Therapeutic Nutrition*, 15th ed. New York: Macmillan Publishing Co., Inc., 1977, chap. 4.

Scrimshaw, N. S.: "Nature of Protein Requirements: Ways They Can Be Met in Tomorrow's World," *J. Am. Dietet. A.*, **54**:94–102, 1969.

Williams, C. D.: "The Story of Kwashiorkor," *Nutr. Rev.*, **31**:334–40, 1973.

FATS

"The fat of the land." The word "fat" brings to mind such ideas as wealth, prosperity, and well-being; likewise, the word makes one think of such rich foods as pastries, cookies, cakes, ice cream, butter, cream, and oil. But fat is also associated with overweight, and more recently with heart disease. *Lipid* is another term for fats and fatlike substances, including phospholipids and sterols.

FATTY ACIDS AND TRIGLYCERIDES

Fats are composed of three chemical elements: carbon, hydrogen, and oxygen. Fats contain much smaller proportions of oxygen than do carbohydrates. Some specialized kinds of fats, called *compound lipids* also contain other elements, for example, phosphorus and nitrogen in phospholipids.

Most fats are *triglycerides;* that is, they are formed from three molecules of *fatty acids* attached to one molecule of *glycerol.* About 20 fatty acids are commonly found in foods. Each fatty acid consists of a short or long chain of carbon atoms attached to an acid group. *Short-chain* fatty acids contain 4 to 6 carbon atoms; *medium-chain* fatty acids contain 8 to 10 carbon atoms; and *long-chain* fatty acids contain 12 to 20 or more carbon atoms.

Long-chain fatty acids may be saturated, monounsaturated, or polyunsaturated. *Saturated* fatty acids are those having single bonds between the carbon atoms (see Fig. 6–1). They cannot take up any hydrogen. Myristic, palmitic, and stearic acids are three examples of such fatty acids; they are abundant in animal fats, including beef and mutton fat, butter, and others. Coconut oil, although liquid, consists mostly of lauric acid, a saturated fatty acid.

52

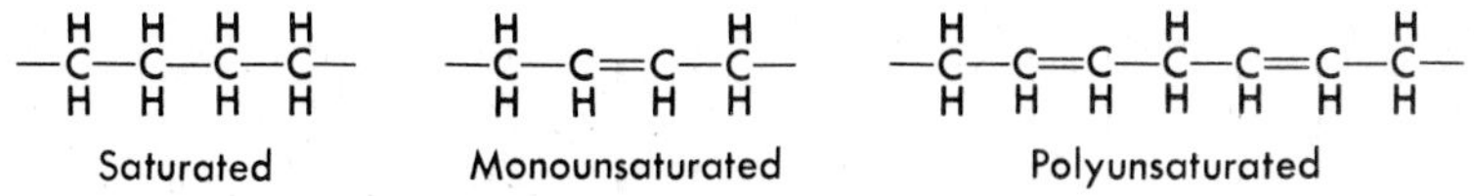

FIGURE 6-1 Fatty acids with one bond between all carbon atoms are saturated; those with a double bond between two or more carbon atoms are unsaturated.

A *monounsaturated* fatty acid is one in which two of the carbon atoms are joined by a double bond. This means that a hydrogen atom could be added to each of the carbon atoms at the double bond. Oleic acid is the most abundant monounsaturated fatty acid. Olive oil is especially high in oleic acid, but most fats contain generous amounts of this fatty acid.

A *polyunsaturated* fatty acid is one in which two or more double bonds are present. Thus, each of four or more carbon atoms could take up a hydrogen atom. *Linoleic* acid has two double bonds and is the most common of the polyunsaturated acids; it is abundant in most vegetable oils.

PROPERTIES

Fats are insoluble in water, but soluble in ether, chloroform, benzene, and acetone. In the blood circulation they are held in solution by being attached to proteins (lipoproteins).

The flavor and hardness of a food fat depend upon the kinds and amounts of the fatty acids that are present. Food fats are a mixture of saturated and unsaturated fatty acids. For convenience a food fat is called *saturated* if it contains more saturated than polyunsaturated fatty acids; such fats are solid. If polyunsaturated fatty acids exceed the saturated fatty acids, the food fat is said to be *polyunsaturated;* such fats are liquid, such as oils, or very soft, such as some special type margarines. By dividing the amount of polyunsaturated fatty acids in a food by the amount of saturated fatty acids, one can obtain the P/S ratio; for example, 4 gm polyunsaturated fatty acid and 2 gm saturated fatty acid gives a P/S ratio of 2.

Hydrogenation is the addition of hydrogen to the carbon atoms in unsaturated fats to produce a solid fat. Regular margarines and many cooking fats are prepared from vegetable oils by this process. As might be expected, the addition of hydrogen increases the proportion of saturated fatty acids.

Fats become rancid if they are exposed to air and light. The change is more rapid at high temperatures. Many manufacturers add antioxidants to food fats to lengthen the time that they may be kept.

FOOD SOURCES

Some fats are "visible," as in butter, shortenings, oils, and between and around muscle fibers in meat. Others are "invisible," as in milk, egg yolk, and food mixtures. The meat and milk groups furnish about half of the fat

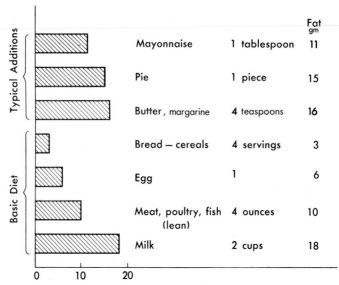

FIGURE 6–2 The fat content of a diet is rapidly increased with the addition of margarine or butter, salad dressings, and most desserts. See Table 4–2 (p. 37) for calculation of the Basic Diet.

in our diets. Visible fats and oils are the next important source of fats. The vegetable-fruit group (except olives and avocado) and the bread-cereal group are very low in fat. The fat content of the basic diet is shown in Fig. 6–2.

The important way by which fats contribute to the calories of the diet is shown in Table 6–1.

The food sources of specific categories of lipids follow.

High in saturated fatty acids
    Whole milk, cream, ice cream, cheeses made from whole milk, egg yolk
    Medium fat or fatty meats: beef, lamb, pork, ham
    Bacon, beef tallow, butter, coconut oil, lamb fat, lard, regular margarine, salt pork,
        hydrogenated shortenings
    Chocolate, chocolate candy, cakes, cookies, pies, rich puddings
High in polyunsaturated fatty acids
    Vegetable oils: safflower, corn, cottonseed, soybean, sesame, sunflower
    Salad dressings made from the above oils: mayonnaise, French, and others
    Special margarines: liquid oil listed first on label
    Fatty fish: salmon, tuna, herring
Sources of cholesterol
    High: egg yolk, liver, sweetbreads, brains, kidney, heart, fish roe, shrimp
    Moderate: whole milk, whole-milk cheeses, cream, ice cream, butter, meat, poultry,
        fish, clams, crab, oysters, scallops
    Low: non-fat milk, cheeses made from skim milk, nonfat yogurt
    Absent: egg white; plant foods

TABLE 6–1 COMPARISON OF FAT CONTENT and CALORIES

	Total Fat gm	kcal
Skim milk, 1 cup	Trace	90
Whole milk, 1 cup	9	160
Half milk and half cream, 1 cup	28	325
Tossed salad	Trace	20
Tossed salad with 2 tablespoons blue cheese dressing	16	170
Bread, 1 thin slice	1	65
Bread, 1 slice with 1 pat butter	5	100
Baked potato, one	Trace	90
Baked potato with 2 tablespoons sour cream	4	140
Lamb chop, lean, one	6	140
Lamb chop, lean with fat, one	33	400

FUNCTIONS

Triglycerides account for most of the fat in food and in the body. Normally, about 95 per cent of the fat in food is digested and absorbed. (See Chapter 3.) Fats, as we all know, are important sources of calories; each gram contributes 9 kcal. It is quite normal for the body to have deposits of fat (adipose tissue) that serve as a continuing supply of energy each and every hour. In fact, if we had no reserves of fat in the body whatsoever, we would need to eat much more frequently in order to provide a continuous supply of energy. Judging by the frequency and degree of obesity, fat can be stored in almost unlimited quantity.

Fat is said to be *protein-sparing* because its availability reduces the need to burn protein for energy. Carbohydrates and proteins in excess of body needs are also changed into fatty tissue, just as fat in the diet contributes to these stores.

In addition to providing energy, fats are essential (1) to maintain the constant body temperature by providing effective insulation underneath the skin; (2) to cushion the vital organs, such as the kidney, against injury; (3) to facilitate the absorption of the fat-soluble vitamins A, D, E, and K; (4) to provide satiety and to delay the onset of hunger; and (5) to contribute to flavor and palatability of the diet.

Essential fatty acids. *Linoleic acid,* a long-chain polyunsaturated fatty acid must be present in the diet because it cannot be synthesized in the body. In the body it is converted to *arachidonic acid* which is essential for normal growth and skin health. Safflower, sunflower, corn, cottonseed, and soybean oils are good sources of linoleic acid.

Phospholipids. These are fats in which a phosphorus-nitrogen compound has been substituted for one of the fatty acids in the triglyceride molecule. The diet contains some phospholipids, and the body readily makes them. *Lecithin* is the most abundant of these. Phospholipids are important in brain and nervous tissue. They also assist in the absorption of fats from the small intestine and in the transport of fats in the blood.

Lipoproteins. By being attached to proteins fats can be held in solution in the blood circulation and carried to the tissues. The lipoproteins are synthesized primarily in the liver. They contain varying amounts of triglycerides, cholesterol, phospholipids, and protein, and are classified according to their composition. (See Chapter 25.)

Cholesterol. Cholesterol is a white waxy substance related to fats, but very different in chemical structure. It is a normal constituent of the tissues, but is especially important in the formation of brain and nervous tissues. It serves as a precursor of vitamin D; that is, cholesterol in the skin can be changed into active vitamin D by exposure to the ultraviolet rays in sunlight. Cholesterol is closely related to the sex hormones and to the hormones of the adrenal gland. Excess cholesterol is removed from the body in the bile.

The body can manufacture cholesterol to meet its needs from fats, carbohydrates, and amino acids. Beyond infancy there does not appear to be any need to supply cholesterol in the diet.

DAILY ALLOWANCES

The requirement for linoleic acid can be met if 1 to 2 per cent of the calories are derived from appropriate fats; that is, 15 to 25 gm fat daily in the adult diet. Other than this there is no specific quantity of fat that is needed. Throughout the world the fat intake varies widely. For example, people in some Asian and African nations consume as little as 10 to 20 per cent of their calories from fat, whereas other people, such as Eskimos, eat large quantities of fat.

On the average, Americans obtain more than 40 per cent of their calories from fat. However, as you would expect, the intake varies widely. Some people eat many fried foods, pastries, rich desserts, cream, salad dressings, butter, and margarine, while others consume very little of these high-fat foods. A typical cholesterol intake ranges from 500 to 800 mg daily, but the American who consumes two eggs or more a day plus large servings of meat and other cholesterol-rich foods may ingest in excess of 1000 mg cholesterol daily.

Many scientists and clinicians agree with the recommendations set forth in the Dietary Goals:

1. Include not more than 30 per cent of calories from fat.
2. Decrease saturated fats to no more than 10 per cent of calories; increase polyunsaturated fats to about 10 per cent of calories.
3. Restrict cholesterol to about 300 mg per day.

To bring about these changes in the diet, the following steps are taken: skim milk and skim-milk cheeses instead of whole milk and whole-milk cheeses; moderate portions of low-fat meats, poultry, fish; 3 to 4 eggs per week; oils, margarines, salad dressings high in polyunsaturated fatty acids. Such changes in the diet can be readily made with available foods in the market; they are palatable, safe, and potentially beneficial.

CLINICAL PROBLEMS

Because fats are a concentrated source of calories, it is very easy to consume calories in excess of one's needs. Thus, the person who uses extra teaspoons of butter, margarine, or salad dressing—not to mention fat-rich sauces and desserts—may rapidly find obesity to be a problem.

Fats and oils do not provide protein, minerals, and vitamins. As their intake is increased, it becomes more difficult to obtain these essential nutrients without exceeding the caloric limit.

Diets rich in saturated fat and/or in cholesterol tend to lead to increased serum cholesterol levels. Some estimates indicate that at least half of all Americans have serum cholesterol levels that are above desirable levels. The elevation of blood lipids is associated with increased incidence of coronary heart and blood vessel disease. (See Chapter 25.) An association has also been made between high-fat intakes and the incidence of cancer of the colon and of the breast, but more evidence is needed to establish this with certainty. In diseases of the gallbladder and pancreas fats are poorly tolerated. (See Chapter 30.)

SOME FALLACIES AND FACTS

1. *Fallacy.* Fried foods are hard to digest.
   Fact. Digestion of fried foods is as complete as that of other foods. However, because fat coats the food particles, the digestion of fried foods takes somewhat longer.
2. *Fallacy.* Mineral oil is a good substitute for regular oil in low-calorie salad dressings.
   Fact. Mineral oil is not absorbed through the intestinal wall and thus provides no calories. However, it interferes seriously with the absorption of fat-soluble vitamins A, D, E, and K. Therefore, it should never be used in food preparation.
3. *Fallacy.* Vegetable oils without additives are more nutritious than those preserved with an antioxidant.
   Fact. The unsaturated fatty acids in vegetable oils are rapidly oxidized in the absence of antioxidants; this results in rancidity of the oil. Tocopherols (vitamin E)

are among the most effective antioxidants, and any excess in the oils enters into the normal metabolism of vitamin E.

4. *Fallacy*. Vegetable oils are less fattening than solid fats.

Fact. Oils and solid fats are equally high in calories; that is, each gram of fat from either source furnishes 9 kcal.

5. *Fallacy*. Sour cream is lower in calories than sweet cream.

Fact. Sour cream has the same number of calories as the sweet cream from which it is made. Usually sour cream is made from light cream.

6. *Fallacy*. Lecithin supplements should be added to the diet in order to meet the needs for synthesis of brain and nervous tissue.

Fact. The liver readily manufactures lecithin to fully meet the needs for cell membranes and for the synthesis of nervous tissues.

REVIEW QUESTIONS AND PROBLEMS

1. What is meant by lipid, saturated fat, polyunsaturated fat, linoleic acid, hydrogenated fat, cholesterol?

2. What chemical elements are present in fats?

3. If a diet contains 90 gm fat, how many kilocalories are provided?

4. List six functions of fats.

5. List the sources of fat that you had in your diet yesterday. Which of these sources furnished linoleic acid? What foods did you eat that contained cholesterol?

6. A person complains that a meal that included fried chicken, French fried potatoes, and apple pie was "heavy." What does he probably mean by this? How do you explain this feeling?

7. A person tells you that he is not going to eat any more eggs, milk, or butter because they are high in cholesterol. How would you respond to this?

8. Examine the labels on several brands of margarine. Which of these brands is the best source of polyunsaturated fatty acids?

REFERENCES

Alfin-Slater, R. B.: "Fats, Essential Fatty Acids, and Ascorbic Acid," *J. Am. Dietet. A.*, 64:168–70, 1974.

Grollman, A.: "A Common Sense Guide to Cholesterol," *Today's Health*, **44**:3, August 1966.

Holt, P. A.: "Fats and Bile Salts: Physiologic Considerations," *J. Am. Dietet. A.*, 60:491–95, 1972.

Robinson, C. H., and Lawler, M. R.: *Normal and Therapeutic Nutrition*, 15th ed. New York: Macmillan Publishing Co., Inc., 1977, chap. 6.

7

CARBOHYDRATES

All people of the world depend upon carbohydrate-rich foods as the principal source of calories. In the United States carbohydrates furnish less than half of the calories, whereas in some countries of the world as much as four fifths of the calories are obtained from carbohydrate. The carbohydrate-rich plants are easily grown, give a large yield of food per acre, keep rather well, and are less expensive than foods of animal origin. The foods are highly acceptable in a great variety of ways and are easily digested and used in the body.

NATURE AND CLASSIFICATION

By a complex process known as *photosynthesis* all green plants use energy from the sun, water from the soil, and carbon dioxide from the air to make carbohydrate. All carbohydrates contain the chemical elements carbon, hydrogen, and oxygen. The hydrogen and oxygen are present in the same proportions as found in water.

Table 7–1 shows a common classification of carbohydrates. The single and double sugars are often referred to as "simple" carbohydrates, while the polysaccharides including starches and dietary fibers are designated as "complex" carbohydrates.

PROPERTIES

Carbohydrates may be ranked in decreasing order of sweetness: fructose, sucrose, glucose, lactose, dextrin, and starch. Regardless of their sweetness, all carbohydrates furnish 4 kcal per gram. Only a small amount of honey, which

59

TABLE 7–1 CLASSIFICATION OF CARBOHYDRATES

Class	Examples	Some Food Sources
Monosaccharides (single sugars)	Glucose (dextrose, grape sugar, corn sugar, blood sugar)	Fruits, vegetables, corn syrup, honey
	Fructose (levulose, fruit sugar)	Fruits, vegetables, corn syrup, honey
	Galactose	Occurs only from the hydrolysis of lactose
Disaccharides (double sugars)	Sucrose	Cane, beet, maple sugar; small amounts in fruits, vegetables
	Maltose	Malting of cereal grains; acid hydrolysis of starch
	Lactose	Milk only
Polysaccharides (complex carbohydrates)	Starch	Grains and grain foods, legumes, potatoes and other root vegetables, green fruits
	Glycogen (animal starch)	Liver and muscle of freshly killed animals; freshly opened oysters
	Dextrin	Partial breakdown of starch by heat or in digestion
	Dietary fiber* cellulose hemicellulose gums mucilages pectins	Bran of cereal grains, fruits and fibers of fruits and vegetables, nuts, legumes. Pectin occurs in ripe fruits such as apples, citrus fruits

* Lignin is also a dietary fiber occurring in plant materials, but is not a carbohydrate.

is rich in fructose, can be eaten at one time. If one needs to increase the caloric value of a glass of lemonade, for example, he could use about twice as much glucose as sucrose. Lactose is only about one seventh as sweet as sucrose.

Sugars vary greatly in their solubility. Glucose is less soluble than sucrose; when making up a beverage it should be stirred well so that the sugar will not settle to the bottom. Lactose is now seldom used in beverages because of its poor solubility, its higher cost, and its tendency to irritate the intestinal tract when taken in large amounts.

Starches are bland in flavor and not sweet. A green banana is high in starch; as it ripens, the starch is changed to glucose and the sweetness is thereby increased. When corn ripens, it becomes less sweet as the sugars are converted to starch.

The thickening property of starch is well known, as in the making of cornstarch pudding or the cooking of a breakfast cereal such as oatmeal. When mixed with water and cooked, the starch absorbs water, and the mixture thickens.

SOURCES

Cereal grains, legumes, roots, and sugars are the principal sources of carbohydrate. When you are planning diets, you should consider not only the amount of carbohydrate in the food but also the contributions of other nutrients made by a given food.

Cereal grains and breads are the outstanding source of carbohydrate amongst the Four Food Groups. Rice is the leading staple food of the world, being especially prominent in Asian diets. Wheat ranks second and is the staple cereal in parts of India, the Middle East, Russia, Western Europe, and America. Rye, oats, and millet are important cereals in some dietaries of the world. Corn is favored in Central and Latin America.

The cereal grains and breads are important for their caloric contribution because of the amounts that are eaten daily. They also contribute protein, and if whole-grain or enriched they furnish significant amounts of thiamin, riboflavin, niacin, and iron. (See Fig. 7–1.)

Enrichment is a legal term used by the U.S. Food and Drug Administration to apply to the addition of specific amounts of thiamin, riboflavin, niacin, and iron. Most white flour and bread is now enriched. Look for the word "enriched" on labels for breads, pastas, breakfast cereals, cornmeal, or rice.

Fruits and vegetables vary widely in their content of carbohydrate. Potatoes, sweet potatoes, taro, plantain, breadfruit, and cassava furnish significant amounts of carbohydrate and calories to the diets of some peoples. Some fruits such as bananas and dried fruits, and some vegetables such as fresh corn, peas, and lima beans are relatively high in carbohydrate. Much of the carbohydrate in vegetables is in the form of starch, but there are also varying amounts of naturally occurring sugars. Ripe fruits contain sucrose, fructose, and glucose; unripened fruits contain some starch.

Milk is unique in that it is the only dietary source of lactose. Each cup contains 12 gm; thus the daily intake of this naturally occurring sugar would be 24 to 48 gm lactose, depending upon the amount of milk consumed. Cheeses contain only traces of lactose.

Meat, poultry, and fish contain no carbohydrate. The small amount of glycogen present in fresh liver and oysters has usually disappeared before the food reaches the consumer. Legumes and peanuts are fair sources of carbohydrate.

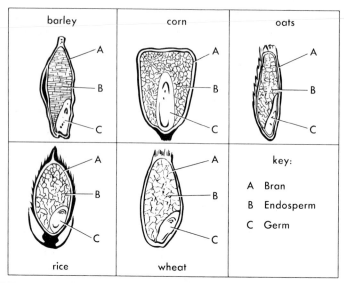

FIGURE 7–1 (A) The bran layer contains fiber, some B-complex vitamins, and iron. (B) The endosperm consists mainly of starch and some protein. This is the part used for refined flours and cereals. (C) The germ contains some carbohydrate, protein, and fat; minerals, especially iron; thiamin and other B vitamins, and vitamin E. Whole-grain flours, breads, and cereals include all three layers of the grain. *(Cereal Institute, Inc., Chicago.)*

Sugars and sweets. Sugars, candies, jellies, jams, sweetened beverages, cakes, cookies, and pastries supply important amounts of carbohydrate to the diet. Unlike the foods in the Four Food Groups the sugars are deficient in minerals, vitamins, and protein; they are sometimes referred to as "empty-calorie" foods. Honey, brown sugar, and raw sugar furnish the same amount of carbohydrate and calories, gram for gram, as do cane and beet sugars. Moreover, they are just about as lacking in minerals and vitamins as are the cane and beet sugars, and there is no merit in substituting one for the other.

Dietary fiber refers to the structural parts of plants and includes cellulose, hemicellulose, and lignin. Gums, mucilages, and pectins are also included as dietary fibers although they may not seem to be fibrous in nature. Dietary fibers are not digested by the enzymes of the gastrointestinal tract. However, bacteria in the colon bring about some fermentation and breakdown of the dietary fibers. The bran coating of cereal grains is high in fiber. Legumes and vegetables such as celery, cabbage, asparagus stalks, and the skins of fruits are important sources of fiber.

FUNCTIONS

Glucose, fructose, and galactose are the end products of carbohydrate digestion (see Chapter 3). These single sugars are absorbed from the small intestine into the portal circulation and are carried to the liver.

The form of sugar in the blood is glucose. The blood glucose is rapidly withdrawn by the cells of all body tissues, and is constantly replaced by the liver. The hormone insulin is the primary regulator of the level of sugar in the blood. As soon as the blood sugar rises, the pancreas is stimulated to produce insulin. Three important functions are performed by insulin: (1) the utilization of glucose for energy by the tissues; (2) the conversion of glucose to glycogen in the liver; and (3) the conversion of glucose to fat, as a reserve store of energy.

The amount of carbohydrate in the body at any given moment is about 300 gm (¾ lb) or less. Some of this is present in the blood, and the greater amount is stored in the liver and muscles as glycogen. Any carbohydrate in excess of immediate body needs is converted into fat. Carbohydrate has many functions in the body, such as these:

1. The chief function of carbohydrate is to provide energy to carry on the work of the body and heat to maintain the body's temperature. Glucose is the only form of energy used by the central nervous system, but other tissues also use fats for energy. Glucose and oxygen are carried by the blood to the tissues. In a complex manner involving many enzymes and intermediate reactions, glucose is oxidized to yield the following results:

$$\text{glucose} + \text{oxygen} = \text{energy} + \text{carbon dioxide} + \text{water}.$$

When tissues require much energy for their work, oxidation of glucose will proceed at a rapid rate. If you run, for example, you begin to breathe rapidly. You are then providing additional oxygen to combine with the extra glucose to meet this energy need. The carbon dioxide produced in this reaction is a waste product that is removed through the lungs. The water that results may be reused by the body in a number of ways or may be eliminated by the kidneys, skin, and lungs.

2. Carbohydrate spares protein. This means that the body need not burn protein from the diet or from body stores to meet energy needs when carbohydrate is available. Carbohydrates also furnish chemical elements that can be combined with nitrogen to manufacture nonessential amino acids.

3. The complete oxidation of fats requires some carbohydrate. When too little carbohydrate is available, some fatty acids known as ketones accumulate. This condition is seen in poorly regulated diabetic patients, and is known as *diabetic acidosis* or *coma*. (See Chapter 23.)

4. Nervous tissue, cartilage, and a number of body compounds contain carbohydrate. DNA and RNA, the genetic materials in each cell, contain the monosaccharide *ribose*. This sugar does not need to be in the diet because the body makes its own supply. Another carbohydrate-containing compound is heparin which controls blood clotting.

5. Lactose favors the growth of certain intestinal bacteria that synthesize

some of the B-complex vitamins. Lactose also increases the absorption of calcium and phosphorus.

6. Dietary fiber can absorb and hold water. This aids in normal elimination by the formation in the colon of a softer, bulkier stool.

7. Starches and sugars give flavor and variety to the diet, a value that should not be minimized.

DAILY NEEDS

The exact carbohydrate needs of the body have not been established. It is well known that some people in the world maintain good health with extremely high intakes of carbohydrate while others are equally healthy on diets very low in carbohydrate. Generally, the daily diet should contain not less than 100 gm carbohydrate. This is more than sufficient to supply the glucose needed by the central nervous system and for the effective oxidation of fats. (See Fig. 7–2.)

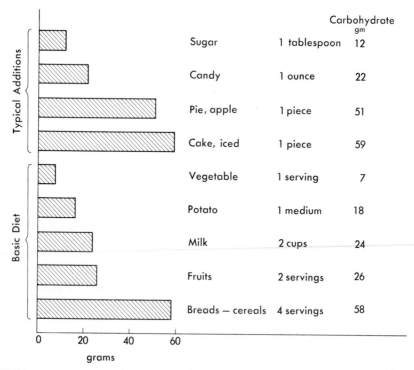

			Carbohydrate gm
Sugar	1 tablespoon		12
Candy	1 ounce		22
Pie, apple	1 piece		51
Cake, iced	1 piece		59
Vegetable	1 serving		7
Potato	1 medium		18
Milk	2 cups		24
Fruits	2 servings		26
Breads — cereals	4 servings		58

grams

FIGURE 7–2   Desserts and sweets are typical additions to the Basic Diet for additional calories. Some additions provide few nutrients other than carbohydrate. See Basic Diet, Table 4–2 (p. 37) for calculations.

Typical American diets furnish 46 per cent of calories from carbohydrate: 22 per cent from complex carbohydrates, 6 per cent from naturally occurring sugars, and 18 per cent from processed sugars. The United States Dietary Goals (see p. 38) recommend that the carbohydrate intake be increased to about 58 per cent of calories with the following specific goals:

1. Increase consumption of complex carbohydrates and naturally occurring sugars to about 48 per cent of calories.

2. Reduce consumption of refined and processed sugars to about 10 per cent of calories.

CLINICAL PROBLEMS

Nutritive adequacy. The Dietary Goals suggest that processed sugar intake be reduced to about 10 per cent of total calories. Why is this important? Perhaps the greatest single problem associated with a high sugar intake is that sugar contributes only carbohydrate and calories. Thus, with a high sugar intake it is necessary to get all the protein, minerals, and vitamins from other foods and still stay within the caloric requirement. By substituting complex carbohydrates for sugars, the mineral and vitamin content of the diet is improved.

Obesity. Sugar in coffee, honey on waffles, a candy bar, a soft drink sweetened with sugar, jam on bread, a piece of cake—all of these contribute carbohydrate and calories. It is very easy to eat sufficient amounts of these sugar-rich foods that the caloric intake exceeds the requirement. Thus, obesity results. For example, if you were to drink one 12-ounce can of a soft drink each day beyond your caloric requirement, the daily caloric excess would be 145 kcal. In one month the weight gain would be 0.56 kg (1.2 lb) or 3.7 kg (8 lb) in a year. Using sugar-rich foods in moderation, within one's caloric requirement, remains a good rule.

Dental caries. Dentists usually warn their patients about the effects of sugars on tooth decay. Bacteria in the mouth digest sugars, leaving plaque and acids that lead to tooth decay. Two factors are especially important. (1) Chewy sweets stick to the teeth for long periods so that bacteria have ample time to grow and produce decay. On the other hand, a sweetened beverage leaves less sugar in contact with the teeth and the harmful effect is lower. (2) Frequent snacking with sweets provides many opportunities for bacterial growth and increases tooth decay. Two practical rules thus apply: reduce the number of times during the day when sweets are consumed; and brush teeth after each meal. If brushing is not practical, rinse the mouth vigorously with water after consuming sweets.

Lactose intolerance. Some ethnic groups (including blacks, native Americans, Orientals, and others) produce insufficient lactase in the intestinal tract to digest lactose. As a result they have symptoms of flatulence, abdominal cramping, and diarrhea. Except in congenital lactase deficiency which is rare, the inability to digest lactose usually appears in late childhood or adulthood. Infants and young children of all population groups are almost always able to tolerate sufficient milk in their diets to meet nutritional needs. In some young children from ½ to 1 cup of milk may be tolerated at the time, while larger amounts produce symptoms of intolerance. (See also Chapter 29.)

Hypoglycemia—a current fad.   Claims are often made that eating a high-carbohydrate diet is a cause of hypoglycemia (low blood sugar). However, hypoglycemia is seldom seen in people who eat diets much higher in carbohydrate than do most Americans. Hypoglycemia, in itself, is a symptom, not a disease. Its presence can be determined only by measuring the level of blood sugar under controlled conditions. There is no scientific evidence that symptoms such as fatigue, allergies, depression, abnormal child behavior, drug addiction, alcoholism, nervous breakdown, and others are caused by hypoglycemia.

Hypoglycemia does occur in certain clinical conditions such as (1) following removal of the stomach, (2) severe liver disease, (3) tumor of the pancreas, and (4) very occasionally in adolescents as a functional disorder. Because the treatment varies for each of these conditions, the cause of the hypoglycemia must first be determined. (See also Chapter 24.)

Fiber.   It can be said with some assurance that increasing the fiber content of the diet aids in normal bowel elimination. Many physicians have found that a high-fiber diet is helpful in preventing recurrences of diverticulitis. (See p. 282.) Much more research must be carried out before there is proof that a low-fiber diet increases the risk of colon cancer, heart disease, and several gastrointestinal disorders. Also, there is no present proof that a high-fiber diet will reduce the risk of these diseases.

REVIEW QUESTIONS AND PROBLEMS

1. Define these terms: photosynthesis, galactose, cellulose, dextrin, maltose, enrichment, legume, monosaccharide, carbohydrate, starch, glycogen.

2. List the foods you ate yesterday. Which of these are important sources of carbohydrate? Which are important sources of fiber? Which are "empty-calorie" foods?

3. Outline the steps in the digestion of a carbohydrate meal, including the names of the enzymes, the site of their activity, and the digestion products that result. (Review Chapter 3.)

4. You sometimes find that a glass of fruit juice quickly makes you feel better. How can you explain this?

5. List four functions of carbohydrates in the body.

6. How many kilocalories would be provided by 250 gm carbohydrate?

7. Why is fiber important? What foods would you increase in the diet for more fiber?

8. Using Table A-1 compare the carbohydrate value of 1 piece of layer cake, 1 fresh peach, ½ cup cooked rice, 1 piece of apple pie, 1 sweet potato, 1 teaspoon sugar, 1 sweet roll, ½ cup spinach, 1 candy bar, 1 cup blueberries.

REFERENCES

Burkitt, D. P., *et al.:* "Dietary Fiber and Disease," *J.A.M.A.,* **229:**1068–74, 1974.

Council on Foods and Nutrition: "Fortification of Flour and Bread with Iron," *J.A.M.A.,* **223:**322, 1973.

Graham, D. M., and Hertzler, A. A.: "Why Enrich or Fortify Foods?" *J. Nutr. Educ.,* 9:166–68, 1977.

Leveille, G. A.: "Dietary Fiber," *Food and Nutrition News,* **47** (3), February 1976. (National Live Stock and Meat Board)

Mayer, J.: "The Whole Wheat Story," *Family Health,* 8:45, May 1976.

Robinson, C. H., and Lawler, M. R.: *Normal and Therapeutic Nutrition,* 15th ed. New York: Macmillan Publishing Co., Inc., 1977, chap. 5.

ENERGY METABOLISM

Fuel and Energy

Probably no aspect of nutrition is more discussed than that of calories. People say they "eat" too many calories or not enough calories. They associate calories with their weight. We need to know what we mean by calories, how many calories we need each day, and which foods are good and poor sources of calories.

Every engine requires fuel. The automobile runs only so long as it has a supply of gasoline. The furnace heats the house only when oil, gas, or coal is fed into it. The human body, sometimes likened to an engine, requires fuel to carry on all of its activities and to keep it warm. Every moment of our lives some energy is being used by the body—for every breath we draw, every beat of the heart, the blinking of the eyelid, the lifting of the heavy weight, or any activity whatsoever. The carbohydrate, fat, and protein in the foods we eat are the potential sources of energy for all body activities. Unlike the engine, the body will draw upon its own substance when no food is provided.

CALORIE, A UNIT OF ENERGY

Strictly speaking, we don't eat "calories." Just as we can measure length in centimeters or inches and weight in kilograms or pounds, so we can measure energy values of foods or energy needs of the body in units called *calories* or *joules*. The calorie or joule is a measure of heat. By definition, one large calorie, more correctly called a *kilocalorie* (kcal), is the amount of heat required to raise the temperature of 1000 gm of water by 1° C. In nutrition the large calorie is always used, whether it is written with a small "c" *calorie*, or a capital "C" *Calorie*, or as a *kilocalorie*. It is 1000 times as great as the small calorie unit used in chemistry and physics.

The international unit for energy is the *joule*. One kilocalorie is equal to 4.184 kilojoules. Presently, food tables and energy needs of people are expressed as calories, but gradually with other metric conversions the energy values will be in terms of joules.

The energy value of food is measured in the laboratory with an instrument called a *bomb calorimeter*. The caloric values for foods obtained with this instrument must be corrected to allow for some losses that occur in the feces and urine. In the body, these are the corrected values for pure carbohydrate, fat, and protein:

Carbohydrate	4 kcal (17 kj) per gram
Fat	9 kcal (38 kj) per gram
Protein	4 kcal (17 kj) per gram

If we know the carbohydrate, fat, and protein values of a food or diet we can easily calculate the caloric value. For example, the caloric value of one cup of milk would be calculated thus:

12 gm carbohydrate	x 4 kcal =	48
9 gm fat	x 9 kcal =	81
9 gm protein	x 4 kcal =	36
	Total kcal	165

You will see that this calculation is quite close to the actual value listed in Table A-1, Appendix A. Ordinarily we don't need to make such calculations because tables of caloric values are readily available.

Energy Needs of the Body

The body uses glycogen, simple sugars, fatty acids, glycerol, and amino acids to supply energy. The breakdown of these substances requires numerous steps and is exceedingly complex. The rate of breakdown depends upon the total daily energy requirement: the basal metabolism, the amount of voluntary activity, the influence of food, and the needs for growth.

BASAL METABOLISM

Basal metabolism, sometimes called the "cost of living," accounts for more than half of the energy requirements of most people. It includes the involuntary activities of the body (activities over which we have no control) while resting but awake. The breathing, the beating of the heart, the circulation of the blood, the metabolic activities within the cells, the keeping of muscles in good tone, and the maintenance of the body temperature require energy.

For measuring the basal metabolism the following conditions are observed: (1) the individual is awake but lying quietly in a comfortable room; (2) he is in the *postabsorptive* state; that is, he has had no food for 12 to 16 hours; (3) his body temperature is normal; and (4) he is not tense or emotionally upset.

For his basal metabolism the adult requires about one kilocalorie per kilogram per hour. Thus, a woman weighing 55 kg (121 lb) would have a basal metabolism of approximately 1320 kcal ($1 \times 55 \times 24$). A man weighing 70 kg (154 lb) would have a basal metabolism of 1680 kcal ($1 \times 70 \times 24$).

Several factors affect the rate of basal metabolism. The first of these is *body size.* The larger a person is, the greater is the amount of lean muscle tissue and the greater is the skin surface area. Thus a tall, well-built man has a greater skin surface and will have a higher basal metabolism than a short, fat man of the same weight.

The amount of *muscle tissue* has an effect on the basal metabolism. An athlete with firm muscles has a higher rate than a nonathlete with poorly developed, flabby muscles. Usually men have a higher rate than women, because men, as a rule, have more muscle tissue, and women have more deposits of fat.

Rapid *growth* increases the basal metabolism greatly. Infants in proportion to body size have a very high rate of metabolism. The metabolism is also high during the rapid growth period of adolescence and the last trimester of pregnancy when the fetus is greatly increasing in size.

After the *age* of 25 years the metabolism declines about 2 per cent for each ten years. Thus, at 65 years the basal metabolism would be about 92 per cent of the metabolism of a young adult. Many men and women become overweight during middle age because they fail to reduce their caloric intake as their metabolism goes down.

The *thyroid* gland produces thyroxine, an iodine-containing hormone that regulates the rate of energy metabolism. If too much thyroxine is produced, the metabolism will increase; if too little thyroid hormone is manufactured, the metabolism will be correspondingly lower. The level of protein-bound iodine (PBI) in the blood is now widely used by physicians in place of the basal metabolism test to determine the activity of the thyroid.

VOLUNTARY ACTIVITY

Our daily work may well vary from sitting at a desk to bedside nursing, active housework, or hard manual labor. In our leisure time we might choose to watch television, take a leisurely walk, or go swimming or dancing. The

TABLE 8–1   CALORIE EXPENDITURE FOR VARIOUS TYPES OF ACTIVITIES

*Type of Activity**	*Kcal per Hour*
Sedentary activities, such as: Reading; writing; eating; watching television or movies; listening to the radio; sewing; playing cards; and typing, miscellaneous office work, and other activities done with sitting that requires little or no arm movement	80 to 100†
Light activities, such as: Preparing and cooking food; doing dishes; dusting; handwashing small articles of clothing; ironing; walking slowly; personal care; miscellaneous office work and other activities done while standing that require some arm movement; and rapid typing and other activities done while sitting that are more strenuous	110 to 160
Moderate activities, such as: Making beds; mopping and scrubbing; sweeping; light polishing and waxing; laundering by machine; light gardening and carpentry work; walking moderately fast; other activities done while standing that require moderate arm movement; and activities done while sitting that require more vigorous arm movement.	170 to 240
Vigorous activities, such as: Heavy scrubbing and waxing; handwashing large articles of clothing; hanging out clothes; stripping beds; other heavy work; walking fast; bowling; golfing; and gardening	250 to 350
Strenuous activities, such as: Swimming; playing tennis; running; bicycling; dancing; skiing; and playing football	350 and more

* During sleep the average caloric expenditure would range from 50 to 65 kcal per hour.

† These values include the basal metabolism. The lower level of calories is typical for women; the upper level is more appropriate for the average man.

L. Page, and L. J. Fincher, *Food and Your Weight.* Washington, D.C.: Home and Garden Bulletin No. 74, U.S. Department of Agriculture, 1964, p. 4.

kind of physical activity in which we engage, and the amounts of time spent in each activity, determine the amount of energy the body uses. It is difficult to assign exact values to any activity because individuals vary widely in the efficiency with which they use their bodies. Average values for common activities are grouped in five categories in Table 8-1. One can readily see why a typist, classed as sedentary, requires fewer calories than the moderately active homemaker who might be doing some gardening in addition to her housework.

Mental effort, as in studying, is a sedentary activity and the effort expended in solving a paper problem requires little caloric expenditure. If you are studying and nibbling foods all the while, it is certain that you are consuming far more calories than are needed for your mental effort. Of course, if you are tense or move about quite a bit while you study, this would have some effect on increasing your caloric need.

INFLUENCE OF FOOD

The digestion, absorption, and metabolism of food increase the total caloric requirement. This is really the cost of preparing nutrients for their use by the cells. It is sometimes referred to as *specific dynamic action*. It is highly variable and amounts to about 6 to 10 per cent of total caloric need.

ENERGY ALLOWANCES

The recommended daily allowances for kilocalories are shown in Table 8-2. At best, these recommendations can be only approximate because of individual variations. For persons who are lighter or heavier than the reference individual, the allowances would be decreased or increased. Women who have average physical activity require about 35 kcal per kilogram (16 kcal per pound), and men with average physical activity require about 38 kcal per kilogram (17 kcal per pound). The allowances for persons who are sedentary would be decreased, while those for persons engaged in hard physical labor would be much more.

The allowances for infants and for children are very high in proportion to their body size so that there is ample energy for growth as well as the high level of physical activity. Note, for example, that the 30-kg child between 7 and 10 years requires about 2400 kcal—a level that is more than his mother needs and only 300 kcal less than his father needs. (See Fig. 8–1.)

Ordinarily, no calorie adjustments need to be made for climate. Most Americans live in well-heated buildings in winter and wear warm clothing. Many people now also work in air-conditioned buildings in the summer.

TABLE 8–2   RECOMMENDED DAILY ALLOWANCES FOR ENERGY

Age Years	Weight kg	lb	Energy kcal	Age Years	Weight kg	lb	Energy kcal
Infants				Females			
0.0–0.5	6	13	kg × 115	11–14	46	101	2200
0.5–1.0	9	20	kg × 105	15–18	55	120	2100
				19–22	55	120	2100
Children				23–50	55	120	2000
1–3	13	29	1300	51–75	55	120	1800
4–6	20	44	1700	76 +	55	120	1600
7–10	28	62	2400				
				Pregnancy			+ 300
Males				Lactation			+ 500
11–14	45	99	2700				
15–18	66	145	2800				
19–22	70	154	2900				
23–50	70	154	2700				
51–75	70	154	2400				
76 +	70	154	2050				

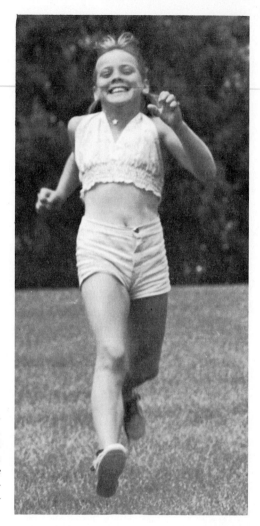

FIGURE 8–1 Vigorous physical activity increases the energy requirement. Throughout life physical activity should be encouraged as one way to maintain normal weight. (Department of Public Welfare, Commonwealth of Pennsylvania, and Mr. James L. Flanigan 3rd photographer.)

Meeting Energy Needs

DIETARY GOALS

In the United States about 45 per cent of total calories in the diet come from carbohydrate; 40 per cent or more of calories come from fat; and about 12 to 15 per cent of calories come from protein. The Dietary Goals recommend that a better distribution would be as follows:

1. About 48 per cent of calories from complex carbohydrates; no more than 10 per cent of calories from processed and refined sugars.

2. About 30 per cent of calories from fat, with no more than 10 per cent from saturated fats.

These recommendations would mean that Americans would derive more of their calories from foods of the grain group and less from sugars and sweets. They would reduce their consumption of fats, including fatty meats, fat-rich foods of all kinds, as well as visible fats.

ENERGY VALUE OF FOODS

The caloric value of many foods is given in Table A-1, Appendix A. If you will examine this table you will find that you could draw some general conclusions about the caloric value of food groups. Some foods contain much water and some fiber and are low in calories. Vegetables and fruits, as a class, are in this group. The variation in calories between a tomato, for example, and a sweet potato lies in the much greater carbohydrate content of the sweet potato. Fresh fruits are much lower in calories than canned or frozen fruits, which have been packed in syrup.

Many foods contain little water but appreciable amounts of carbohydrate: flour, cereal foods, bread, sugar, candy, jellies, and others. Weight for weight these foods rank much higher in calories than vegetables and fruits.

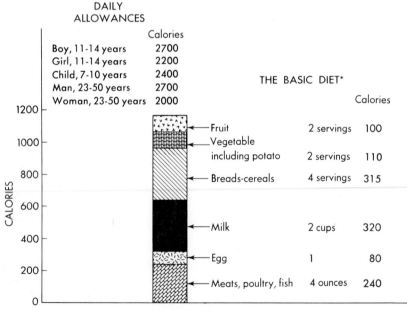

FIGURE 8–2 The Basic Diet furnishes a little more than half of the energy requirements for girls and women. The full energy requirement is met by eating additional foods from the Four Food Groups and by including fats, sugars, and desserts. See Table 4–2 (p. 37) for complete calculation.

The highest concentration of calories occurs in foods that contain much fat. Lean meat, poultry, and fish are moderate in calorie content, but fatty meats and fish are high in calories. Oils, butter, margarine, cooking fats, and cream are concentrated sources of calories because of their high fat content.

Many cooked foods are higher in calories because of the ingredients used and the method of preparation. Cakes, cookies, pies, and pastries contain much flour, sugar, shortening, eggs, and milk, and are, of course, high in calories. A piece of lean meat may be only moderately high in calories if it is broiled, but if it is dipped in egg, crumbs, and then fried, the calorie value could be twice as high. Deep-fat fried foods are, generally speaking, high in calories.

Alcohol.   One gram of pure alcohol furnishes 7 kcal. One can of beer (12 oz) contains 150 kcal, one martini (1 ½ oz gin) about 120 kcal, and one glass of dessert wine (3 ½ oz) 140 kcal. Thus, for many people alcoholic beverages supply significant amounts of energy.

Energy value of the Basic Diet.   The recommended number of servings from the Four Food Groups supplies almost 60 per cent of the energy needs of the average woman. Note in Fig. 8–2 that the milk and meat groups are roughly equal in their calorie contribution; likewise, the vegetable-fruit group and the bread-cereal group are about equal in their contribution.

SOME FALLACIES AND FACTS

1. *Fallacy.* Potatoes, bread, meat, and milk are fattening. Grapefruit is not fattening.

   Facts. No single food can be called fattening or nonfattening. A calorie from one food is the same as a calorie from another food. Some foods provide more calories than others. One becomes overweight only if the total calorie intake is greater than the calorie expenditure of the body.

2. *Fallacy.* Boiled potatoes are more fattening than baked potatoes.

   Facts. Potatoes of the same weight will have the same number of calories whether boiled or baked. The hidden calories in the form of butter, or sour cream, would rapidly increase the number of calories.

3. *Fallacy.* Polyunsaturated fats are lower in calories than saturated fats.

   Facts. Gram for gram, all pure fat—polyunsaturated or saturated—contain the same number of calories. One tablespoon of whipped butter or whipped margarine will have fewer calories than 1 tablespoon regular butter or margarine because air has been whipped into it. But gram for gram, or pound for pound, the whipped fats would contain the same number of calories as the regular fats.

4. *Fallacy.* Toast has fewer calories than bread.

   Facts. The caloric content of a slice of bread does not change with toasting. The bread has lost some weight in toasting because it has lost some of its water content.

CLINICAL PROBLEMS

Nutritive adequacy.   Many people meet or exceed their energy requirement by selecting excessive amounts of foods rich in sugars and/or fats. Others also consume varying amounts of alcoholic beverages. The sugars, fats, and alcoholic beverages furnish only traces of minerals and vitamins. They are often referred to as "empty-calorie foods," or "junk foods." They are low in *nutrient density* which is another way of saying that the food supplies a high proportion of the person's caloric need but only a low proportion of the nutrient needs. Unless most of the calories for the diet are selected from a variety of foods in the Four Food Groups, the diet is likely to lack some of the essential nutrients.

Weight control.   For the adult the best guide to the calorie requirement is the body weight. If the amount of energy needed by the body is less than the amount of energy supplied by the diet, the extra energy will be stored as fat, and the individual will gain weight. This is the problem that many men and women face. On the other hand, insufficient energy in the diet to meet body needs means that the adipose tissue will be used up, and thus weight is lost.

The adult in good health and who has a desirable body weight should aim to keep his weight constant. If people will weigh themselves regularly and will learn to avoid many hidden calories, to refuse second servings, to select low-calorie snacks, and to engage in a regular program of exercise, the maintenance of weight is not difficult. If a pound is gained, the effort should be made to lose it promptly so that there is no accumulation from month to month and year to year. (See also Chapter 22.)

REVIEW QUESTIONS AND PROBLEMS

1. What is meant by a kilocalorie? What is a bomb calorimeter?

2. What is measured when a person is having a basal metabolism test? What conditions are necessary for such a test? What would be your approximate basal metabolism?

3. List ten foods you especially like. Without looking up the calorie values, which would you rate as high in calories? Check your classification with the actual calorie values in Table A-1, Appendix A.

4. Keep a record of your food intake for one day. Calculate the caloric value of these foods.
    a. Compare your caloric intake with the allowance stated for you in Table 8–2. Give reasons for differences.
    b. List the foods in your diet that are low in nutrients. What changes, if any, should you make in your choice of calories?

5. Keep a record of your activities for 24 hours. Classify these activities according to the groups in Table 8–1. Calculate your approximate caloric expenditure.

6. What is the best guide for determining whether you are obtaining your caloric requirement?

REFERENCES

Konishi, F.: "Food Energy Equivalents of Various Activities," *J. Am. Dietet. A.,* **46:**186–88, 1965.

Page, L., and Fincher, L. J.: *Food and Your Weight*. HG 74, Washington, D.C.: U.S. Department of Agriculture.

Robinson, C. H., and Lawler, M. R.: *Normal and Therapeutic Nutrition*, 15th ed. New York: Macmillan Publishing Co., Inc., 1977, chap. 7.

MINERAL ELEMENTS

NATURE AND DISTRIBUTION

Mineral elements are inorganic substances as contrasted to such organic compounds as proteins, fats, carbohydrates, and vitamins. They are found in all body tissues and fluids. They occur in foods as salts; for example, sodium chloride. They may also be combined with organic compounds; for example, iron in hemoglobin, and sulfur in almost all proteins. Unlike carbohydrates, fats, and proteins, mineral elements do not furnish energy.

Unlike vitamins, the mineral elements are not destroyed in food preparation. However, they are soluble in water so that some loss will occur if cooking liquids are discarded.

It is often said that valuable things come in small packages. About 15 to 20 mineral elements account for only 4 per cent of the body weight; that is, 2 to 3 kg (5 to 6 lb) in the average adult. They vary in amount from 1000 to 1500 gm calcium, which alone accounts for one half of all mineral matter in the body, to 20 to 25 mg iodine, to cobalt which is present in such minute traces that measurement is difficult. Yet the absence of any one of these elements can cause serious problems. An excess of some of them can be toxic.

A summary of the kinds and average amounts of mineral elements in the body is presented in Table 9–1. *Macronutrients* are those major elements that occur in the largest amounts, whereas *micronutrients* or *trace* elements are found in very small amounts indeed.

TABLE 9–1   MINERAL ELEMENTS IN THE ADULT BODY

	Per Cent of Body Weight	Man gm	Principal Locations in Body
Macronutrients			
Calcium (Ca)	1.5–2.2	1050–1540	99% in bones and teeth
Phosphorus (P)	0.8–1.2	560– 840	80–90% in bones, teeth
Potassium (K)	0.35	245	Fluid inside cells
Sulfur (S)	0.25	175	Associated with protein
Chlorine (Cl)	0.15	105	Fluid outside cells
Sodium (na)	0.15	105	Fluid outside cells
Magnesium (Mg)	0.05	35	60% in bones and teeth
Micronutrients			
Iron (Fe)	0.004	2.8	Chiefly in hemoglobin; stores in liver and other organs
Manganese (Mn)	0.0003	0.21	
Copper (Cu)	0.00015	0.11	
Iodine (I)	0.00004	0.02	Thyroid gland
Fluorine (F)			Bones and teeth
Zinc (Zn)			
Molybdenum (Mo)			
Selenium (Se)			
Cobalt (Co)			Part of vitamin B_{12} molecule
Chromium (Cr)			

Present and possibly essential: cadmium, nickel, silicon, tin, vanadium.
Present but not known to be essential: aluminum, arsenic, barium, boron, bromine, gold, lead, mercury, strontium

Calculations based on elementary composition of body as stated by H. C. Sherman, *Chemistry of Food and Nutrition*, 8th ed. Macmillan Publishing Co., Inc., 1952, p. 227.

GENERAL FUNCTIONS

For convenience mineral elements are often discussed separately. However, within the body they function together in building body tissues and in the regulation of body metabolism. Some of the important ways in which mineral elements function together are discussed below. Specific functions will also be listed under the headings for each element.

Bone formation.   Bone consists of a soft, pliable, but tough protein material into which minerals are deposited. Most of the calcium, phosphorus, and magnesium, and smaller amounts of other mineral elements, are deposited in the bones and teeth. During the last two months of pregnancy most of the ossification of the bones of the fetus occurs. The infant at birth has a well-formed skeleton, but the bones are still quite soft. Throughout childhood, adolescence, and into the early twenties the bones continue to harden as well as to grow in length and in diameter. The individual who has ample calcium, phosphorus, and protein in his diet during the growing years will be taller than the one who is poorly nourished.

As well as providing the framework for the body, bones serve as a storehouse for the mineral elements they contain. They are never fixed for life. The blood can withdraw mineral elements from the bone according to the daily soft-tissue and fluid needs of the body. These withdrawals are ordinarily replaced from the diet.

Tooth formation. Teeth, like bones, contain a ground substance of protein. The tooth enamel and dentine are hard substances containing appreciable amounts of calcium and phosphorus. The first teeth form in the fetus at the fourth to sixth week of pregnancy and begin to calcify by the twentieth week. The permanent teeth calcify soon after birth up to about three years of age. Wisdom teeth may calcify as late as eight to ten years of age. The teeth are fully mineralized before they erupt. The enamel and dentine are not supplied with blood vessels. Therefore, a decayed tooth cannot repair itself, so that proper care of the teeth once they have erupted is vital.

Soft tissues contain many mineral elements in their structure, including potassium, sulfur, phosphorus, iron, and others.

Vitamins, enzymes, and hormones. Minute amounts of mineral elements are constituents of the various regulatory compounds. Sulfur is a part of the thiamin molecule and cobalt is present in the vitamin B_{12} molecule. Zinc is part of the enzyme (carbonic anhydrase) that releases carbon dioxide from the red blood cells. Iodine is present in the thyroxine molecule.

Some mineral elements are needed to change an inactive enzyme to its active form; for example, calcium activates pancreatic lipase, an enzyme that splits fats in the digestive process. In other instances a mineral element is necessary to *catalyze* (speed up) a reaction. Copper is needed to incorporate iron into the hemoglobin molecule, just as zinc is necessary for the formation of insulin by the pancreas.

Nervous response and muscle contraction. Body fluids contain exact amounts of sodium, potassium, calcium, and magnesium. These elements control the passage of materials into and out of the cells. They regulate the transmission of the nerve impulses, and the contraction of the muscles.

Water balance. The balance of fluid between the inside and the outside of each cell depends in large part upon the correct concentrations of sodium and potassium. Sodium occurs primarily in the extracellular fluid, and potassium is found chiefly in the intracellular fluid. (See Chapter 10.)

Acid-base balance. The body fluids are maintained at a constant pH at all times. The pH is a measure of the acidity or alkalinity. The role of mineral elements in this function is discussed further in Chapter 10.

DYNAMIC EQUILIBRIUM

Body tissues are continuously changing—taking up nutrients, synthesizing new compounds, and releasing waste materials. Even bones, which many people mistakenly think of as fixed materials, are changing; they take up nutrients to replace those that are lost and to maintain stores for release to the blood circulation. Even with this constant change the body maintains, in health, a fine balance often referred to as *dynamic equilibirum* or *homeostasis.*

One way in which balance is maintained is by the release of stored mineral elements, for example, from the liver and bones. This balance is regulated by hormones that respond to very slight changes in the blood levels. Another way by which balance is achieved is to control the absorption of a nutrient according to the body's need. The per cent of absorption of calcium and iron is low. But if the body needs more calcium or iron, the rate of absorption increases, for example, during growth. By regulating the amount of these minerals absorbed, the small intestine protects the body against overload. Still another mechanism of control is through excretion by the kidney. Almost all of the sodium in the diet is absorbed from the intestinal tract into the blood circulation. But if the sodium is in excess of the body need—which it usually is—the amount not needed is rapidly excreted in the urine.

TOXICITY

Although many mineral elements are absolutely necessary for a great variety of functions, some of these can be toxic if they are consumed in excessive amounts. Among these are copper, fluorine, iodine, iron, manganese, selenium, and zinc. The levels of these trace elements found in a mixed diet furnish essential needs but are below levels of toxicity. The danger of toxicity arises (1) when supplements such as iron pills are used in excess, (2) when mistakes are made in substituting one compound for another, or (3) when workers in industrial plants are exposed to toxic levels of substances. From time to time there are reports of children opening a bottle of iron-containing pills and consuming sufficient amounts to become ill. Some years ago a worker mistook salt for sugar and added it to infant formulas; some infants died from the excess salt.

Macronutrients

CALCIUM

Functions. About 99 per cent of the body calcium is found in the bones and teeth where it is combined with phosphorus and other elements to give rigidity to the skeleton. The bones also serve as the storehouse for calcium needed for a number of cellular functions. Calcium is required for the complex process of blood coagulation. Together with other elements it regulates the passage of materials into and out of cells; controls the transmission of nerve messages; brings about the normal contraction of muscles, including the heart; activates enzymes such as pancreatic lipase; and aids in the absorption of vitamin B_{12}.

Utilization.   Calcium absorption from the gastrointestinal tract is regulated according to the body needs for maintenance and growth. The daily absorption ranges from 10 to 40 per cent of the dietary intake. A child who is growing rapidly absorbs a greater proportion of the calcium in his diet than the adult who simply needs to maintain the proper level of calcium in the bones and soft tissues.

Since calcium salts are more soluble in acid solution, most of the absorption takes place from the upper small intestine. Three hormones control the levels of calcium in the blood. When the blood calcium level falls below normal levels, *parathormone* is secreted by the parathyroid gland. This hormone stimulates the kidney to change vitamin D to its active form, another hormone. *Active vitamin D* increases the absorption of calcium from the intestine, and also releases calcium from bone so that the blood level rises to normal level. If the blood calcium level is too high, *calcitonin* is secreted by the thyroid gland. This shuts off the action of the parathyroid and thus brings the calcium level of the blood to normal range.

Daily allowances.   The calcium allowance for schoolchildren and adults throughout life is 800 mg. During periods of rapid growth in teenagers and during pregnancy and lactation the calcium allowance is 1200 mg. (see Table 4–1, p. 32).

Food sources.   Any kind of milk—fresh whole, skim, evaporated, dry, yogurt, or buttermilk—is an equally good source of calcium. Hard cheeses such as American and Swiss are excellent. You would need to eat 1½ cups of ice cream or cottage cheese to get the same amount of calcium as that in one cup of milk. Cream cheese and butter, although dairy products, are not sources of calcium.

Kale, turnip greens, mustard greens, and collards are good sources of calcium. Broccoli, cabbage, and cauliflower rate as fair sources. Such other greens as spinach, chard, and beet greens contain oxalic acid, which combines with calcium in the intestines to form an insoluble salt. This insoluble compound cannot be absorbed into the blood. Therefore, these greens should not be counted on for calcium, but they do not affect the utilization of calcium from other foods.

Among the fruits, oranges contribute some calcium, although oranges cannot take the place of milk. Canned salmon is a fairly good source of calcium if the tiny bones are eaten. Clams, oysters, lobster, dried beans, and peas are moderate sources, but these foods are not eaten often enough to make an appreciable contribution. Meats and cereal foods are poor sources. (See Fig. 9–1.)

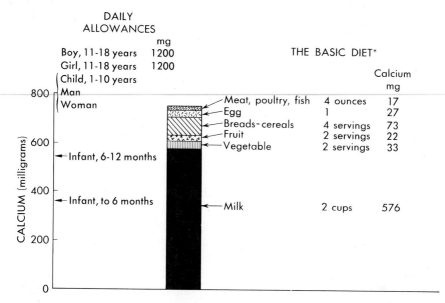

FIGURE 9-1 Milk furnishes about three fourths of the calcium allowance for adults. The addition of 1 to 2 cups for boys and girls supplies their greater needs during growth. See Table 4-2 (p. 37) for complete calculation.

Clinical problems. Calcium deficiency becomes evident only after years of inadequate intake. A dietary deficiency does not lower the blood calcium since the bones will supply the amounts needed. As much as 30 to 40 per cent of bone calcium is lost before changes can be detected by x-ray.

Long periods of immobilization such as those following an injury or being bedfast increase calcium excretion, and many of these persons are in negative calcium balance. Rickets, now rarely seen in infants and children in the United States, is a deficiency more directly related to vitamin D lack, but calcium and phosphorus metabolism are also involved.

Periodontal disease (changes in the structure of the gums) is believed to be an early sign of bone change. About 14 million women and a lesser number of men in the United States, chiefly in the later years of life, have *osteoporosis*. The older person experiences shorter stature, bone pain and susceptibility to fractures. Osteoporosis is a disease of complex causes, including faulty steroid production after menopause. Some research workers have shown that it occurs more often in nonmilk drinkers.

PHOSPHORUS

Probably no mineral element has more functions than phosphorus. It is essential for (1) building bones and teeth, (2) phospholipids that regulate the absorption and transport of fats, (3) DNA (deoxyribonucleic acid) and RNA (ribonucleic acid), which are nucleic acids essential for protein synthesis and genetic coding, (4) ATP (adenosine triphosphate) and ADP (adenosine diphosphate), which are necessary for storing and releasing energy according to the body needs, (5) enzymes that are required to utilize carbohydrates, fats, and proteins, and (6) buffer salts in the regulation of acid-base balance.

The phosphorus allowances for individuals of various ages are the same as those for calcium. (See Table 4–1, p. 32.) If the diet supplies enough calcium and protein, it will furnish enough phosphorus. Milk, meat, poultry, fish, egg yolk, legumes, and nuts are rich sources.

MAGNESIUM

About 60 per cent of the body magnesium is found in the bones and teeth. Together with other mineral elements, magnesium regulates nervous irritability and muscle contraction. Magnesium activates many enzymes including those involved in energy metabolism. Like calcium, the salts of magnesium are rather insoluble, and much of the dietary magnesium is not absorbed. Most absorption occurs from the upper gastrointestinal tract.

The adult allowance for magnesium is 300 to 350 mg per day. Magnesium is a constituent of the chlorophyll of plants; so one would expect green leaves to be rich in this mineral element. Nuts, cereal grains, and seafoods are especially rich in magnesium.

Dietary deficiency of magnesium is not likely. However, some disease states give rise to symptoms of deficiency. Patients with diabetic acidosis, chronic alcoholism, kwashiorkor, and severe malabsorption diseases sometimes show the characteristic symptoms of tremor and nervous irritability.

SULFUR

Sulfur is present in three amino acids: methionine, cystine, and cysteine. Thus, it is present in all proteins in the body. Connective tissue, skin, hair, and nails are especially rich in sulfur. Also, thiamin and biotin which are B-complex vitamins and coenzyme A contain sulfur in their molecules.

No recommended allowance has been set for sulfur, nor has any deficiency in human beings been observed. A diet that is adequate in protein supplies liberal amounts of sulfur.

Micronutrients

IRON

Functions.   The total content of iron in the adult body is only 3 to 5 gm. Most of this iron is present in hemoglobin, a protein that consists of an iron-containing compound, *heme*, attached to a protein, *globin*. Hemoglobin is carried in the circulation in the red blood cells. It picks up oxygen in the lungs and transports the oxygen to the tissues so that oxidation reactions can take place in the cells. From the cells the hemoglobin carries carbon dioxide to the lungs to be exhaled.

Myoglobin is an iron-containing protein similar to hemoglobin and is present in muscle tissue. Iron is also a constituent of many enzymes that are required for the use of glucose and fatty acids for energy.

Utilization.   Iron salts are relatively insoluble, and the proportion absorbed from the gastrointestinal tract is small and varies widely. The amount absorbed depends upon the body's need for iron. The well-nourished adult absorbs only 5 to 10 per cent of the iron in his diet, but somewhat larger percentages are absorbed by children during periods of rapid growth, by pregnant women, and by people who have anemia.

Iron salts are more soluble in acid, so most of the absorption takes place from the upper part of the small intestine. The amount of iron absorbed depends also upon the food source. In general, *heme* iron (that is, iron occurring in meats) is much more efficiently absorbed than is *nonheme* iron (from plant foods.) Vitamin C improves the absorption of iron, as do also the organic acids present in some fruits. The iron in plant foods is somewhat less absorbed than that in animal foods. Antacid medications interfere with the absorption of iron.

Iron is used very economically by the body. When the red blood cells are destroyed after their normal life-span of about 120 days, the hemoglobin is broken down. The iron that is released is used over and over again.

Small amounts of iron are lost daily in perspiration, in the sloughing of cells from the skin and mucosal membranes, in hair and nail clippings, and through excretion in the urine. These losses account for 0.5 to 1 mg iron per day. Menstrual losses are about 15 to 30 mg per month, or an average of 0.5 to 1 mg per day.

Daily allowances.   The allowance for the well-nourished woman is 18 mg iron per day, whereas that for the healthy man is 10 mg. Infants and children need liberal intakes of iron to take care of the expanding blood circulation as they grow. (See Table 4–1, p. 32.)

Food sources.   Foods in the meat group are good sources of available iron, any kind of liver or organ meat being especially rich. (See Fig. 9–2.) Oysters and clams are rich in iron but other seafoods are somewhat lower than meat. Although egg yolk contains an appreciable amount of iron, much of this iron is not absorbed from the intestine. Legumes and nuts are fairly rich in iron.

Dark green leafy vegetables of all kinds are especially rich in iron. Fruits are fair contributors. Dried prunes, apricots, peaches, and raisins are rich in iron, but their infrequent use means that the daily intake is not importantly affected.

Whole-grain or enriched breads, cereals, and pastas supply appreciable amounts of iron if eaten in quantity. The milk group supplies very little iron.

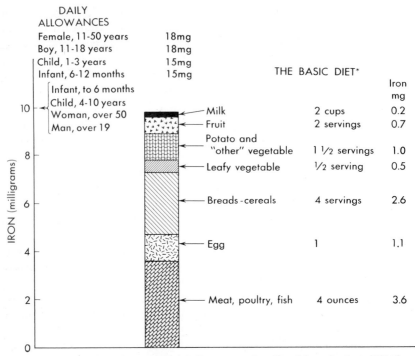

DAILY
ALLOWANCES

Female, 11-50 years	18mg
Boy, 11-18 years	18mg
Child, 1-3 years	15mg
Infant, 6-12 months	15mg

THE BASIC DIET*

		Iron mg
Milk	2 cups	0.2
Fruit	2 servings	0.7
Potato and "other" vegetable	1 1/2 servings	1.0
Leafy vegetable	1/2 serving	0.5
Breads-cereals	4 servings	2.6
Egg	1	1.1
Meat, poultry, fish	4 ounces	3.6

Infant, to 6 months
Child, 4-10 years
Woman, over 50
Man, over 19

IRON (milligrams)

FIGURE 9–2 The Basic Diet supplies sufficient iron for the adult male. It is difficult to meet the recommended allowances for women and children unless fortified foods or dietary supplements of iron are used. See Table 4–2 (p. 37) for complete calculation.

From Figure 9–2 it becomes evident that the Four Food Groups do not furnish enough iron for the girl or woman. In fact, typical diets in the United States can be counted on to furnish about 6 mg iron per 1000 kcal. During periods of rapid growth in teenage girls and during pregnancy iron supplementation is desirable.

Clinical problems. Iron-deficiency anemia is widespread in the United States. Mild anemia occurs in vulnerable groups who have had a diet low in iron for some time: infants fed principally on milk formulas without iron supplement; teenagers whose food selection is poor; and women who have had several pregnancies without iron supplementation. In severe iron-deficiency anemia, blood loss from the gastrointestinal tract should be suspected; for example, a bleeding ulcer, ulcerative colitis, or the losses that accompany parasite infestation such as hookworm. It is also necessary to take into account the frequency with which persons make blood donations, and any extraordinary menstrual losses.

Iron deficiency can be detected before the stores become sufficiently depleted to lower the hematocrit and hemoglobin levels. Symptoms are often absent in mild anemias. As the deficiency becomes more severe there is insufficient hemoglobin to carry oxygen to the tissues. With physical effort the individual becomes very tired, looks pale, and may have a poor resistance to infection. Iron-deficiency anemia is most effectively treated with iron salts. It is not practical to provide iron by diet alone since it is very difficult to achieve intakes of more than 15 to 20 mg. Such levels are far too low for recovery from an existing anemia.

Hemosiderosis is an excessive accumulation of iron in the liver, lungs, pancreas, heart, and other tissues. Sometimes it is a genetic defect that permits excessive absorption of iron. It could also result from overuse of iron supplements, but is not a problem with usual American diets.

IODINE

Most of the body iodine is present in the thyroid gland, but all cells contain minute traces. Iodine is a constitutent of two hormones, *thyroxine* and *thyroglobulin.* These hormones (1) regulate energy metabolism, (2) are involved in the synthesis of protein and cholesterol, and (3) facilitate the conversion of carotene to vitamin A.

Iodine is rapidly absorbed from the gastrointestinal tract and stored in the thyroid gland. Intakes in excess of body needs are promptly excreted in the urine.

The allowance for iodine for men and women is 150 mcg (see Table 4–1, p. 32). Foods grown along the seacoast, saltwater fish, and shellfish are good sources. Breads to which iodates have been added as a dough conditioner are also good sources. The most reliable way to ensure an adequate intake of iodine is through the use of iodized salt.

Clinical problems. A deficiency of iodine leads to a decreased production of thyroxine, and, in turn, a lowered rate of energy metabolism. In an attempt to produce more thyroid hormones the thyroid gland enlarges. This condition is called *simple* or *endemic goiter.* In a mild deficiency the only symptom noted is a slight enlargement of the thyroid gland, visible at the neckline. However, if the condition persists, the woman who has a simple goiter and who fails to get sufficient iodine during pregnancy will be unable to supply the fetus with its needs; thus, the baby is more severely affected than its mother was. When the deficiency is severe, growth is retarded and mentality is dulled.

Simple goiter, once frequently seen in the midwestern states where the soil content of iodine is low, now occurs rarely in the United States. The use of iodized salt is credited with this decline. Endemic goiter is still a major problem in some Central and South American countries, Asia, and Africa.

ZINC

About 2 to 3 gm zinc are found in the body. Like iron, zinc is absorbed according to body need. Zinc is important for these functions: (1) normal growth and sexual maturation; (2) as part of an enzyme that transfers carbon dioxide from the tissues to the lungs; (3) the production of insulin by the pancreas; (4) the synthesis of proteins; and (5) normal sensitivity to taste.

The adult allowance for zinc is 15 mg, and for children is 10 mg. Zinc is widely distributed in animal and plant foods that are good sources of protein: meats, eggs, liver, seafood, legumes, nuts, peanut butter, milk, and whole-grain cereals. People who eat a normal diet adequate in protein are not likely to lack zinc. Some vegetarian diets provide zinc levels lower than desirable.

Clinical problems. In Iran and Egypt where diets have been extremely low in zinc as well as inadequate in other respects, children have been dwarfed, and sexual development has been retarded. In the United States growth in some children was improved when zinc supplements were given.

Zinc deficiency leads to diminished sensitivity to taste (hypogeusia) and to a decrease in odor sensitivity (hyposmia). Patients with zinc deficiency often complain of a foul odor in the nasopharynx, and a metallic taste. They also complain about the saltiness, sourness, sweetness, or bitterness of foods. Zinc supplementation in such patients has resulted in improved appetite. Wound healing is also more prompt following surgery when supplements are given to depleted patients.

FLUORIDE

Fluorine exists in the body in compounds called fluorides. Minute amounts of fluoride enter into the complex calcium salts that form tooth enamel. The fluoride-containing calcium salt is more resistant, and tooth decay has decreased as much as 60 percent in communities where the water supply has contained sufficient fluoride. Fluorides may also be useful in maintaining bone structure. A lesser incidence of osteoporosis has been observed in persons living in areas with fluoridated water.

Fluoride is best provided in the water supply. Many major cities and hundreds of smaller communities now add 1 part fluoride to 1 million parts water (about 1 mg per quart). This inexpensive, safe, and effective public health measure for the protection of the teeth deserves the fullest public support. Alternatives to the use of a fluoridated community water supply are bottled fluoridated water, topical applications of stannous fluoride by a dentist together with use of fluoride toothpaste, or administration of fluoride tablets under a dentist's supervision.

In some parts of the world natural supplies of drinking water contain over 1.5 parts fluoride per million parts of water. People who live in these areas have *mottled* teeth; that is, their teeth have a chalky white appearance and later become discolored. Such teeth are resistant to decay, and no signs of other health changes have occurred in these people.

OTHER TRACE ELEMENTS

A number of trace elements function primarily as parts of enzymes or vitamin molecules, or as catalysts for chemical reactions. They include:

Chromium: involved in carbohydrate metabolism
Cobalt: a constituent of vitamin B_{12}
Copper: a catalyst for hemoglobin formation
Manganese: enzyme systems; normal bone structure; blood formation
Molybdenum: enzyme systems
Selenium: related to activity of vitamin E

The amounts of these elements required by the body are not known, but at any rate they are very small. The mixed diet supplying adequate amounts of other nutrients will furnish sufficient amounts of these elements.

SOME FALLACIES AND FACTS

1. *Fallacy.* A diet low in calcium leads to nervousness.
   Fact. When the diet is inadequate, calcium is readily withdrawn from the bones to supply the minute amounts needed to regulate the response of the nerves. There is no evidence that a low-calcium intake leads to nervousness.
2. *Fallacy.* Cocoa and chocolate interfere with the absorption of calcium.
   Fact. The amounts of cocoa and chocolate normally eaten do not interfere with the absorption of calcium. Although they contain some oxalic acid, one would need to eat abnormally large amounts of chocolate and cocoa to have any noticeable effect. Hot cocoa, chocolate pudding, and chocolate milk are quite appropriate in the menus of children as well as adults. However, the child should not be given these foods so often that he refuses to take regular milk.
3. *Fallacy.* Foods purchased in American markets are likely to be lacking in important trace elements.
   Fact. The wide variety of foods used in the diet supplies ample amounts of all trace elements known to be needed except iodine and fluorine. See discussion on pp. 87 and 88. Farmers use chemical and organic fertilizers in order to realize high yields of foods that are excellent in nutritive quality. Present-day techniques of food processing retain most of the nutritive values.

A summary of the mineral elements and review questions appear at the end of Chapter 10.

REFERENCES

American Dietetic Association: "Policy Statement on Fluoridation," *J. Am. Dietet. A.,* 64:68, 1974.
Cohen, N. L., and Briggs, G. M.: "Trace Minerals in Nutrition," *Am. J. Nurs.,* 68:807–11, 1968.

Council on Foods and Nutrition: "Iron Deficiency in the United States," *J.A.M.A.*, **203:**407–14, 1968.

Finch, C. A.: "Iron Metabolism," *Nutr. Today,* 4:2–7, Summer 1969.

Kidd, P. S., *et al.:* "Sources of Dietary Iodine," *J. Am. Dietat. A.,* **65:**420–22, 1974.

Mayer, J.: "Trace Elements: Pinning Down the Facts," *Family Health,* 7:43, May 1975.

Underwood, E. J.: "Trace Element Imbalances of Interest to the Dietitian," *J. Am. Dietet. A.,* **72:**177–79, 1978.

FLUID AND ELECTROLYTE BALANCE

Two of the important functions of mineral elements mentioned in Chapter 9 are the maintenance of water balance and acid-base balance. These functions will be further described in this chapter together with a discussion of sodium and potassium, which are especially concerned in the maintenance of these balances.

Water

Next to oxygen, water is most important to life. We can survive, at best, for only a few days without water; persons who have been lost in the desert have sometimes perished within 24 hours.

DISTRIBUTION

About 50 to 60 per cent of the total body weight is made up of water. The proportion varies somewhat, with fat persons having less body water than lean persons. Infants and young children have more body water than older persons.

About three fourths of the water in the body is within the cells; this is referred to as *intracellular* fluid. The remaining water is in the blood and lymph circulation and in the fluids around the cells and tissues. This is called *extracellular* fluid.

91

FUNCTIONS

Every cell in the body contains water. Muscle tissue contains as much as 80 per cent, fat tissue about 20 per cent, and bone about 25 per cent water.

Water is the solvent for materials within the body. The foods we eat are digested by enzymes in an abundance of digestive juices; the nutrients are carried in solution across the intestinal wall; the blood transports nutrients to all body tissues; materials dissolved in water are transported across the cell membranes; chemical reactions take place in the presence of water; and body wastes are carried by the blood for elimination by the kidneys, lungs, skin, and bowel.

Water is also a lubricant, for it avoids friction between moving body parts. Water regulates the body temperature through its evaporation from the skin, thus giving a cooling effect. On very humid days we feel uncomfortable because water does not evaporate very readily.

NORMAL WATER LOSSES

Water is lost from the body through the kidneys, skin, lungs, and bowel. Usually, most of the water is lost in the urine. The amount of urine is related to the daily intake of water and other fluids, and varies from about 600 to 2000 ml. Because the nitrogenous and other materials must be kept in solution, about 600 ml urine is the minimum or *obligatory* excretion.

An appreciable amount of water is lost through the skin by *insensible* and *visible* perspiration. Insensible perspiration is so called because one is not aware of it; it evaporates as rapidly as it is formed. On the other hand, with vigorous activity, especially in warm weather, we lose much additional water through visible perspiration. A baseball player, for example, might lose 3 to 5 liters of fluid through perspiration. Appreciable amounts of urea, salts, and traces of other mineral elements are also lost in the visible perspiration. When we perspire a great deal, the urine volume is reduced.

The adult loses about 350 ml water in the air exhaled through the lungs. The amount of water lost in the feces is small, averaging about 100 to 150 ml daily.

WATER REQUIREMENT

The daily water requirement is about 1 ml per kcal; a requirement of 2000 kcal necessitates a water intake of 2000 ml. Infants have proportionately greater water losses, and should be allowed about 150 ml (5 oz.) water for each 100 kcal. Thirst is a good guide for adequate fluid intake, except for sick persons and for infants.

TABLE 10-1 WATER CONTENT OF FOODS

	Water Per Cent		Water Per Cent
Milk	87	Fruits and vegetables	70–95
Egg	74	Bread	35
Cooked meat, poultry, fish		Dry cereals, crackers	3–7
Well done	40–50	Cooked cereals	60–85
Medium to rare	50–70	Nuts, fats, sweets	0–10
Cheese, hard	35–40		

SOURCES OF WATER

The fluids we drink account for the chief intake of water. There is no harm in drinking water with meals provided it is not used to wash foods down without chewing them.

Foods contribute a fair amount of water, as many be seen from Table 10-1.

Water also results from the oxidation of glucose, fatty acids, and amino acids. The amount of water produced in the body from metabolism is about 300 to 450 ml daily.

WATER BALANCE

Ordinarily the water sources to the body and the water losses from the body are in balance, as the following example shows:

Sources of Water	ml	Losses of Water	ml
Water, tea, coffee	1100	Urine	1200
Milk (2 cups)	420	Feces	100
"Solid" foods	480	Skin and lungs	1000
Metabolic water	300		2300
	2300		

CLINICAL PROBLEMS

Dehydration results when the intake is less than the body needs. This can occur when, for some reason, there is no food or fluid intake, or when the losses from the body are abnormally high: excessive perspiration because of marked activity in hot weather; severe diarrhea; vomiting; fever with increased losses through the skin; hemorrhage; severe burns with the accompanying water losses from the skin; uncontrolled diabetes with frequent urination. Dehydration is a serious medical problem requiring prompt attention. Fluids are given by mouth when possible; intravenous fluids are given when the patient is unable to take sufficient fluid by mouth. In dehydration there has often been loss of electrolytes as well so that these will require replacement with the water.

Edema is the accumulation water in the body. It occurs when the body is unable to excrete sodium in sufficient amounts. This is not unusual in diseases of the heart when the circulation is impaired, or when the kidneys are unable to excrete wastes normally. Edema also occurs following prolonged protein deficiency, because the tissues are no longer able to maintain normal water balance.

Electrolytes

DISTRIBUTION

Electrolytes are chemical compounds that can break up into their ions when dissolved in water. They are called electrolytes because they carry electrical charges. *Cations* carry positive electrical charges; *anions* carry negative electrical charges. For example, salt (NaCl) dissociates to sodium (Na^+), a cation; and chloride (Cl^-), an anion. The total cations are exactly equal to the total anions in an electrolyte solution. Electrolytes are essential for the regulation of water and acid-base balance.

The electrolytes in body fluids are measured in units called milliequivalents (mEq). The normal electrolyte composition of blood plasma and interstitial fluid is shown in Table 10–2. Note that the cations exactly balance the anions. Note also that the principal cation in blood plasma and interstitial fluid is sodium, and the principal anion is chloride. Within the cells, however, the principal cation is potassium, and the chief anion is phosphate.

In health the concentrations of the electrolytes in the extracellular fluid and in the intracellular fluid are maintained within very narrow ranges. Very little sodium enters into the cell, and very little potassium leaves the cell into

TABLE 10–2 ELECTROLYTE COMPOSITION OF BLOOD PLASMA

Cations	mEq per Liter	Anions	mEq per Liter
Sodium (Na^+)	142	Chloride (Cl^-)	103
Potassium (K^+)	5	Bicarbonate (HCO_3^-)	27
		Phosphate (HPO_4^{--})	2
Calcium (Ca^{++})	5	Sulfate (SO_4^{--})	1
		Organic acids$^-$	6
Magnesium (Mg^{++})	3	Proteinate$^-$	16
Total	155	Total	155

the interstitial fluid or the blood plasma. A change in the level of any of the electrolytes in the blood plasma has great significance in deciding upon the correct treatment in various disease conditions.

SODIUM

About half of the body sodium is found in the extracellular fluid. Another 40 per cent is present in bone, and not over 10 per cent in the intracellular fluid. Sodium helps to maintain the fluid and acid-base balance of the body; in the transmission of nerve impulses; in the absorption of glucose; in the relaxation of muscle cells; and in the maintenance of permeability of cell membranes.

Utilization. Sodium in the diet is almost completely absorbed from the gastrointestinal tract. Any excess is rapidly excreted in the urine. A person who is perspiring heavily will lose much sodium through the skin. The amount of sodium that is excreted is regulated by adrenal hormones that exert control over the kidneys. When the sodium intake is high, the excretion by the kidneys is increased; but if the body stores of sodium, or the dietary supply is low, only traces of sodium will be excreted.

Sources. A typical American diet based on the Four Food Groups would furnish about 500 gm sodium, if no salt or other sodium-containing compound were added. About three fourths of this sodium is present in foods from the milk and meat groups. With a few exceptions, the fruit-vegetable and bread-cereal groups are low in sodium.

The chief source of sodium in the diet is salt. It is used not only in food preparation and at the table, but it is present in considerable amounts in many processed foods such as ham, bacon, luncheon meats, smoked poultry and fish; pickles, olives; catsup, meat sauces, relishes; snack foods such as potato chips, pretzels, and many crackers. Other sodium compounds such as monosodium glutamate (MSG), baking powder, and baking soda also contribute important amounts of sodium.

Requirement. For the normal healthy adult the sodium requirement is quite low—about 500 mg (1250 mg salt). Greater intakes would be needed by laborers or athletes engaged in vigorous physical activity in very hot, humid climates.

Salt is an acquired taste. The sodium intake of Americans varies widely from about 3 to 8 gm (7.5 to 20 gm salt). This is far in excess of needs.

Clinical problems. In some individuals a high intake of salt over a lifetime is believed to increase the likelihood of hypertension. Most physicians recommend that their patients who have hypertension reduce their sodium intake to about 2 to 3 gm per day (5 to 7 gm salt). This moderate restriction is in addition to any anti-hypertensive medications that are prescribed.

The Dietary Goals propose that all persons restrict their salt intake to 5 gm daily. This permits light salting of food in its preparation, but eliminates the use of salt at the table, and also the use of foods that are high in salt content. Although such restriction of salt over a lifetime might reduce the risk of hypertension, there is no guarantee that such benefit would take place. On the other hand, this level of restriction is a safe approach and still permits a palatable diet.

When the kidney or heart is not functioning normally, sodium may accumulate in the tissues and water will also be held (edema). The need for diets restricted in sodium is fully discussed in Chapter 26. Dietary deficiency of sodium does not occur. However, excessive perspiration, severe vomiting or diarrhea, or diseases of the adrenal gland may lead to depletion of body sodium.

POTASSIUM

Just as sodium is the principal mineral element in fluids surrounding the cells, so potassium is the principal mineral element within the cell. Potassium is essential for the synthesis of proteins, for enzyme functions within the cells, and for maintenance of the fluid balance. A small amount of potassium is also found in the extracellular fluid, and aids in the regulation of muscle contraction and nervous irritability.

Sources. Most diets supply liberal amounts of potassium. Among the rich sources are meats, potatoes, peanut butter, dried fruits, oranges, grapefruit, tomatoes, bananas, carrots, and celery.

Clinical problems. The exact requirement for potassium is not known. Dietary deficiency does not normally occur. However, persons who take diuretics have an increased excretion of potassium in the urine, and they need to emphasize potassium-rich foods in their diets to make up for these losses. Severe vomiting, diarrhea, and diabetic acidosis may also lead to potassium deficiency. Some of the symptoms are nausea, vomiting, apprehension, listlessness, muscular weakness, abnormalities in cardiac rhythm, and respiratory failure.

Hyperpotassemia (high blood potassium) is a complication in severe dehydration, adrenal insufficiency, and renal failure. Numbness of the face, tongue, and extremities, muscle weakness, and cardiac arrhythmia are observed. Cardiac failure may occur. Diets low in protein and potassium and high in carbohydrate are used in these conditions. (See Chapter 27.)

Acid-Base Balance

pH

The pH is a measure of acidity or alkalinity. A pH of 7.0 is exact neutrality. A pH below 7 indicates acid; the lower the number, the greater the acidity. A pH above 7 indicates alkalinity; the higher the number, the greater the alkalinity.

Body fluids are maintained at a pH ranging between 7.35 and 7.45, which is slightly alkaline. A pH of 7.0 to 7.2 is abnormally low; it is called *acidosis* in relation to the normal level. It is seen in uncontrolled diabetic patients who are excreting large quantities of ketones (see Chapter 23). It also occurs in severe starvation, and in renal failure.

A pH above 7.5 is labeled as *alkalosis*. It results when there is prolonged, severe vomiting so that there is much loss of stomach acid. Alkalosis also occurs with excessive ingestion of soluble antacids such as sodium bicarbonate because such compounds are rapidly absorbed form the gastrointestinal tract.

REACTION OF FOODS

Some foods are potentially *alkali-producing* because they contain important amounts of calcium, sodium, potassium, and magnesium. Other foods are *acid-producing* because they contain greater amounts of sulfur, chlorine, and phosphorus than they do of the alkali-producing elements. Still other foods are low in mineral elements and are considered to be neutral.

Acid-producing: meat, poultry, fish, eggs, cheese, legumes, cereal foods, corn, almonds, chestnuts, coconut, prunes, plums, cranberries
Alkali-producing: fruits, vegetables, milk, peanuts, walnuts, Brazil nuts
Neutral: butter, margarine, oils, cooking fats, sugar, syrup, starch, tapioca

Certain fruits such as lemons, grapefruit, oranges, and peaches contain organic acids that give a sour (acid) taste. These acids are weak and they do not increase the acidity of the stomach. The hydrochloric acid in the stomach is a strong acid that is useful for the digestion of proteins. The organic acids in fruits are oxidized, just as are the carbohydrates, to yield energy, carbon dioxide, and water.

Plums, cranberries, and prunes contain an organic acid that is not metabolized by the body. The excretion of this acid increases the acidity of the urine; therefore, these fruits are sometimes recommended with other acid-producing foods to help counteract the formation of certain types of renal calculi.

REGULATION OF ACID-BASE BALANCE

A number of acids are normally produced in the metabolism of foodstuffs. The body has several efficient mechanisms for taking care of these acids so that the normal acid-base balance is not disturbed.

A principal acid produced in metabolism is carbonic acid. This is released through the lungs by exhalation of carbon dioxide. When the carbon dioxide content of the blood increases, the individual breathes more rapidly and more deeply to get rid of more carbon dioxide.

Minerals function in *buffer* salts. A buffer is a substance that can react

TABLE 10–3 SUMMARY OF MINERAL ELEMENTS

Element	Function	Utilization	Daily Allowances Food Sources
Calcium	99% in bones, teeth Nervous stimulation Muscle contraction Blood clotting Activates enzymes	10 to 40% absorbed Aided by vitamin D and lactose; hindered by oxalic acid Parathyroid hormone regulates blood levels	RDA, adults: 800 mg Milk, cheese, ice cream Mustard and turnip greens Cabbage, broccoli Clams, oysters, salmon
Phosphorus	80–90% in bones, teeth Acid-base balance Transport of fats Enzymes for energy metabolism; protein synthesis	Vitamin D favors absorption and use by bones Dietary deficiency unlikely	RDA, adults: 800 mg Milk, cheese, ice cream Meat, poultry, fish Whole-grain cereals, nuts, legumes
Magnesium	60% in bones, teeth Transmit nerve impulses Muscle contraction Enzymes for energy metabolism	Salts relatively insoluble Acid favors absorption Dietary deficiency unlikely	RDA, adults: 300–350 mg Milk, meat, green leafy vegetables, legumes, whole-grain cereals
Sodium	Extracellular fluid Water balance Acid-base balance Nervous stimulation Muscle contraction	Almost completely absorbed Body levels regulated by adrenal; excess excreted in urine and by skin	Safe, adequate: 1100–3300 mg Table salt Baking powder, soda Milk, meat, poultry, fish, eggs
Potassium	Intracellular fluid Protein and glycogen synthesis Water balance Transmit nerve impulse Muscle contraction	Almost completely absorbed Body levels regulated by adrenal; excess excreted in urine	Safe, adequate: 1875–5625 mg Ample amounts in meat, cereals, fruits, fruit juices, vegetable
Iron	Mostly in hemoglobin Muscle myoglobin Oxidizing enzymes for release of energy	5–20% absorption Acid and vitamin C aid absorption Daily losses in urine and feces Menstrual losses Anemia is common	RDA, men: 10 mg women: 18 mg Organ meats, meat, fish, poultry Whole-grain and enriched cereal Green vegetables; dried fruits
Iodine	Form thyroxine for energy metabolism	Chiefly in thyroid gland Deficiency leads to endemic goiter	RDA: 150 mcg Iodized salt Shellfish, saltwater fish
Fluorine	Prevent tooth decay		Fluoridated water
Zinc	Enzymes for transfer of carbon dioxide Taste; protein synthesis	Little likelihood of deficiency or excess	RDA, adults: 15 mg Plant and animal proteins are good sources

with an acid or an alkali without much change occuring in the pH. The sodium phosphate and carbonate buffer systems are important. Proteins are also good buffers.

The kidneys are the final regulators of acid-base balance. When excess acid is being produced, the kidneys secrete a highly acid urine, so that little change takes place in the pH of the blood. The kidneys also synthesize the ammonium (NH_4^+) ion which can combine with acid so that the body loses less of its sodium.

The healthy individual maintains acid-base balance regardless of the composition of his diet. Moreover, there is no evidence that shows the merits of an acid-producing or alkali-producing diet. In certain pathologic conditions such as renal failure or renal calculi these characteristics of the diet may be adjusted.

REVIEW QUESTIONS AND PROBLEMS

1. Define these terms: insensible perspiration, water balance, ossification, pH, osteoporosis, fluoridation, endemic goiter.

2. List the ways in which water assists in making the nutrients of food available to the cells of the body.

3. Record your fluid intake for one day. Include water, tea, coffee, soft drinks, milk, fruit juices, and soup.

4. What reasons might account for edema? For dehydration?

5. Which mineral elements are listed in the Recommended Dietary Allowances? What are your daily allowances? How do these compare with those of a 14-year-old girl?

6. What other mineral elements are known to be essential for human nutrition? Why are there no allowances listed in the table of Recommended Dietary Allowances?

7. What is meant by intracellular fluid? By extracellular fluid? What mineral elements would you expect to find in each?

8. What mineral elements are especially important for each of the following: building hemoglobin; construction of bones and teeth; function of the thyroid gland; maintenance of water balance; release of energy from fats, carbohydrates, and proteins.

9. A woman patient asks you why it is important to drink milk. What would you tell her?

10. Write a menu for one day, including foods from the Four Food Groups. Do not use liver. Calculate the iron content of your menu. Adjust the menu so that it includes 18 mg iron.

11. What is meant by anemia? What lack in the diet may cause it?

12. Of what importance is fluorine? How is it best supplied?

13. List three acid-producing foods; three alkali-producing foods.

REFERENCES

Abbey, J. C.: "Nursing Observations of Fluid Imbalances," *Nurs. Clin. North Am.*, 3:77–86, March 1968.

Fenton, M.: "What to Do about Thirst," *Am. J. Nurs.,* 69:1014–17, 1969.

Grant, M. M., and Kubo, W. M.: "Assessing the Patient's Hydration Status," *Am. J. Nurs.,* 75:1306–11, 1975.

Sharer, J. E.: "Reviewing Acid-base Balance," *Am. J. Nurs.,* 75:980–83, 1975.

VITAMINS: INTRODUCTION AND
FAT-SOLUBLE VITAMINS

Introduction to Vitamin Study

Undoubtedly the discovery of vitamins in the twentieth century will go down in history as one of the major factors in the improvement of health of people throughout the world. The fact that these substances in such small amounts affect the course of health in so many ways has also led to widespread abuse of them. Many people, lacking full understanding of how vitamins function, place emphasis upon vitamin intake from one source or another, while ignoring other equally important nutrients. Other people somehow expect that a vitamin pill will solve many nutritional problems. Let us now look at some of the facts concerning vitamins.

DEFINITIONS

Vitamins are chemical compounds of an organic nature that occur in minute quantities in foods and are necessary for life and growth. Many, but not all, are components of enzymes. As enzymes they facilitate the use of the energy nutrients. Vitamins are important regulators of the synthesis of countless body compounds.

Vitamins are generally classified as fat-soluble and water-soluble. But within each of these broad classes the vitamins differ in their chemical structure, their distribution in foods, and in their functions. Moreover, each vitamin deficiency is specific in its characteristics.

101

Precursors or *provitamins* are compounds that can be changed into the active vitamin.

Avitaminosis means "without vitamins." It denotes a deficiency or lack of sufficient vitamin to carry out normal body functions. Some deficiencies are so mild that a diagnosis can be made only by biochemical tests of the blood and urine. As deficiencies become more severe, clinical signs typical of the specific vitamin lack begin to appear.

Hypervitaminosis is an excessive accumulation of a vitamin in the body leading to toxic symptoms. Excessive intakes of vitamins A and D can be toxic.

Vitamin *antagonists* or *antivitamins* are substances that interfere with the functioning of a vitamin.

MEETING DAILY NEEDS

Values for five vitamins are given for commonly used foods in Table A–1, Appendix A. Most foods are poor sources of vitamin D and hence no values are published. Analyses have been made for a number of B-complex vitamins not included in Table A–1, but the nurse is rarely required to refer to these data. The diet that supplies sufficient thiamin, riboflavin, and niacin will also furnish enough of the other B factors.

In selecting food sources for vitamins we should keep in mind (1) how much of a given food we would ordinarily eat, (2) how often the food is eaten, and (3) how stable the vitamin may be after processing or cooking. Parsley is an excellent source of vitamin A, but it will make little difference in the average diet, because it is so often left on the plate or, when eaten, is consumed in such small amounts. A raw fruit might be a good source of ascorbic acid but might contain little of the vitamin after drying or canning.

Wheat germ, dried yeast, and fish-liver oils are rich sources of several vitamins but are generally regarded as dietary supplements rather than basic items of the diet. Liver and other organ meats are outstanding sources of vitamin A and B-complex vitamins; yet their contribution to the diet will be important only if these foods are included on a fairly regular basis—for example, once a week.

VITAMIN SUPPLEMENTS

For the healthy individual, the diet that includes recommended levels of the Four Food Groups together with some oils for vitamin E will meet the needs for vitamins.

Supplements of vitamins A and D, when taken over a period of time, could result in toxic symptoms. Supplements of the water-soluble vitamins in excess of body need will be excreted in the urine. Thus, they are a waste of money.

Vitamin supplements are indicated when the diet, through illness or ignorance, has been inadequate over a long period of time. In such circumstances the vitamin in a concentrated form is a rapid form of therapy. Equally important is dietary counseling so that the affected individual makes the necessary changes in his diet.

Vitamin supplements are indicated in some specific disease conditions: pancreatitis, ulcerative colitis, sprue, cystic fibrosis; and following surgery or injury from burns. In these situations the intake is usually much greater than that supplied by a diet alone. The physician prescribes the kinds and amounts of vitamins that are to be taken.

Fat-Soluble Vitamins

VITAMIN A

Nomenclature.   Preformed vitamin A exists in three forms: retinol, retinal, and retinoic acid. The precursors of vitamin A are alpha-, beta-, and gamma carotene and cryptoxanthin.

Function.   Vitamin A is important (1) for the normal structure of the bones and teeth; (2) for the maintenance of the epithelium or outer layer of the skin, and the mucous membranes that line the nose and respiratory tract, the mouth and gastrointestinal tract, the eyes, the genitourinary tract, and the glands of secretion; and (3) for the formation of *visual purple*, which enables the retina of the eye to adapt to dim light.

Bile is essential for the absorption of carotenes from the intestines. Mineral oil can seriously interfere with the absorption of vitamin A; if it is used as a laxative, it should not be taken near mealtimes. The liver stores vitamin A, and well-nourished individuals usually have a sufficient supply to last for several months.

Recommended allowances.   Vitamin A is measured in retinol equivalents (R.E.) and international units (I.U.). The latter designation will no longer be used when food tables have been converted to retinol equivalents.

The allowance for vitamin A from 11 years throughout life is 1000 R.E. (5000 I.U.) for males, and 800 R.E. (4000 I.U.) for females. During pregnancy and lactation the allowances are increased to 1000 R.E. and 1200 R.E., respectively. Intakes ranging from 400 R.E. (2000 I.U.) to 700 R.E. (3300 I.U.) are recommended for infants and children.

Sources.   With the many good sources of vitamin A or its precursor, there is little excuse for an inadequate intake. The liver of any animal—beef, veal, pork, lamb, chicken, turkey—is a rich source. For those who like it, liver once a week or every ten days will go far toward ensuring the full weekly allowance. Fish-liver oil are excellent sources, but are not generally consumed as foods.

Whole milk, cream, butter, and whole-milk cheeses are good sources of vitamin A. One egg yolk furnishes one tenth of the daily allowance of the adult. Fortified margarine contains the same levels as butter.

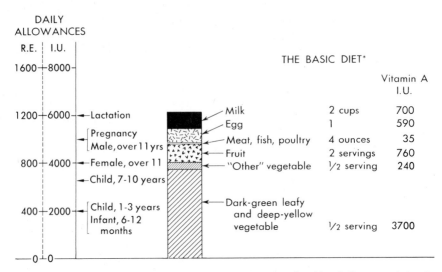

FIGURE 11–1 The Four Food Groups of the Basic Diet provide a liberal allowance of vitamin A. Note the contributions made by dark-green leafy and deep-yellow vegetables. Breads, cereals, and white potato do not provide vitamin A. See Table 4–2 (p. 37) for complete calculation.

Dark green leafy vegetables and deep yellow vegetables and fruits are rich in carotene, which can be converted into vitamin A by the intestinal wall. Among the carotene-rich foods are carrots, sweet potatoes, pumpkin, yellow winter squash, cantaloupe, yellow peaches, apricots, spinach, kale, turnip greens, dark salad greens, broccoli, and green asparagus. (See Fig. 11–1.)

Toxicity. Toxic effects of vitamin A have been observed in children and adults when supplements of 25,000 to 50,000 I.U. have been taken daily for several months. The symptoms include nausea, vomiting, abdominal pain, failure to grow in children or weight loss in adults, drying and scaling of the skin, thinning of the hair, swelling and tenderness of the long bones, joint pains, and enlargement of the liver and spleen. The condition is corrected when the individual stops taking the supplement, although recovery may require weeks.

Clinical problems. Some estimates of dietary intakes indicate that one diet in every four may not provide the recommended allowances for vitamin A. However, in the United States vitamin A deficiency symptoms are not widely prevalent. When they do occur they are generally mild. In diseases of malabsorption such as pancreatitis, celiac disease, or cystic fibrosis the absorption is often sufficiently impaired to produce some signs of deficiency. When diets are low in fat, or when there is inadequate bile production, the absorption of vitamin A may be significantly reduced.

Night blindness (nyctalopia) is a form of vitamin A deficiency sometimes seen in the United States. It is experienced when the visual purple is slowly reduced in the eye because of lack of vitamin A. The affected person has difficulty in adjusting to the glare of automobile headlights or in trying to find a seat in a darkened theater, for example.

Skin changes and infections caused by lack of vitamin A are rarely seen in the United States, but are fairly prevalent in the Far East. With the lack of the vitamin the skin becomes *keratinized* (dry and scaly). Soft, moist epithelium normally offers protection against bacteria, but when it becomes dry and hard, infections of the respiratory tract, the mouth, the eye, and the genitourinary tract occur easily. Additional vitamin A does not provide further protection against infection to individuals who are well nourished, but it would be indicated for those persons whose vitamin A store has become depleted. *Xerophthalmia* is the severe eye disease caused by changes in the epithelium of the eye and is the cause of some blindness in the Orient.

VITAMIN D

Nomenclature. There are about ten forms of vitamin D. The two most common forms are *ergocalciferol* (vitamin D_2) and *cholecalciferol* (vitamin D_3). Precursors of vitamin D are ergosterol in plants and 7-dehydrocholesterol in the skin.

Utilization. Being fat-soluble, vitamin D is absorbed with fats. It is transported through the lymph circulation to the liver. Vitamin D in foods occurs in an inactive form. The liver accomplishes the first step and the kidney the second step in converting vitamin D to an active form. In its active form vitamin D behaves as a hormone; this is the only known example of a vitamin functioning as a hormone.

Functions. Active vitamin D aids in the absorption of calcium and phosphorus from the gastrointestinal tract; promotes the mineralization of bones and teeth; and regulates the normal level of calcium in the blood by releasing calcium from bone as it is needed. The regulation of calcium and phosphorus metabolism is also dependent upon the hormones parathormone and calcitonin. (See Chapter 9.)

Meeting daily needs. An allowance of 10 mcg (400 I.U.) vitamin D as cholecalciferol is recommended for infants, children, and adolescents; 5 mcg for men and women over age 22. Adults probably get enough vitamin D through exposure of the skin to sunlight. However, clothing, soot, fog, and window glass cut off the ultraviolet light and prevent the change of the precursor in the skin to the active vitamin. People who work at night and sleep in the day, invalids who do not get out in the sun, and people who wear religious habits may require a vitamin D supplement.

Sources. Foods are not good sources of vitamin D except when they are fortified. Almost all fresh milk or evaporated milk is fortified with 400 I.U. vitamin D to the quart or tall can, thus providing the daily needs during growth, pregnancy, and lactation.

Toxicity. Large doses of vitamin D—20,000 to 100,000 I.U.—have severe effects including loss of appetite, vomiting, diarrhea, fatigue, growth failure, and drowsiness. The blood calcium level is increased, and calcium salts are deposited in the soft tissues, including the blood vessels, heart, and kidney tubules. Kidney stones may form.

As little as 1800 I.U. of vitamin D given daily may be mildly toxic, with some of the symptoms listed above being observed. Thus, if an infant is receiving vitamin D concentrate, it is important to measure the intake carefully, and also to avoid the use of fortified milk or other foods that might contain vitamin D.

Clinical problems. Rickets is the deficiency disease seen in children who fail to get enough vitamin D. Calcium and phosphorus are inadequately deposited in the bones. The soft, pliable bones yield to pressure, the joints enlarge, and

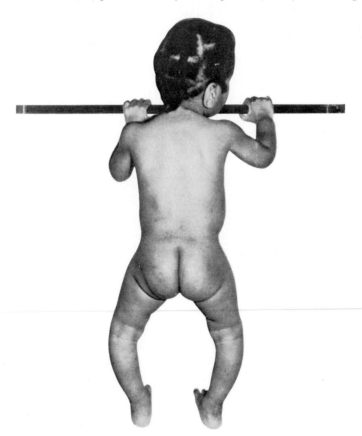

FIGURE 11-2 Early skeletal deformities of rickets often persist throughout life. Bowlegs that curve as shown here indicate that the weakened bones have bent as a result of standing. *(Dr. Rosa Lee Nemir and the Upjohn Company, Kalamazoo, Michigan)*

there is delayed closing of the skull bones. The child may have an enlarged skull, chest deformities, spinal curvature, and bowed legs. (See Fig. 11–2.)

Premature infants are more susceptible to rickets than full-term infants. The use of vitamin-D formulas, or the vitamin-D supplements if the infant is breast fed, account for the rarity of rickets in the United States.

Osteomalacia or adult rickets is sometimes seen in women of the Orient who have had a grossly inadequate intake of calcium, phosphorus, and vitamin D and who have had several pregnancies.

Osteodystrophy often occurs in severe renal disease because the kidney is unable to convert vitamin D to its active form. As a result the absorption of calcium is reduced. The level of calcium in the blood is lowered, which in turn leads to release of calcium from the bones. If allowed to continue the bones lose so much calcium that they become very fragile. The impairment of vitamin D function is accompanied by increased activity of the parathyroid hormone and also by the retention of phosphorus. The correction of the faulty vitamin D-calcium-phosphorus metabolism requires delicate dietary adjustment as well as appropriate medication.

VITAMIN E

Vitamin E activity is possessed by a number of compounds known as *tocopherols.*

Functions. Although vitamin E has been known since the 1920s its functions are still poorly understood. The principal role of vitamin E appears to be as an antioxidant. By accepting oxygen, vitamin E can prevent the oxidation of vitamin A in the intestinal tract, thus making vitamin A available for body use. Vitamin E also reduces the oxidation of the polyunsaturated fatty acids, thereby helping to maintain normal cell membranes. It protects the red blood cell against hemolysis. Vitamin E is required by animals, and presumably by humans, for the normal reproductive processes. It may have some function in the aging of cells.

Dietary allowances. The recommended allowance for vitamin E, expressed as alpha-tocopherol equivalents (T.E.), is 10 mg for men and 8 mg for women.

Food sources. Vitamin E is widely distributed in foods, with vegetable oils (corn, soy, safflower, cottonseed), shortening, and margarines furnishing about two thirds of the day's intake. Whole-grain cereals, legumes, nuts, and dark green vegetables are also good sources. Some commercial use is made of tocopherols as an additive to prevent or retard oxidation and rancidity.

Clinical problems. Deficiency of vitamin E in humans is unlikely except when diets are grossly lacking in many other nutrients. In infants with protein-calorie malnutrition vitamin E deficiency has been noted by increased hemolysis of red blood cells and a macrocytic anemia. The possibility of deficiency should be considered in premature infants and in patients who have a defect in the absorption of fats and fat-soluble vitamins.

Perhaps the chief problem associated with vitamin E is that many exaggerated and unproven claims have been made in the treatment of disease conditions. There is no reliable evidence that supports the claims that vitamin E is effective for the treatment or cure of muscular dystrophy, acne, ulcers, rheumatic fever, heart disease, and reproductive disorders. It is fortunate that vitamin E has not been shown to be toxic in view of the overuse of the vitamin as a result of these false claims.

VITAMIN K

Vitamin K is also known as the *antihemorrhagic* vitamin. *Menadione* and *phylloquinone* are compounds with vitamin K activity.

Functions.   Vitamin K is needed for the formation of prothrombin, a substance necessary for blood clotting.

Intestinal bacteria normally synthesize a substantial amount of vitamin K. Because vitamin K is fat soluble, absorption is facilitated in the presence of bile. Small amounts of vitamin K are stored in the liver, heart, skin, muscles, and kidney.

Meeting daily needs.   The requirement for vitamin K is not known. Green leaves are an excellent source of the vitamin. Cereals, fruits, and nonleafy vegetables are rather poor sources.

Clinical problems.   Because of intestinal synthesis there is little likelihood of vitamin K deficiency in normal individuals. Some newborn infants have a tendency to hemorrhage because the intestinal bacteria are not yet sufficiently developed for synthesis of the vitamin. Hence, vitamin K preparations are sometimes given to the infant.

Hemorrhage can also result if there is interference with the synthesis of vitamin K or with its absorption. Oral sulfa drugs and antibiotics are known to reduce bacterial growth in the intestine so that there is less synthesis of the vitamin. In diseases of malabsorption, hemorrhage can be a complicating factor since the absorption of vitamin K is reduced.

Dicumarol is a vitamin K antagonist. It counteracts the effect of vitamin K in the formation of prothrombin and thus prevents blood clotting. It has been effective in treating circulatory diseases in which blood clots tend to form and that might endanger the patient's life. Patients who are given dicumarol must be monitored closely to avoid excessive bleeding.

SOME FALLACIES AND FACTS

1. *Fallacy.* A vitamin A supplement will help to prevent infections.

Facts. A diet planned to furnish the recommended allowance for vitamin A will help to maintain healthy mucous membranes. Such membranes resist invasion by disease-

TABLE 11-1 SUMMARY OF FAT-SOLUBLE VITAMINS

Vitamins	Metabolism and Function	Deficiency or Excess	Meeting Body Needs
Vitamin A precursors: Carotenes	Bile needed for absorption of carotenes Mineral oil prevents absorption Stored in liver Bone and tooth structure Healthy skin and mucous membranes Vision in dim light	Night blindness Lowered resistance to infection *Severe:* drying and scaling of skin; eye infections; blindness Overdoses are toxic: skin, hair, and bone changes	Men: 1000 R.E. (5000 I.U.) Women: 800 R.E. (4000 I.U.) Liver, kidney Egg yolk, butter, fortified margarine Whole milk, cream, cheese Dark green leafy and deep yellow vegetables Deep yellow fruits
Vitamin D precursors: Ergosterol in plants 7-dehydrocholesterol in skin	Some storage in liver Active form produced by kidney Function as hormone in absorption of calcium and phosphorus Calcification of bones, teeth	*Rickets* Soft bones Enlarged joints Enlarged skull Deformed chest Spinal curvature Bowed legs *Osteomalacia* in adults (infrequent in U.S.) Even small excess is toxic	Infants, children, adolescents, and pregnant women: 10 mcg (400 I.U.) Fortified milk Concentrates: calciferol, viosterol Fish-liver oils Exposure to ultraviolet rays of sun
Vitamin E tocopherols	Prevents oxidation of vitamin A in intestine Protects red blood cells Limited stores in body Polyunsaturated fats increase need	Deficiency not a problem in humans	Men: 10 mg α T.E. Women: 8 mg α T.E. Salad oils, shortenings, margarines Whole grains, legumes, nuts, dark leafy vegetables
Vitamin K	Forms prothrombin for normal blood clotting Dicumarol is an antagonist	Hemorrhage, especially in newborn infants, and biliary tract disease	No recommended allowances Synthesis by intestinal bacteria Dark green leafy vegetables

producing organisms. An intake of vitamin A above the body's requirement does not enable the mucous membranes to give additional protection.

2. *Fallacy.* Vitamins from food sources are better than those from synthetic sources.

Facts. Each vitamin has a definite chemical composition. Thus, 1 milligram of vitamin from a food source or from a concentrate has exactly the same behavior in the body. But good dietary planning eliminates the need to spend additional money for vitamin pills. There are, of course, legitimate uses for vitamin pills in disease conditions. (See p. 102.)

3. *Fallacy.* Night blindness is always caused by lack of vitamin A.

Fact. There are a number of causes of night blindness. An increased intake of vitamin A will not correct the condition if the cause is other than vitamin A lack.

REVIEW QUESTIONS AND PROBLEMS

1. Explain the meaning of each of these terms: antagonist, antivitamin, avitaminosis, calciferol, carotene, ergosterol, keratinization, menadione, precursor, provitamin, rickets, tocopherol, xerophthalmia.

2. If an individual is on a very low-fat diet, what effect might this have on the fat-soluble vitamins?

3. State the vitamin most directly concerned with each of the following items and indicate the relationship of the vitamin: visual purple, blood clotting, healthy skin, formation of bones and teeth, normal mucous membranes, carotene, ergosterol.

4. If your intake of vitamins A and D is more than you need, what happens to the excess?

5. Keep a record of your own diet for two days. Which foods provided you with vitamin A? What improvements are needed, if any?

6. Examine the labeling on fresh milk, evaporated milk, nonfat dry milk, and margarines. What information do you find concerning vitamins A and D?

7. What problems may arise if an individual uses vitamin A and D supplements in additon to an adequate diet?

REFERENCES

Committee on Nutrition Misinformation, Food and Nutrition Board: "Supplementation of Human Diets with Vitamin E," *Nutr. Rev.,* **31:**327–28, 1973.

Committee on Nutrition Misinformation, Food and Nutrition Board: "Hazards of Overuse of Vitamin D," *Nutr. Rev.,* **33:**61–62, 1975.

Hodges, R. E.: "Vitamin E and Coronary Heart Disease," *J. Am. Dietet. A.,* **62:**638–42, 1973.

Palmisano, P. A.: "Vitamin D: A Reawakening," *J.A.M.A.,* **224:**1526, 1973.

Robinson, C. H., and Lawler, M. R.: *Normal and Therapeutic Nutrition,* 15th ed., New York: Macmillan Publishing Co., Inc., 1977, chap. 10.

Russell, R. M., *et al.:* "Hepatic Injury from Chronic Hypervitaminosis A Resulting in Portal Hypertension and Ascites," *N. Engl. J. Med.,* **291:**435–40, 1974.

12

ASCORBIC ACID | THIAMIN | RIBOFLAVIN | NIACIN | VITAMIN B₆ | VITAMIN
B₁₂ | FOLACIN | OTHER B-COMPLEX VITAMINS | SOME FALLACIES AND
FACTS • Summary of Water-Soluble Vitamins

WATER-SOLUBLE VITAMINS

ASCORBIC ACID

Functions.   Ascorbic acid (vitamin C) is essential for building *collagen*, the connective tissue protein that "cements" the cells and tissues together. The effect of this material is to provide firm tissues of all kinds: strong blood vessels, teeth firmly held in their sockets, and bones firmly held together.

Ascorbic acid improves the absorption of iron from the intestines; it is needed to convert folacin to folinic acid (see p. 120); it is required for the formation of hormones such as thyroxine and adrenaline and probably the steroid hormones; it participates in the metabolism of amino acids; and it is essential in wound healing.

Body stores.   With an adequate diet the body maintains a normal saturation of vitamin C in the tissues. The greatest concentration occurs in the adrenal gland and the eyes. With an adequate intake, the stores in the adult body range between 600 and 1500 mg. If an individual consumed no vitamin C, this store would be used up in 20 to 50 days, assuming that he needed 30 mg per day. During this time symptoms would begin to develop as described below.

The kidney helps to regulate tissue storage. When the tissues are depleted, very little ascorbic acid will be excreted. When the tissues are saturated, the excess intake will be excreted.

Recommended allowances.   A minimum intake of 10 mg ascorbic acid daily will prevent scurvy, but higher intakes are recommended for optimum health. The recommended allowance for adults is 60 mg; of infants, 35 mg; and for children, 45 mg. (See also Table 4–1, p. 32.)

111

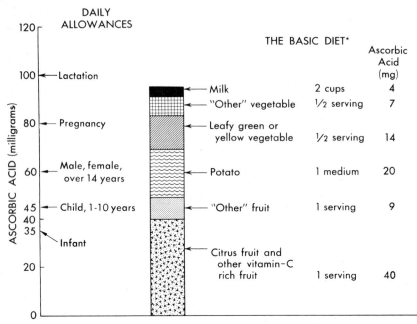

DAILY ALLOWANCES

THE BASIC DIET*

		Ascorbic Acid (mg)
Milk	2 cups	4
"Other" vegetable	½ serving	7
Leafy green or yellow vegetable	½ serving	14
Potato	1 medium	20
"Other" fruit	1 serving	9
Citrus fruit and other vitamin–C rich fruit	1 serving	40

ASCORBIC ACID (milligrams)

120

100 ◄— Lactation

80 ◄— Pregnancy

60 ◄— Male, female, over 14 years

45 ◄— Child, 1-10 years
40
35 ◄ Infant

20

0

FIGURE 12–1 The Basic Diet furnishes more than the ascorbic acid allowance for all age categories. Note the absence of the meat group and the bread-cereal group. For complete calculations of the Basic Diet see Table 4–2, p. 37.

Food sources. Ascorbic acid is sometimes called the "fresh-food" vitamin. It occurs in the growing parts of the plant, but it is absent from the dormant seed. Only the vegetable-fruit group contributes to the vitamin C intake. (See Fig. 12–1.) Human milk from a healthy mother supplies sufficient amounts for the young infant. Pasteurized milk contains only traces.

Raw fresh fruits and vegetables all contain vitamin C, but some foods are more outstanding than others. Oranges, grapefruits, tangerines, limes, and lemons are especially rich. Cantaloupe, strawberries, guava, and fresh pineapple are good sources. Blueberries, peaches, apples, pears, and banana are lower in vitamin C; if they are eaten in large amounts, they may be important for this vitamin.

The dark green leafy vegetables so rich in carotene are also important for ascorbic acid. Tossed salad, or freshly prepared cabbage slaw, or fresh tomatoes are excellent sources. Broccoli is one of the outstanding sources; one serving, even after cooking, is equal in vitamin content to that of an orange.

Potatoes and sweet potatoes contain much less vitamin C, but it is sometimes said that "the lowly potato has prevented more scurvy than the lordly orange." This statement applies, of course, to those people who include appreciable amounts of fresh potato in the daily diet and who exercise care in proper preparation so that the vitamin is retained.

Canned and frozen citrus juices and fruits and tomato juice contain almost as much ascorbic acid as the fresh fruit. Cooked or canned nonacid fruits and vegetables lose more of the ascorbic acid. Frozen vegetables and fruits contain most of the vitamin C of the fresh product. On the other hand, dried foods contain only traces. Some food processors now add ascorbic acid to dehydrated potatoes, apple juice, and other foods. Labels should be read for this information.

Food preparation. Of all the water-soluble vitamins, ascorbic acid is most easily destroyed. Therefore, if precautions are taken to preserve vitamin C, the retention of other vitamins is also assured in most instances.

1. Ascorbic acid is highly soluble in water. The following rules apply:

   a. Avoid soaking vegetables in large amounts of water.

   b. Cook in the smallest practical amount of water. For most vegetables, fresh or frozen, it is not necessary to cover with water, but to use just enough water to keep from scorching. A cover is necessary when small amounts of water are used.

   c. Whenever practical, use the cooking liquids in sauces for vegetables, or in gravies or soups. They may not contain much ascorbic acid, but they will retain some mineral elements.

2. The oxidation of ascorbic acid increases rapidly as the temperature is increased.

   a. Store fruits and vegetables in a cool place; use promptly.

   b. Use the shortest cooking time—just enough for vegetables to be tender, yet crisp.

3. The oxidation of ascorbic acid increases when fruits and vegetables are cut, since cutting releases the enzymes.

   a. If foods must be cut, do this just before serving or cooking.

4. Ascorbic acid is destroyed in the presence of alkali.

   a. Do not use baking soda to retain green color in vegetables such as spinach, broccoli, or peas.

Clinical problems. Severe body stress increases the need for ascorbic acid, sometimes to very high levels. Among these are burns, fractures, and surgical procedures. Patients with tuberculosis, pneumonia, or rheumatic fever also require greater amounts.

Some drug therapies increase the excretion of vitamin C: sulfonamides, salicylates, indomethacin, and adrenal steroids. Cigarette smoking also increases the excretion of ascorbic acid.

In recent years many people have greatly increased their vitamin-C intake to as much as 1 to 5 gm daily, in the belief that these huge dosages (20 to 100 times the RDA) would prevent or lessen colds. While a normal tissue saturation of vitamin C is helpful in reducing the risk of infection, it has not been clearly shown that these huge (megadose) amounts of vitamin C provide any further benefit. More research is needed to prove or disprove the claims. It should be pointed out that use of such large amounts of vitamin C, or any other vitamin, is not primarily a diet problem, but a use of a vitamin as a drug.

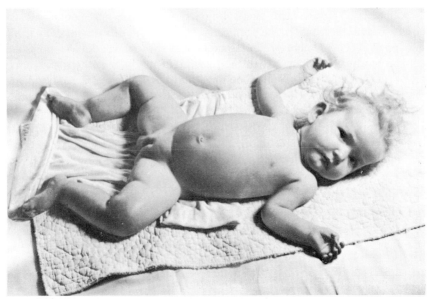

FIGURE 12-2 Infants who have been bottle-fed but who have not received a supplement of vitamin C will have scurvy. They assume this position because of the pain and tenderness of the skin. *(Dr. Bernard S. Epstein and the Upjohn Company, Kalamazoo, Michigan.)*

Severe deficiency of ascorbic acid leads to *scurvy*. This was the disease that figured so importantly in the sea journeys of explorers in the sixteenth century and accounted for the death of so many sailors. Scurvy is characterized by easy bruising and hemorrhaging of the skin, loosening of the teeth, bleeding of the gums, and disruption of the cartilages that support the skeleton.

Scurvy is occasionally seen in infants who have had a cow's milk formula for several months without vitamin C supplements. One of the outstanding symptoms found in the infant is the extreme tenderness of the skin to touch. (See Fig. 12-2.)

THIAMIN

Functions. Thiamin (vitamin B_1) is a coenzyme in many enzyme systems. These are involved principally in the breakdown of glucose to yield energy. Thiamin also aids in the formation of *ribose*, a sugar that is an essential constituent of DNA and RNA, the carriers of the genetic code. The adequate functioning of thiamin maintains healthy nerves, a good mental outlook, a normal appetite, and good digestion.

Meeting daily needs. The thiamin allowance is 0.5 mg per 1000 kcal. Thus, an adult whose calorie allowance is 2000 would need 1.0 mg thiamin daily. For older adults 1.0 mg is allowed even though the calorie intake may be less than 2000.

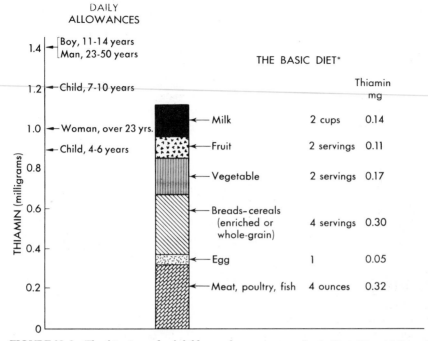

FIGURE 12–3   The thiamin needs of children and women are met by the Basic Diet. Additional foods from any of the Four Food Groups to satisfy the calorie requirement will also fulfill the thiamin need. See Table 4–2 (p. 37) for complete calculation.

Each of the Four Food Groups contributes importantly to the daily thiamin intake. (See Fig. 12–3.) Meats, especially pork and liver, are rich in thiamin and account for about one fourth of the average intake. Dry beans and peas, peanuts, peanut butter, and eggs are good sources.

Enriched and whole-grain breads and cereals supply about one third of the daily thiamin intake. Although individual foods of the fruit-vegetable and milk groups contain lower concentrations of thiamin, the intake of recommended amounts of foods from these groups accounts for about 40 per cent of the daily need.

Clinical problems.   The symptoms of thiamin deficiency occur because the tissue cells are unable to receive sufficient energy from glucose. Therefore, they cannot carry out their normal functions. Early symptoms of thiamin deficiency include fatigue, irritability, depression and moodiness, poor appetite, a tingling and numbness of the legs, and poor tone of the gastrointestinal tract together with constipation. As you know, such symptoms could result from many other causes. At this stage of deficiency a diagnosis pointing to lack of thiamin as the cause would require laboratory tests.

Severe thiamin deficiency in the United States is rare. It occurs occasionally in alcoholics who fail to get an adequate diet over a period of time. Deficiency may also occur when there has been protracted vomiting or diarrhea, or following infections or surgery when dietary intake has been inadequate.

Beriberi, sometimes called "rice-eater's disease" because it is often seen in people whose chief diet is refined rice, is the severest form of thiamin deficiency. It is still seen in some areas of the Orient. The symptoms include polyneuritis (disease of the nerves, especially of the legs and hands), heart disease, and edema. Infants are sometimes seen with beriberi when their mothers have had a grossly inadequate diet so that their milk does not protect the baby.

RIBOFLAVIN

Functions. Riboflavin is a constituent of a group of enzymes called *flavoproteins*. As with thiamin, these enzymes are necessary in the breakdown of glucose to form energy. It is important to remember that the function of riboflavin in the release of energy is different from the function of the thiamin-containing enzymes. In other words, one vitamin cannot replace another; they might be considered as part of a team.

Riboflavin is essential for a healthy skin and for good vision in bright light. If the individual ingests more riboflavin than his body needs, the urinary excretion will increase; if the intake is inadequate, the body maintains its supply very carefully and the urinary excretion will practically stop.

Meeting daily needs. The requirement for riboflavin is related to the calorie and protein intake. The recommended allowance for the reference woman is 1.2 mg and for the reference man is 1.6 mg. The allowances are somewhat higher in proportion to body size for growing children and during pregnancy and lactation.

About half of the intake of riboflavin daily is furnished by milk alone. Cheese is a good source, although some of the vitamin has been lost in the whey. Important but smaller contributions are made by meat, especially organ meats, dark green leafy vegetables, and enriched cereal foods. (See Fig. 12–4.)

Riboflavin is stable to heat, acid, and oxidation. There is less loss in cooking than with thiamin or ascorbic acid. When exposed to light riboflavin is rapidly destroyed; thus, exposing milk in clear-glass bottles to sunlight for a few hours leads to considerable loss.

Clinical problems. Riboflavin deficiency leads to *cheilosis*, a cracking of the skin at the corners of the lips and scaliness of the skin around the ears and nose. There may be redness and burning as well as itching of the eyes, and extreme sensitivity to strong light.

NIACIN

Functions. Niacin is also required for the stepwise breakdown of glucose to yield energy. Thus, if niacin, or thiamin, or riboflavin is missing, the metabo-

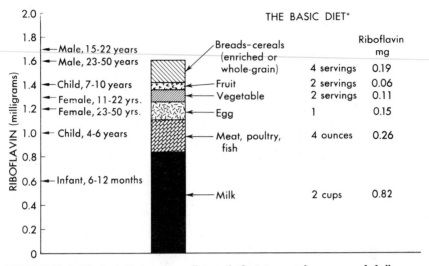

FIGURE 12–4 The basic diet supplies sufficient riboflavin to meet the recommended allowances for all groups except teen-age boys. Note the importance of the milk and meat groups. See Table 4–2 (p. 37) for complete calculation.

lism will fail at the point of the missing enzyme. Niacin is essential for a healthy skin, normal function of the gastrointestinal tract, and maintenance of the nervous system.

Meeting daily needs. The recommended niacin allowance is 6.6 mg per 1000 kcal. This can be supplied by preformed niacin in the diet and by tryptophan, an essential amino acid that is a precursor of niacin. Each 6 gm protein in the diet supplies about 60 mg tryptophan which is equal to 1 mg niacin.

The Basic Diet (see Fig. 12–5) supplies 13 mg niacin from food. In addition, the protein of the diet furnishes 720 mg tryptophan or 12 mg niacin; thus, the diet is equal to 25 mg niacin—about twice the daily need of the reference woman. Excess niacin in the diet is excreted and not stored.

The meat group, especially organ meats and poultry, is the chief source of preformed niacin. Dark green leafy vegetables and whole-grain or enriched breads and cereals are fair sources. Milk contains little preformed niacin. All good sources of complete proteins, including milk, cheese, eggs, meat, poultry, and fish, are good sources of the precursor tryptophan. Niacin is more stable to cooking procedures than thiamin or ascorbic acid.

Clinical problems. Niacin deficiency is not likely to be common in the United States because most people have a liberal protein intake. The protein-rich foods are good sources of preformed niacin, and also of the niacin precursor, tryptophan.

Pellagra, the deficiency disease resulting from lack of niacin, was once preva-

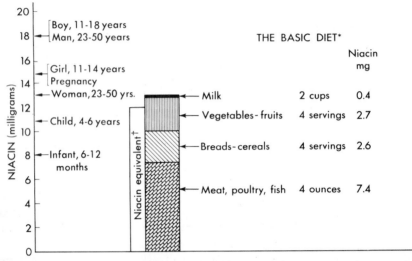

FIGURE 12–5   The niacin available from tryptophan in the Basic Diet is about 12 mg. The preformed niacin from the meat and bread-cereal groups brings the total well above the needs for all age groups. See Table 4–2 (p. 37) for complete calculation.

lent in the United States, especially among people of extreme poverty. Dermatitis, especially of the skin exposed to the sun, soreness of the mouth, swelling of the tongue, diarrhea, and mental changes including depression, confusion, disorientation, and delirium are typical of the advancing stages of the disease, which ends in death if not treated. The disease is sometimes referred to as the "4 D's"—dermatitis, diarrhea, dementia, and death.

VITAMIN B$_6$

Functions.   Three forms of vitamin B$_6$ exist: pyridoxine, pyridoxal, and pyridoxamine. The functions of vitamin B$_6$ are closely related to protein metabolism: the synthesis and breakdown of amino acids; the conversion of tryptophan to niacin; the production of antibodies; the formation of heme in hemoglobin; the formation of hormones important in brain function; and others.

Meeting daily needs.   More vitamin B$_6$ is required when diets are high in protein. The adult allowance is 2.0 mg for women and 2.2 mg for men.

Meat, especially organ meats, whole-grain cereals, soybeans, peanuts, and wheat germ are rich sources. Milk and green vegetables supply smaller amounts.

Clinical problems.   Several drugs interfere with the use of vitamin B$_6$. Isoniazid used for the treatment of tuberculosis binds vitamin B$_6$ so that it cannot be utilized by the body. If the intake of vitamin B$_6$ is not increased, neurologic problems may occur. Penicillamine, a drug used in the treatment of Wilson's disease, and renal dialysis increase the loss of the vitamin in the urine. In these conditions supplements of vitamin B_6 are recommended. Blood levels of vitamin B_6 are lowered in pregnancy and with the use of contraceptives. Although supplements restore the blood levels to a normal range, there has been no clear-cut evidence that there is any change in physiologic state.

Some years ago vitamin B_6 deficiency was diagnosed in infants who had received a formula in which vitamin B_6 had been inadvertently destroyed by high heat. These infants had a reduced growth rate, nervous irritability, anemia, and convulsions; they recovered promptly when adequate vitamin B_6 was provided. Today all commercial infant formulas supply sufficient vitamin B_6 to meet the infant's needs.

VITAMIN B_{12}

Functions. Of all vitamins, vitamin B_{12} is the most complex. The trace mineral cobalt is an essential part of the molecule. Vitamin B_{12} is required for the maturation of the red blood cells in the bone marrow; for the synthesis of proteins; and for the metabolism of nervous tissue.

Absorption and storage. The absorption of vitamin B_{12} is much more complex than that for other B-complex vitamins. The stomach produces a protein-carbohydrate substance called *intrinsic factor*. Vitamin B_{12} is attached to intrinsic factor and is carried to the ileum from which it is absorbed. In the absence of intrinsic factor vitamin B_{12} cannot be absorbed.

The liver stores most of the vitamin B_{12}. On an adequate diet, the storage in the adult may be sufficient to provide the body's needs for as much as 3 to 5 years.

Meeting daily needs. For adults 3 mcg vitamin B_{12} is recommended daily; 0.5 to 1.5 mcg for infants, 2 to 3 mcg for children, and 4 mcg during pregnancy and lactation.

Milk, eggs, cheese, meat, fish, and poultry supply ample amounts of vitamin B_{12} even though the intakes of these animal foods may be relatively low. Plant foods supply no vitamin B_{12} and use of an exclusively vegetarian diet for a long period of time will lead to symptoms of deficiency.

Clinical problems. Pernicious anemia is the disease resulting from vitamin B_{12} deficiency. It is a genetic defect with an absence of intrinsic factor; hence the vitamin B_{12} in the diet cannot be absorbed. Patients with pernicious anemia have a macrocytic type of anemia; that is, the red blood cells are large and reduced in number. There are frequent complaints of sore mouth, poor appetite, and gastrointestinal disturbances. The nervous system is affected so that the individual shows poor coordination in walking, for example; his mental processes may also be affected. Parenteral injections of vitamin B_{12} effectively control the condition; they must be used throughout the life of the patient.

Patients who have been subjected to surgical removal of the stomach also exhibit signs of vitamin B_{12} deficiency after a period of months or years if they are not given parenteral injections of vitamin B_{12}. If children are given an exclusive plant diet, there is slowing of growth; this is the only situation in which dietary deficiency of vitamin B_{12} occurs.

FOLACIN

Functions. Folacin, like other B vitamins, is a component of specific enzymes. These are required for the formation of DNA and heme in the red blood cells, and for the metabolism of specific amino acids. Although both folacin and vitamin B_{12} are needed for the formation of red blood cells, one cannot replace the other.

Meeting daily needs. The recommended allowance of folacin is 400 mcg for adults and 100 to 300 mcg for children.

The word "folacin" is derived from *folium* meaning green leaf. Thus, green, leafy vegetables are a good source. Other good sources include organ meats, meat, poultry, fish, and whole-grain cereals. Folacin is rapidly destroyed in prolonged cooking, with high temperatures as used in food processing, and with prolonged storage periods.

Clinical problems. Folacin deficiency is relatively uncommon. It does occur because of (1) lack in the diet, or (2) failure to absorb folacin in diseases of malabsorption, especially sprue. The principal characteristic of folacin deficiency is a macrocytic anemia. A sore mouth and diarrhea are often present.

During pregnancy a macrocytic anemia because of folacin deficiency is sometimes observed. Apparently the folacin needs of the fetus are high. Elderly persons who have had a diet low in folacin for a long period of time sometimes have a folacin deficiency.

The absorption of folacin is reduced in alcoholism, and with the use of antitubercular drugs and some anticonvulsants. Contraceptives also increase the requirement for folacin. Methotrexate, a powerful antitumor treatment, is also an antagonist to folacin.

OTHER B-COMPLEX VITAMINS

Biotin occurs in extremely minute amounts in the body and in foods. It is required for many enzymes that participate in the metabolism of carbohydrates, fats, and amino acids. It is closely related to folacin and pantothenic acid in its activities.

The adult allowance for biotin is 100 to 200 micrograms. Average diets supply 100 to 300 mcg daily. A protein, *avidin*, found in raw egg white is an antagonist to biotin. The protein combines with biotin in the small intestine and prevents the absorption of the vitamin. However, the amount of egg white that needs to be ingested to bring about this effect is far in excess of the number of eggs that would be eaten in a day. No deficiency of biotin has been observed on typical American diets.

Pantothenic acid. This vitamin is part of a complex enzyme known as *coenzyme A.* This enzyme is an important key to the breakdown of carbohydrates and fats to produce energy. It is also involved in the synthesis of fatty acids, cholesterol, and steroid hormones; in the synthesis of heme in the hemoglobin molecule; and in the formation of acetylcholine, a compound needed for the transmission of nervous impulses.

The adult allowance for pantothenic acid is 4 to 7 mg. The word pantothenic means "from everywhere" and the vitamin is widely distributed in foods. Deficiency of pantothenic acid occurs only when there is severe deficiency of other vitamins. Meat, whole-grain cereals, and legumes are rich in the vitamin; milk, fruits, and vegetables contain moderate amounts.

SOME FALLACIES AND FACTS

1. *Fallacy.* When properly planned, vegetarian diets will supply all nutrients required.
   Fact. If no animal foods whatsoever are eaten, the diet will not supply sufficient vitamin B_{12}. Lacto-ovo-, and lacto-vegetarian diets, on the other hand, will furnish ample amounts of vitamin B_{12}.
2. *Fallacy.* Raw milk is a better source of vitamins than pasteurized milk.
   Facts. During pasteurization some vitamin C is lost, but milk is not a good source of this vitamin—even if raw milk is used. There is practically no loss of other

TABLE 12–1   SUMMARY OF WATER-SOLUBLE VITAMINS

Vitamins	Metabolism and Function	Deficiency	Meeting Body Needs
Ascorbic acid Vitamin C	Form collagen Teeth firm in gums Hormone synthesis Resistance to infection Improve iron absorption	*Scurvy:* Bruising and hemorrhage Bleeding gums Loose teeth	Adults: 60 mg Citrus fruits Strawberries, cantaloupe Tomatoes, broccoli Raw green vegetables
Thiamin Vitamin B_1	Healthy nerves Good digestion Normal appetite Good mental outlook Breakdown of glucose for energy	Fatigue Poor appetite Constipation Mental depression Neuritis of legs *Beriberi:* Polyneuritis Edema Heart failure	0.5 mg per 1000 kcal Pork, liver, other meats, poultry Dry beans and peas, peanut butter Enriched and wholegrain bread Milk, eggs

TABLE 12–1 (*Continued*)

Vitamins	Metabolism and Function	Deficiency	Meeting Body Needs
Riboflavin Vitamin B₂	Enzymes for protein and glucose metabolism Fatty acid synthesis Healthy skin Normal vision in bright light	*Cheilosis:* Cracking lips Scaling skin Burning, itching, sensitive eyes	Men: 1.6 mg Women: 1.2 mg Milk, cheese Meat, poultry, fish Dark green leafy vegetables Enriched and whole-grain breads
Niacin	Enzymes for energy metabolism Normal digestion Healthy nervous system Healthy skin Tryptophan a precursor: 60 mg = 1 mg niacin	*Pellagra:* Dermatitis Sore mouth Diarrhea Mental depression Disorientation Delirium	6.6 mg per 1000 kcal Meat, poultry, fish, Dark green leafy vegetables Whole-grain or enriched breads, cereals Tryptophan in complete proteins
Vitamin B₆ Pyridoxine, pyridoxal, pyridoxamine	Enzymes for protein metabolism Conversion of tryptophan to niacin Formation of heme	Gastrointestinal upsets Weak gait Irritability Nervousness Convulsions	Women: 2.0 mg Men: 2.2 mg Meat, whole-grain cereals, dark-green vegetables, potatoes
Vitamin B₁₂ Cobalamin	Formation of mature red blood cells Synthesis of DNA, RNA Requires intrinsic factor from stomach for absorption	Pernicious anemia: lack of intrinsic factor, or after gastrectomy Macrocytic anemia; neurologic degeneration	Adults: 3 mcg Animal foods only: milk, eggs, meat, poultry, fish
Folacin	Active form is folinic acid Maturation of red blood cells Synthesis of DNA, RNA Not a substitute for vitamin B₁₂	Macrocytic anemia in pregnancy, sprue	Adults: 400 mcg Deep green leafy vegetables, meats, fish, poultry, eggs, whole-grain cereals

vitamins by pasteurization. The most important reason for pasteurization of milk is to destroy pathogenic organisms that might be present.

3. *Fallacy.* Pernicious anemia is caused by lack of vitamin B_{12} in the diet.

Facts. Pernicious anemia is caused by a lack of intrinsic factor, a genetic defect. Because of this defect, even large amounts of the vitamin in the diet cannot be used. These patients require vitamin B_{12} by injection.

4. *Fallacy.* A supplement of vitamin-B complex will provide an individual with additional energy.

Facts. Vitamins do not furnish calories, hence they are not a source of additional energy. B-complex vitamins are needed for the enzymes that bring about breakdown of carbohydrates and fats to furnish energy. A diet that meets the recommended allowances supplies ample amounts to form these enzymes. Supplements will not further improve the use of carbohydrates and fats.

REVIEW QUESTIONS AND PROBLEMS

1. Define each of the following terms: anti-pernicious anemia factor, beriberi, biotin, cheilosis, cyanocobalamin, dermatitis, extrinsic factor, folacin, macrocytic, niacin equivalent, pellagra, pyridoxine, scurvy.

2. Which vitamins are most directly concerned with each of the following: scurvy, wound healing, healthy skin, pellagra, normal red blood cells, breakdown of glucose for energy, intercellular substance for firm skeletal structure, tryptophan, bleeding gums?

3. If your daily intake of ascorbic acid, thiamin, riboflavin, or niacin is greater than your body needs, what happens to the excess?

4. What vitamins are added to flours and cereal foods through the enrichment program? Collect labels of several enriched foods and evaluate them according to your daily need for these vitamins.

5. Suppose a person is allergic to citrus fruits. What foods could you recommend to meet the day's needs for ascorbic acid?

6. Record your own food intake for two days. Which foods in your diet are providing you with riboflavin; niacin; thiamin; ascorbic acid? What changes do you need to make to improve your intake?

7. Normally you do not need to be concerned about the food sources for B-complex vitamins other than thiamin, riboflavin, and niacin. Explain why this is true.

REFERENCES

Erhard, D.: "The New Vegetarians," *Nutr. Today,* 8:4–12, November–December 1973.

"Controversy over Megavitamins," *Am. J. Nurs.,* 77:1614, 1977.

Fawns, H. T.: "Discovery of Vitamin C. James Lind and the Scurvy," *Nurs. Times,* 71:872–75, 1975.

Mayer, J.: "The Battle over Vitamin C," *Family Health,* 9:26–28, April 1977.

Sherlock, P., and Rothschild, E. O.: "Scurvy Produced by a Zen Macrobiotic Diet," *J.A.M.A.,* 199:794–98, 1967.

Vaisrub, S.: "Vitamin Abuse," *J.A.M.A.,* 238:1762, 1977.

PRACTICAL PLANNING FOR
GOOD NUTRITION

13

Meal Planning | BASIC CONSIDERATIONS IN MEAL PLANNING | FOUR FOOD
GROUPS | ADAPTATIONS FOR DIETARY GOALS | MEAL PATTERNS   •   **Nutrition**
for Older Persons | NUTRITIONAL NEEDS | PROBLEMS OF FOOD INTAKE |
DIETARY PLANNING | COMMUNITY PROGRAMS   •   **Pregnancy** | NUTRITION
BEFORE PREGNANCY | DEVELOPMENT DURING PREGNANCY | NUTRITIONAL
ALLOWANCES | DIETARY PLANNING | CLINICAL PROBLEMS   •
Lactation | SOME FALLACIES AND FACTS

MEAL PLANNING FOR ADULTS

The purposes of this unit are to consider the particular emphases on nutritional requirements that must be made in each phase of the life cycle, to study ways by which food habits can be improved, and to learn something about meal planning, food safety, and how to interpret information available to consumers. These are practical aspects of nutrition that will be of equal value to you either in your personal and family life or in your professional career.

Meal Planning

BASIC CONSIDERATIONS IN MEAL PLANNING

A family may sit down, day by day, at the same table and partake of the same choice of food with apparently different results. A six-year-old boy seems to grow slowly, the teenage boy may be a foot taller and 15 lb heavier in a year's time, one parent may gain weight, and the other maintains constant weight. The six-year-old is often finicky about his food, the teenager never seems to get filled up, and the parent whose weight never changes appears to have a hearty appetite. If there are toddlers, preschool children, or grandparents at this table, the homemaker makes particular adaptations for them and yet tries to keep the meal as uniform as possible. Many factors enter into meal planning, some of which are summarized in Table 13–1.

127

TABLE 13-1 BASIC CONSIDERATIONS IN MEAL PLANNING

Factors	Interpretation
Nutritional needs	Include recommended amounts of foods from each of the Four Food Groups.
	Complete the menu for adequate calories from foods that also supply essential nutrients.
	Consider nutritive value of meals away from home so that meal at home makes up for any deficiencies.
Family composition	Make menu adjustments for children of various ages (see Chapter 14), the pregnant woman (see p. 135), the elderly (see p. 133), variations in weight status, or specific health needs.
Food habits	Consider psychologic and cultural meanings of food (see Chapter 15).
Food costs	Plan menus that make use of seasonal foods, advertised specials (see Chapter 17).
Preparation facilities	Working homemakers may have to budget time carefully, as well as money; may need to use more convenience foods.
	Plan menus to make effective use of energy; for example, oven meals.
	Plan for proper storage of foods.
Variety	Within each of the Four Food Groups select as wide a variety of foods as possible.
	Color: use foods that complement each other in color; make judicious use of garnishes; avoid meals of all one color.
	Texture: combine soft with crisp or chewy foods.
	Flavor: combine bland and highly flavored foods; learn to use herbs and spices with a light touch.
	Preparation methods: boiling, stewing, baking, broiling, roasting, frying; with or without sauces.
	Season: heartier foods such as stews or thick soups are more acceptable in winter months; lighter foods in summer, yet retaining same nutritive values.
Satiety	Protein and fat in each meal increase satiety, and reduce hunger between meals. Substantial main courses should be followed with a light dessert such as fruit, rather than a heavy rich pastry.

FOUR FOOD GROUPS

Preceding chapters have emphasized why you need protein, minerals, and vitamins, as well as calories, and have shown how your nutrient needs are substantially met by using the Four Food Groups as a basis for planning. (See Table 4–2, p. 37.) However, when only the specified amounts of the foods from each of these groups are consumed, the caloric intake will range from about 1100 to 1400 kcal—far below the needs of the teenager or adult.

It has often been stated: "First include the specified amounts of each of the Four Food Groups in your diet. Then complete your caloric need by eating any foods you like to maintain your normal weight." This rule may work reasonably well for some people, but it is not necessarily the best advice. It could lead to excessive use of sugars and fats that supply little else than calories. A much better selection to fill the caloric need would include additional amounts of whole-grain or enriched breads, cereals, pastas, legumes, nuts, fruits, and vegetables. These foods supply not only calories, but additional minerals, vitamins, and protein.

The teenage girl and woman must select foods added to the skeleton menu pattern with care because their caloric requirements are lower than those of the man and their iron requirements are much higher. A serving of liver weekly, enriched or whole-grain breads and cereals, frequent use of dried fruits, molasses, and legumes enhance the intake of iron. Nevertheless, the recommended allowance of 18 mg iron is not likely to be met without the use of an iron supplement.

ADAPTATIONS FOR DIETARY GOALS

If the Dietary Goals (see p. 38) are to be incorporated with the Four Food Groups into menu planning, the following changes would need to be made:

Milk group: use skim or low-fat milk. Children may be given whole milk. Use low-fat cheeses. Cheeses made from whole milk may be used occasionally.
Meat group: include not more than 5 oz meat, fish, or poultry daily. Select meats that are lean; trim off visible fat. Use fish and poultry more frequently, and beef, pork, ham, lamb less frequently. Use up to 3 to 4 eggs per week; count one egg as a substitute for 1 oz meat. Legumes and nuts are not restricted; they are a good protein source when combined with grain foods.
Vegetable-fruit group: increase the intake of this group.
Bread-cereal group: substantially increase the intake of this group to meet energy needs and to supply B-complex vitamins and iron.

In addition the goals recommend:

Reduced consumption of sugars, sweets, and foods high in sugar content.
Reduced consumption of fat, especially saturated fat: butter, cream, bacon, lard, hydrogenated fat, visible fat on meats, regular margarines.
Moderate increase in the consumption of polyunsaturated fats: corn, cottonseed, soybean, and safflower oils for cooking, baking, and in salad dressings; soft-type margarines made from these oils.
Reduced intake of salt: omit salting food at the table; reduce the amount of salt added to food in preparation; limited use of very salty foods such as pickles, catsup, meat sauces, pretzels, potato chips, salted fish and meat, and many others.

MEAL PATTERNS

Breakfast. Far too many people skip breakfast, giving such excuses as not being hungry, wishing to lose weight, or not having enough time. Appetite for breakfast is largely a matter of habit; for many people breakfast is the most enjoyable meal of the day. It breaks the night's fast, helps to ensure energy for the morning's work, and reduces irritability. A light breakfast will provide one fourth of the day's calories even if one is reducing. (See Fig. 13–1.) As a matter of fact, people who do not eat breakfast often eat more frequently during the rest of the day, choosing high-calorie snacks, such as pretzels, soft

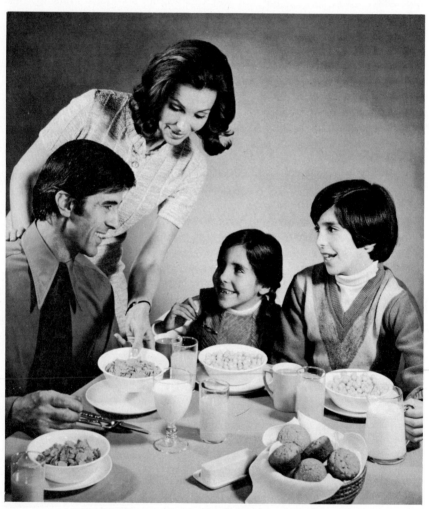

FIGURE 13–1 Schoolchildren and parents start the day right by eating a breakfast that provides one fourth to one third of the recommended allowances. Breakfasts are more enjoyable when the family eats together. *(Cereal Institute, Inc., Chicago.)*

drinks, candy, and so on. Each meal of the day should include some protein food for satiety value and for optimum use of amino acids. Breakfast is a good time to include fruit that is rich in vitamin C, whereas other fruits may be included at lunch and dinner. A good breakfast need take little time to prepare. Two examples of quickly prepared breakfasts are:

Orange juice	Stewed prunes
Wheat flakes with	Soft cooked egg
Skim or low-fat milk	Whole-wheat toast
Toasted English muffin with	Butter or margarine
Soft-type margarine	Coffee, if desired
Coffee, if desired	Milk for children
Milk for children	

Luncheons. The patterns for luncheons vary greatly, depending upon where they are eaten. Children should be encouraged to participate in the school lunch program. Some adults carry a lunch that might include a sandwich, fruit, and a beverage. Variations on this pattern might include a cup of hot soup, some raw vegetables, yogurt, cookies, cake, or pastry. Other adults eat lunch in fast-food restaurants where the choice might consist of a hamburger on bun, French fried potatoes, and a soft drink. Still others might consume a substantial lunch as part of a business conference. The homemaker, far too often, fails to plan a nutritionally satisfactory lunch for herself.

Dinner. The dinner meal customarily includes meat, poultry, fish, or an occasional substitution of a legume dish. White or sweet potato, rice or pasta, plus vegetables, rolls or bread, dessert, and beverage complete the meal. It should be apparent that the dinner include corrections for any deficiencies that may have appeared in the earlier meals. For example, the vegetable should be deep yellow or dark green, leafy at least every other day. If a salad has not appeared at luncheon, one should be included in the evening meal. If the breakfast fruit was not a good source of ascorbic acid, then this might be corrected by such selections as broccoli, or a citrus fruit salad, or cantaloupe for dessert.

Snacks. The coffee break and eating between meals are a well-established custom. Snacks should be planned as part of the daily meals. They should not replace breakfast or lunch. Some people eat snacks to gain weight; others find it easier to lose weight if they have five or six small meals a day rather than three larger meals; still others realize only too late that snacks can be the undoing of effective weight control. Soft drinks, doughnuts, cakes, sweet rolls, pretzels, potato chips, and the like are often a liability, because the additional calories are appreciable although the nutrient contribution is small. More nutritious snacks in increasing order of caloric value are the following:

Raw vegetables—celery and carrot sticks; tomato juice
Fresh fruits and fruit juices

Milk, skim, low-fat, whole
Milk beverages, yogurt
Celery stuffed with peanut butter or cottage cheese
Peanut butter sandwiches
Dried fruits and nuts

Table 13–2 illustrates a day's menu that includes selections from the Four Food Groups together with adaptations for the Dietary Goals.

Nutrition for Older Persons

Aging is a process that covers the entire life-span. The metabolic changes that characterize aging are poorly understood. *Gerontology* is the study of the aging process. *Geriatrics* is the branch of medicine concerned with the prevention and treatment of diseases in older persons.

There is, of course, no specific age that characterizes a person as "old"; some people are "old" at 50 years, and others are "young" at 70 years. About 24 million people in the United States today are over 65 years old. Most of these people are productive, live in their own homes, and enjoy good health. Good nutrition, heredity, and environment play dominant roles in the maintenance of health.

NUTRITIONAL NEEDS

As you well know, it is altogether too common for people to gain weight as they become older. This weight gain is explained in part by a progressively lower basal metabolism after 25 years of age. In addition, older men and women are usually less active than they were in their youth.

The recommended energy allowance at 51 to 75 years for men is 2400 kcal and for women is 1800 kcal. The allowances for thiamin, riboflavin, and niacin are slightly lower to correspond to these lower calorie requirements. The allowances for protein and most minerals and vitamins are the same as for younger adults. (See Table 4–1, p. 32.) Provided that she does not have an anemia, the woman who reaches 51 years can meet her iron needs with a daily intake of 10 mg.

PROBLEMS OF FOOD INTAKE

People over 65 years of age are no more like one another than teenagers are like one another. The nurse is likely to encounter a great variety of problems concerned with adequate nutrition of older persons. She needs to be alert to these problems, and to use ingenuity, patience, and kindness in solving them.

1. Inability to chew is a frequent source of difficulty because of poorly fitting dentures or absence of teeth.

TABLE 13–2 A DAY'S MENU BASED ON THE FOUR FOOD GROUPS

	Suggested Modifications to Meet Dietary Goals
Breakfast	
Honeydew melon	
Shredded wheat	
Milk and sugar	Skim or low-fat milk; no sugar
Scrambled eggs—2	Limit eggs to 3 to 4 per week
Whole-wheat toast	
Butter	Soft-type margarine
Coffee with cream, sugar	Milk in coffee; no sugar
Milk for children	Whole milk for children
Luncheon	
Split pea soup	
Sandwich	
Whole-wheat bread—2 slices	
Cheese—1 ounce	Tuna fish, salmon, or chicken—2 ounces
Ham—1 ounce	
Lettuce	
Mayonnaise	
Apple	
Milk	Skim or low-fat milk
Dinner	
Meat loaf—5 ounces	Prepare with lean ground beef; use 2–3 ounce portion
Baked potato with	
Butter, sour cream	Soft-type margarine; no cream
Parslied carrots	Season carrots with soft-type margarine or corn, soy, cottonseed, or safflower oil
Dinner roll	
Butter	Soft-type margarine
Tossed green salad	
Blue cheese dressing	Oil-vinegar dressing with any of above oils
Cherry pie	Make pie crust with any of above oils; use less sugar in filling
Milk	Skim or low-fat milk
Snack	
Chocolate chip cookies	Dry roasted peanuts or raisins
Orange juice	Orange juice

2. Appetite usually declines in later years because the senses of smell and taste are less acute, the secretion of saliva and gastric juices may be reduced, and the satisfactions of sociability with family and friends may be lacking. Chronic disease and medications often interfere with the appetite.

3. Complaints of heartburn, belching, indigestion, and flatulence are frequent. Specific foods, especially fruits, vegetables, and spicy foods, are often blamed for these effects, but no firm rules can be given that apply to all persons. Thus, one individual experiences discomfort every time he eats onions, and another enjoys onions and tolerates them well. Concern for the individual would omit onion for the former and include them for the latter.

4. Constipation is a common problem of the older individual and is related to the reduction of muscle tone of the gastrointestinal tract and to lessened activity. It is aggravated by eating too many soft, low-fiber foods and failing to drink sufficient fluid.

5. Chronic diseases of the heart, kidney, circulatory system, gastrointestinal tract, and joints impose needs for modified diets (see Unit IV) or interfere with tolerance for foods and ability to manage one's own diet.

6. A lifetime of poor dietary habits contributes to signs of nutritional deficiency including fatigue, anemia, fragility of bones, poor wound healing, and reduced resistance to infection.

7. Living alone, physical handicaps, inability to shop, poor cooking facilities, low income, frustration, boredom, and fear of the future all reduce the desire to eat or the capacity to prepare adequate meals.

8. Faddism and misinformation are responsible for much poor nutrition. Older people are especially likely to fall prey to the food quack who makes promises of good health, vigor, and even cure of disease.

DIETARY PLANNING

The lifetime pattern of eating is not easily changed, and the older woman who has always liked rich desserts or the man accustomed to eating hearty rich foods will find it difficult to adjust to the lower calorie requirements. The Four Food Groups still furnish the basis for meal planning because they provide all the nutrients needed by the older man and woman. (See Table 13–2). Since the Basic Diet provides 1165 kcal (see Table 4–2, p. 37), the woman of 51 years or older will need to restrict her intake of calorie-rich foods lest she rapidly gain weight. Some useful points to keep in mind when planning meals for older persons are noted below.

1. Consider the food likes and dislikes of the individual. Learn to use essential foods in dishes acceptable to the person. For example, milk may be disliked as a beverage but well accepted in puddings, custards, cream soups, and cream sauces, on cereals, and so on.

2. Use fried foods, rich desserts, highly seasoned foods, and strongly flavored vegetables with discretion and according to the patient's tolerance.

3. If chewing is difficult, adjust the meals to include finely minced or chopped meats, soft breads, fruits, and vegetables.

4. Serve four or five small meals when the appetite is poor.

5. Breakfast is the meal most enjoyed by many older persons, and every effort should be made to provide pleasing variety.

6. Dinner at noon rather than in the evening is preferred by some.

7. If coffee and tea produce insomnia, they should be restricted to meals early in the day.

8. Encourage a liberal fluid intake daily. Adjust the fiber content of the diet if constipation is a problem.

COMMUNITY PROGRAMS

The Older Americans Act includes funding for a nutrition program that provides one meal a day for at least five days a week for elderly persons who can come to a center for senior citizens. Each meal is planned to furnish at least one third of the recommended allowances. Provision for modified diets can usually be made in these centers. Nutrition education, periodic health checks, and recreational activities are important components of this program.

Two programs provide meals for persons who are home bound. One of these is federally funded and originates in the centers for older Americans. At least one hot meal is delivered five days a week. In some circumstances arrangements are made for two daily meals, including weekends. "Meals on Wheels" is a program that provides a hot noon meal and a cold evening meal. The program is sponsored by community agencies, for example churches or hospitals. The recipient pays for the meals on a sliding fee scale according to ability to pay.

Pregnancy

The orderly sequence of fetal development and growth, the mechanisms for nourishment of the fetus, the storage of nutrients in anticipation of labor and delivery, and the development of the mammary glands represent a level of anabolism unequaled in any other time of life. All these needs can be met only through a diet planned to meet these increased requirements.

NUTRITION BEFORE PREGNANCY

The young woman who is in good health prior to conception and who maintains good nutrition has the best chance of a pregnancy without complications, a healthy baby, and the ability to nurse. During early pregnancy, often before the woman is even aware that she is pregnant, critical development of the fetus takes place.

Two of every five first babies are born to young women under 20 years of age. These young women must still meet the growth needs of their own maturing bodies as well as the nutritional demands of the fetus. Yet, girls in their teens have, far too often, had diets that were inadequate in calcium, iron, and protein. Pregnant girls under 17 years are in an especially high risk category. They have more frequent complications of toxemia, anemia, and long difficult labor. Babies born to them are more often of low birth weight and have a higher rate of neonatal mortality. Repeated pregnancies before age 20 place both the young woman and the unborn child in an extremely high-risk category. Black women are more vulnerable than white women, probably because of their reduced income and consequently poor diets.

DEVELOPMENT DURING PREGNANCY

During the first two weeks after conception the embryo is fixed in its position in the uterus. The placenta, which is the organ that transfers nutrients from the maternal circulation to the fetus, is well developed early in pregnancy. During the second to eighth weeks there is a rapid development of the skeleton and the organs so that the tiny fetus is a clearly distinguishable human being. By the twelfth week the fetus still weighs only about 30 gm.

The total weight gain during pregnancy should average about 11 kg (24 lb). The weight gain throughout pregnancy should be gradual and steady. During the first trimester a total gain of 0.65 to 1.4 kg (1.4 to 3.0 lb) is normal; for the second and third trimesters a weekly gain of 350 gm (0.8 lb) should be expected. (See Fig. 13–2.)

The weight gain is accounted for in part as follows: fetus, 3300 gm (7½ lb); uterus, 900 gm (2 lb); placenta and membranes, 1450 gm (3 lb); breast tissue, 900 gm; increase in blood volume, 1500 gm. In addition there are considerable stores of protein, fat, calcium, and phosphorus in preparation for delivery and lactation.

NUTRITIONAL ALLOWANCES

The recommended allowances for some of the nutrients for girls and women prior to and during pregnancy and lactation are shown in Table 13–3. (See also Table 4–1, p. 32 for other nutrients required.) If one compares these allowances with the value of the basic diet (Table 4–2, p. 37), it is apparent that calcium, iron, and vitamin D are nutrients that require particular emphasis.

DIETARY PLANNING

The addition of 1½ cups milk to the basic diet pattern meets additional calcium required by the woman, and supplies vitamin A and B-complex vitamins.

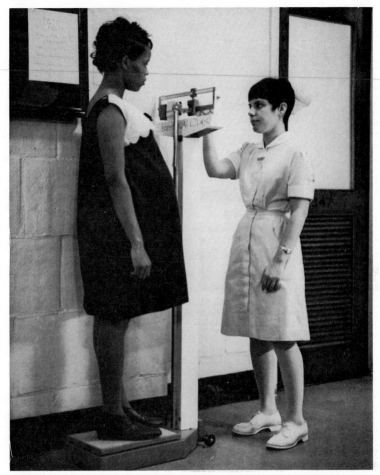

FIGURE 13-2 A steady rate of weight gain should be maintained throughout pregnancy. A total gain of 10 to 12 kg (22 to 26 lb) is normal. *(School of Nursing, Thomas Jefferson University, Philadelphia.)*

The teenage girl needs to consume 5 to 5½ cups milk daily to meet her calcium requirements.

If plain milk is disliked, it may be flavored with chocolate, coffee, molasses, or fruit purées such as strawberry or apricot. Milk may also be used on cereals and in soups and puddings. One ounce of American or Swiss cheese supplies about the same amount of protein and calcium as one cup of milk. Skim milk fortified with vitamins A and D may be substituted for part or all of the whole milk.

The iron allowance cannot be met from foods alone. Ferrous salts to provide 30 to 60 mg iron are usually prescribed by the physician. A supplement of 200 to 400 mcg of folacin is also recommended. Ordinarily it is not necessary

TABLE 13-3 RECOMMENDED DIETARY ALLOWANCES FOR GIRLS AND WOMEN BEFORE AND DURING PREGNANCY AND LACTATION

Nutrient	Girl 15–18 Years	Woman 19 Years and Over	Pregnancy	Lactation
Energy, kcal	2100	2100–2000*	+300	+500
Protein, gm	46	44	+ 30	+ 20
Vitamin A, R.E.	800	800	+200	+400
Vitamin D, mcg	10	5	+ 5	+ 5
Ascorbic acid, mg	60	60	+ 20	+ 40
Thiamin, mg	1.1	1.1–1.0*	+ 0.4	+ 0.5
Riboflavin, mg	1.3	1.3–1.2*	+ 0.3	+ 0.5
Niacin, mg	14	14–13*	+ 2	+ 5
Folacin, mcg	400	400	+400	+100
Vitamin B_{12}, mcg	3.0	3.0	+ 1.0	+ 1.0
Calcium, mg	1200	800	+400	+400
Iron, mg	18	18	Supplemental iron	
Iodine, mcg	150	150	+ 25	+ 50

* The second figure in the range applies to women 23 years and over.
Food and Nutrition Board, National Academy of Sciences, 1979.

to use other mineral or vitamin supplements, providing that the milk used is fortified with vitamin D. Iodized salt should be used instead of plain salt.

CLINICAL PROBLEMS

Mild nausea. Early morning nausea during the first trimester can usually be overcome by eating some high-carbohydrate food, such as dry toast, crackers, or hard candy before arising. Fatty and fried foods should be restricted. Several small meals a day, rather than three large meals, may be more desirable. Fluids should be taken between meals and not at meal time.

Food cravings. Women often experience cravings for certain foods during pregnancy. When these foods are a part of a nutritious diet or don't displace essential foods, these cravings can be satisfied. *Pica*, or craving for abnormal substances such as laundry starch, clay, chalk, or coal, is found among some women, especially in low-income groups. Consuming large amounts of these substances seriously interferes with the intake of nutritious foods, and should be corrected by education and by assuring the means to obtain an adequate diet.

Anemia. Iron-deficiency anemia during pregnancy increases the likelihood of premature birth. The baby at birth is less well supplied with hemoglobin and thus is likely to become anemic during the first year of life. Macrocytic anemia caused by insufficient folacin sometimes occurs in pregnancy. These anemias are prevented or treated by supplements of iron and folacin, respectively.

Constipation is rather common during the latter part of pregnancy. It can usually be avoided by placing more emphasis upon raw fruits and vegetables, some whole-grain breads and cereals, a liberal intake of liquids, and a regular program of exercise.

Toxemia of pregnancy. This condition is characterized by increased blood pressure, swelling of the hands, face, and ankles, and proteinuria. A sudden gain in weight after the twentieth week of pregnancy indicates water retention. The causes of toxemia are little understood, but lack of prenatal care and poverty are associated with the condition. Restriction of calories, protein, and/or sodium have often been tried in the past. These dietary restrictions are no longer considered to be useful, and are potentially dangerous.

Lactation

The lactating woman will produce 550 to 850 ml (20 to 30 oz) of milk each day, representing 20 to 30 gm protein and 400 to 600 kcal. In order to produce this milk, her nutritive allowances are increased as shown in Table 13–3. The calorie needs are best met by choosing more foods from the four food groups. She should continue to consume the amounts of milk recommended for pregnancy.

SOME FALLACIES AND FACTS

1. *Fallacy.* People over 50 years of age have much lower needs for protein, minerals, and vitamins than do younger adults.

Fact. The requirements for most nutrients are the same for adults of any age. Older people need fewer calories and so they must select foods with care to ensure adequate intake of protein, minerals, and vitamins.

2. *Fallacy.* Milk and cheese are constipating, and therefore should be omitted by some older persons.

Fact. Milk and cheese are almost completely digested and leave little bulk. Constipation is corrected by including sufficient amounts of raw fruits and vegetables, whole-grain breads and cereals, and liquids, and not by the omission of milk and cheese.

3. *Fallacy.* As long as the mother receives plenty of vitamins the fetus will receive all of its nutritional needs regardless of the mother's nutritional status.

Fact. Vitamin supplements cannot make up for inadequate intakes of protein, calcium, iron, and other minerals. If the mother is poorly nourished, both mother and baby will be adversely affected.

4. *Fallacy.* The obese pregnant woman should use a low calorie diet so that the baby will be small and delivery will be less difficult.

Fact. Calorie restriction and weight loss are not recommended during pregnancy. Small babies are at greater risk during the early months of life. Weight loss should be planned after the birth of the baby.

5. *Fallacy.* Pregnant women should restrict their salt intake.

Fact. Pregnant women probably have higher requirements for sodium, and salt restriction can be dangerous. The pregnant woman should be allowed to salt her food to taste.

REVIEW QUESTIONS AND PROBLEMS

1. Write a menu for one day that is satisfactory for a healthy young man or woman. How would you change this menu for a 25-year-old pregnant woman? What further changes are necessary for the teenage mother-to-be?

2. Why is good nutrition so important prior to pregnancy?

3. Compare the nutritional needs of a woman of 25 years and of 65 years. How would you adapt the menu you wrote (question 1) for the older woman.

4. As a nurse, what problems might you find in feeding the elderly patient? What measures can you take to meet them?

5. Why is anemia such a serious problem in pregnancy?

6. Describe the normal pattern of weight gain during pregnancy. Why is a low-calorie diet undesirable?

7. What is meant by pica?

8. List five ways to increase milk intake by a person who does not like to drink milk.

REFERENCES

Bozian, M.: "Nutrition for the Aged or Aging," *Nurs. Clin. N. Am.*, 11:169–77, 1976.
Breeling, J. L.: "Are We Snacking Our Way to Malnutrition," *Today's Health*, 48:48, January 1970.
Combs, K. L.: "Preventive Care in the Elderly," *Am. J. Nurs.*, 78:1339–41, 1978.
Elwood, T. W.: "Nutritional Concerns of the Elderly," *J. Nutr. Educ.*, 7:50–52, 1975.
Family Fare: A Guide to Good Nutrition, G 1. Washington, D.C.: U.S. Department of Agriculture.
Goldberg, J.: "The Fast Food Phenomenon," *Family Health*, 7:38, April 1975.
Jacobsen, H. N.: "Nutrition and Pregnancy," *J. Am. Dietet. A.*, 60:26–29, 1972.
Markesbery, B. A., and Wong, W. M.: "Points for Maternity Patients," *Am. J. Nurs.*, 77:1612–14, 1977.
Oakes, G., *et al.:* "Diet in Pregnancy: Meddling with the Normal or Preventing Toxemia?" *Am. J. Nurs.*, 75:1134–36, 1975.
Pinel, C.: "Metabolic Bone Disease in the Elderly," *Nurs. Times*, 72:1046–48, 1976.
Walker, M. A., and Hill, M. M.: *Food Guide for Older Folks*, HG 17, Washington, D.C.: U.S. Department of Agriculture.
Weigley, E. S.: "The Pregnant Adolescent," *J. Am. Dietet. A.*, 66:588–92, 1975.

14

Infant Feeding | GROWTH AND DEVELOPMENT | BREAST FEEDING | BOTTLE FEEDING | SUPPLEMENTARY FEEDINGS | FOOD HABITS • **Preschool and School Children** | NUTRITIONAL NEEDS | FOOD SELECTION AND HABITS | CHILD NUTRITION PROGRAMS • **Preadolescent and Adolescent Youth** | NUTRITIONAL NEEDS | FOOD SELECTION AND HABITS

NUTRITION FOR GROWTH AND DEVELOPMENT

Infant Feeding

GROWTH AND DEVELOPMENT

Infants vary widely in their growth patterns, and it is not wise to compare one infant with another; yet, there is some value in being familiar with typical patterns of development and growth. On the average, infants gain 140 to 225 gm (5 to 8 oz) per week during the first five months, and double their birth weight in this time. For the remainder of the year the weight increase is about 110 to 140 gm (4 to 5 oz) per week; the birth weight is tripled by the age of 10 to 12 months. The initial height of 50 to 55 cm (20 to 22 in.) has increased to 75 cm (30 in.) or more by the end of the first year.

The body content of water at birth is high and that of fat is low. The relative lack of subcutaneous fat and the proportionately high surface area explain why additional precautions must be taken to keep infants warm. The bones are comparatively soft in the newborn baby, but they continue to add mineral substance throughout childhood and adolescence. Teeth begin to erupt at five to six months. By the end of the year the infant will have five to ten teeth.

The baby is born with a large head and short arms and legs. In the first years of life the nervous system continues to develop rapidly so that the brain will have reached 90 per cent of adult size at the age of four years. Severe malnutrition during pregnancy and the first months of life leads to inadequate development of the central nervous system, and the poorly nourished infant and child may never reach his full mental potential.

The newborn infant's stomach has a capacity of about 30 ml, and at one year can hold about 240 ml. The ability to digest protein, simple sugars, and emulsified fats is present at birth in the full-term infant. During the early months of life the production of amylase and lipase increases so that starchy foods and fats may be gradually included.

The kidneys achieve their full functional capacity by the end of the first year. Young infants are unable to excrete high concentrations of waste that might occur if undiluted cow's milk were fed or if the intake of fluid is inadequate.

Normal infants have a hemoglobin level of 17 to 20 gm per 100 ml. This high level protects against anemia until the iron intake is adequate from the diet.

BREAST FEEDING

Most women can nurse their babies if they desire to do so, and if they eat the foods necessary to build up the stores of nutrients for milk production. Breast feeding can convey a sense of satisfaction to the mother, and a safe, protected feeling to the infant. Human milk provides the benefits of easy digestion and desirable rates of growth and development. Women who are unable to breast feed their infants or who must return to employment should never be made to feel guilty if they must choose bottle feeding.

About 15 to 45 ml of a thick, yellowish fluid called *colostrum* is produced during the first few days after delivery. Although this small amount of milk does not provide much nutrient intake, it provides the infant greater protection against infection. Placing the infant at the breast early also helps to stimulate the milk flow.

Self-demand feeding permits the baby to nurse when he is hungry, rather than according to an arbitrary time schedule. The mother soon learns to recognize when the baby is hungry and not crying for relief of some other discomfort. Infants nurse as often as every two hours during the first few weeks, but soon regulate to an approximate three- or four-hour schedule. About the second month the baby begins to sleep through the 2 or 3 A.M. feeding. By five months he usually does not awaken for a feeding at 10 to 11 P.M.

Breast-fed babies should be weaned about the fifth month or later. A bottle or cup feeding is substitued at a convenient feeding time. When the baby has become accustomed to this—after about a week or two—a second bottle or cup is offered. As much as two to three months are needed for full weaning. Breast-fed babies, like bottle-fed babies, require the addition of foods from time to time as discussed later in this chapter.

BOTTLE FEEDING

Nutritional needs. The calorie, protein, mineral, and vitamin needs of the infant are very high in proportion to his body size. See Recommended

TABLE 14–1 COMPOSITION OF HUMAN AND WHOLE COW'S MILK
(PER 100 GM OF MILK)

Nutrient	Human Milk	Whole Cow's Milk	Nutrient	Human Milk	Whole Cow's Milk
Water	87.5	87.69	Ascorbic acid, mg	5.00	1.47
Energy, kcal	70	64	Thiamin, mg	0.014	0.038
Protein, gm	1.03	3.28	Riboflavin, mg	0.036	0.161
Fat, gm	4.38	3.66	Niacin, mg	0.177	0.084
Carbohydrate, gm	6.89	4.65	Pantothenic acid, mg	0.223	0.313
Calcium, mg	32	119	Vitamin B_6, mg	0.011	0.042
Iron, mg	0.03	0.05	Folacin, mcg	5	5
Magnesium, mg	3	13	Vitamin B_{12}, mcg	0.045	0.356
Phosphorus, mg	14	93	Vitamin A, R.E.	64	34
Potassium, mg	51	151	I.U.	241	138
Sodium, mg	17	49			
Zinc, mg	0.17	0.38			

Composition of Foods: Dairy and Egg Products—Raw, Processed, Prepared. Agriculture Handbook No. 8–1, Agriculture Research Service, U.S. Department of Agriculture, 1976.

Dietary Allowances, Table 4–1. The infant under 6 months requires 115 kcal per kg (50 to 55 kcal per lb) and for the remainder of the first year 105 kcal per kg (48 kcal per lb). At these caloric levels the relatively high protein and calcium needs are met by the formula.

To take care of the rapid rate of growth and the expanding blood circulation the infant's iron allowance is 10 mg up to 6 months of age, and 15 mg for the second half of the first year. Particular attention is also called to the need for 35 mg ascorbic acid since this is not always supplied by the formula.

Human and cow's milk compared. Table 14–1 indicates that there are many important differences in the composition of human and cow's milk. Cow's milk contains almost three times as much protein, more than three times as much calcium, and over six times as much phosphorus. Most of the protein in cow's milk is casein, while that in human milk is, for the most part, lactalbumin. Cow's milk furnishes slightly less fat and lactose. Ounce for ounce, both milks supply about 20 kcal.

Proprietary premodified milk formulas comprise about 90 per cent of all formulas used in infant feeding. These formulas have been developed to resemble the composition of human milk. Cow's milk is the usual base for these formulas, but it has been modified in some or all of the following ways: to lower the protein and calcium concentration; to increase the lactose content; to substitute vegetable oil for butterfat, thus furnishing a higher intake of linoleic acid and minimizing the spitting up associated with the butyric acid of butterfat; to adjust the mineral and vitamin levels to meet recommended allowances; and to heat denature the protein so that a soft, flocculent curd results.

Premodified formulas are available (1) as single strength, ready to feed, in quart cans or in 4 oz or 8 oz disposable nursing bottles, (2) as concentrated liquid which is measured into sterilized bottles and diluted with boiled water, and (3) as powdered formula, now seldom used.

Special formulas are also available for therapeutic purposes. For infants who are allergic to milk, nutritionally adequate formulas of soybean or meat base are substitued. Enzyme deficiency such as galactosemia or lactose intolerance requires meat base or amino acid formulas. A low-phenylalanine formula (Lofenalac *) is used for phenylketonuria, an inborn error of metabolism.

Home-prepared formulas are made with fresh whole milk or evaporated milk. To make such formulas comparable to human milk, these changes are required: (1) the milk is diluted with water; (2) cane sugar, corn syrup, or dextrimaltose is added to increase the carbohydrate level; and (3) the formulas are heated to reduce the size of the protein curd and to assure safety from bacterial contamination. Each formula must be calculated to meet the individual infant's needs. Although these formulas may be slightly less expensive than proprietary formulas, their preparation entails precautions in sanitation that may not be adequately observed by mothers who lack education.

SUPPLEMENTARY FEEDINGS

Neither human nor cow's milk will meet the full nutritive needs of the infant during the first year of life. Several factors require consideration when planning for supplementary feedings. (See Fig. 14–1.)

Iron-deficiency anemia is perhaps the most common nutritional problem in the first year of life. Although supplementary foods furnish some iron the amount is usually not enough to meet the needs of the rapidly growing infant. Therefore, many pediatricians recommend that iron-fortified formulas be continued when the infant substitues cup feedings for the bottle. Commercial infant cereals fortified with iron are preferable to family-type cereals that are not as highly enriched.

Salt. Babies, like adults, require some sodium and they respond to the taste of salt. During the early months the formula supplies most of the sodium intake. Thereafter, supplementary foods provide increasing amounts of sodium, often far in excess of needs. Nutritionists have criticized the excessive use of salt for two reasons: (1) the infant becomes accustomed to ingesting higher levels that are continued throughout life, a practice that may have some influence on the incidence of hypertension; (2) the intake of excessive salt increases the excretory load on the kidneys. The sodium level of most proprietary infant foods now comes within the levels recommended by a committee of pediatricians and nutritionists.

* Mead Johnson & Company, Evansville, Indiana.

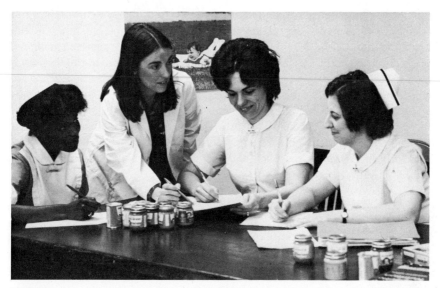

FIGURE 14–1   Nutritionist, student, and staff discuss uses of supplemental foods for infant feeding. *(Handicapped Children's Unit, St. Christopher's Hospital for Children, Philadelphia.)*

Overnutrition is a relatively common problem during the first year, and sometimes sets the pattern for later obesity. It can be prevented by allowing the infant to take what he wants from his bottle feeding rather than urging him to finish it, and by using some moderation in the amounts of supplementary feedings that are given.

Many pediatricians believe that the early introduction of supplementary feedings contributes to overfeeding and excessive weight gain.

Skim-milk formulas should not be used during the first year to reduce the caloric intake. To meet the normal requirements for growth such formulas supply excessively high ratios of protein and carbohydrate. The high protein intake increases the load upon the kidneys for the excretion of nitrogenous products, and a high intake of lactose could contribute to diarrhea.

Baby foods.   Most pediatricians recommend that semi-solid and solid foods be introduced at 3 to 4 months rather than at 6 weeks to 2 months as had been common practice in recent years. This delay results in fewer instances of excessive weight gain.

Many mothers derive much satisfaction from the preparation of foods for the infant. To do this successfully they must have an understanding of the methods for retention of nutritive values and for maintenance of sanitary controls. Also needed is the appropriate equipment for puréeing foods.

Commercially prepared baby foods are generally higher in cost than those prepared at home. For many mothers they possess these advantages; convenience;

safety from bacteriologic contamination; variety; and uniform consistency and composition. The methods of manufacture currently employed result in the high retention of nutritive values, often higher than that achieved in home preparation. Nonetheless, the mother should be aware of the contribution each food makes to the baby's needs. For example, a high-meat dinner will provide considerably less protein than the strained meat.

Sequence of feeding. Practices vary widely on the sequence with which foods are added and on the age of introducing these foods. Some babies need supplements earlier than others; some are ready for changes in texture sooner than others. A typical sequence and suggested daily schedule are shown in Tables 14–2 and 14–3.

TABLE 14–2 SEQUENCE FOR FOOD ADDITIONS TO INFANT'S DIET

Age	Food Addition and Its Nutritive Contribution
2–4 weeks	Vitamins A and D, and ascorbic acid if not supplied in the formula
1 month	Orange juice gradually introduced; start with 1 teaspoon diluted with boiled water. Watch for any signs of allergy. Increase gradually to 3 ounces full strength
3–4 months	Cereal for iron, thiamin, calories; mix precooked cereal with formula; give thin consistency at first; increase to 2 to 5 tablespoons by 7 to 8 months
4–5 months	Mashed ripe banana, applesauce, strained pears, apricots, prunes, or peaches; start with 1 teaspoon and increase to 3–4 tablespoons by one year
4–5 months	Strained asparagus, green beans, carrots, peas, spinach, squash, or tomatoes; start with 1 teaspoon, increasing to 3–4 tablespoons by end of the year
5–6 months	Egg yolk for vitamin A, thiamin, protein; mash hard-cooked egg with a little formula; use ¼ teaspoon at first; avoid egg white since it often gives allergic reaction
5–7 months	Strained meats for protein, iron, B complex
5–8 months	Crisp toast, zwieback, arrowroot cookies, teething biscuits
7–8 months	Baked or mashed potato or enriched pasta for calories and some additional iron and B complex; small amounts
9 months	Peeled raw apple
8–10 months	Chopped vegetables and fruits
10 months	Whole egg; plain puddings, such as custard, Junket

TABLE 14–3 TYPICAL SCHEDULES FOR FIVE-MONTH AND YEAR-OLD INFANTS

Five-Month Infant	Year-Old Infant
6 A.M. Formula, 6–7 oz	6:00 A.M. Orange juice, 3 oz Zwieback
8 A.M. Orange juice, 3 oz	7:30 A.M. Cereal, 2–5 tablespoons Milk, 8 oz * Chopped fruit, 1–2 tablespoons
10 A.M. Formula, 6–7 oz Cereal, 2–3 tablespoons	11:30 A.M. Chopped meat, ½–1 oz or
2 P.M. Formula, 6–7 oz Egg yolk, ½–1 Vegetable, ¼ to 2 table- spoons	Egg, 1 Potato, 2–4 tablespoons Chopped vegetable, 2–4 table- spoons Milk, 8 oz *
6 P.M. Formula, 6–7 oz Cereal, 2–3 tablespoons	5:30 P.M. Cereal or potato, 2–5 table- spoons Milk, 8 oz *
10 P.M. Formula, 6–7 oz	Chopped fruit, 1–2 tablespoons Toast or zwieback

* Iron-fortified formula is recommended throughout the first year.

FOOD HABITS

Good food habits in infancy and childhood will lead in later life to a liking for a wide variety of foods and the willingness to accept change. Parents have a wonderful opportunity as well as a tremendous responsibility for the development of good food habits in the young infant.

1. Hold the young baby while he receives his formula to provide the feelings of satisfaction, security, and warmth. (See Fig. 14–2.)

2. Regulate the feeding schedule to the baby, not to the clock.

3. Introduce only one new food at a time.

4. Give new foods at the beginning of the meal when the baby is hungry.

5. Serve only small portions of a new food; a taste is enough.

6. Don't show your dislike of a food by the expression on your face or by refusing to eat the food yourself.

7. Babies, like adults, are more hungry at some times than others. Don't expect them to finish every bottle or everything at every meal.

8. Expect that the baby will feel his food and be messy. Don't scold him for spilling accidents. (See Fig. 14–3.)

9. Use a cup that does not tip easily, a deep bowl with rounded edges, and a spoon that can be managed by the baby. Provide safe and comfortable seating.

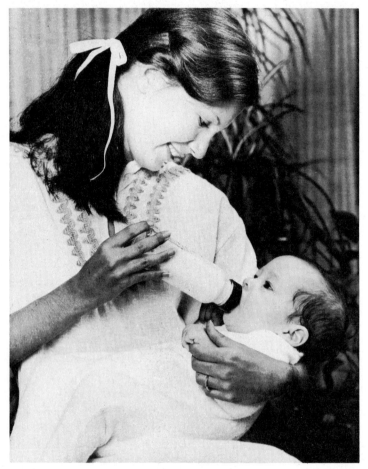

FIGURE 14–2 The infant feels secure when comfortably held by his mother during feeding. *(Ross Laboratories, Columbus, Ohio.)*

Preschool and School Children

NUTRITIONAL NEEDS

Any table of allowances must be interpreted according to the growth pattern of the individual child, the activity, the appetite, and the amount of musculature or body fatness. The growth patterns of children vary widely. Some children, by heredity, are destined to be short and stocky; others, tall and thin. Some children will have their rapid growth spurts at an earlier age than others. If a child does not have a satisfactory nutrient intake he will not reach the full

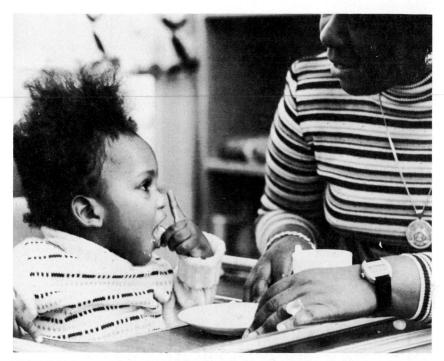

FIGURE 14–3 A toddler enjoys feeding himself. Touching food is important at this stage. *(Handicapped Children's Unit, St. Christopher's Hospital for Children, Philadelphia.)*

growth of his hereditary pattern. The amount of physical activity varies widely and influences the calorie requirements.

During the second year the baby gains 3.5 to 4.5 kg (8 to 10 lb). Following the second birthday and to the ninth year, the increase in height and weight is at a much slower rate; the annual gain in weight is about 2 to 3 kg (4 to 7 lb). The muscles increase in size, the baby fat is lost, the legs become longer, and the bones become harder. There is a great development in motor coordination, in changing body proportions, and in mental development.

The daily allowances for children of one to ten years are relatively high for all nutrients, when the size of the child is taken into account. See Table 4–1 for a complete list of recommended allowances. Seven- to ten-year-old children have calorie needs higher than those of their mothers. Because of the possibility of anemia, additional iron is recommended in the preschool years.

FOOD SELECTION AND HABITS

The Four Food Groups provide the basis for planning the diet for young children. The following list indicates the range in the amounts that are ordinarily eaten.

2 to 3 cups	vitamin D milk
3 to 4 per week	eggs
1 to 4 tablespoons	chopped meat, poultry, fish; some cottage cheese or peanut butter may be substituted
⅓ to ⅔ cup	citrus fruit juice; or whole orange; or twice as much tomato juice
¼ to ½ cup	fruits such as applesauce, peeled apple, apricots, banana, pears, peaches, prunes, etc.
¼ to ½ cup	cooked vegetable; select dark green leafy or deep yellow vegetable at least every other day
1 serving	raw vegetables: carrots, cabbage, tomatoes, lettuce, rutabagas
2 to 4 tablespoons	white or sweet potatoes
⅓ to ⅔ cup	enriched or whole-grain cereal
1 to 3 slices	enriched or whole-grain bread

Few foods need to be omitted entirely from the diet of children, but some discretion in food selection is necessary. The appetite is ordinarily a good guide, but parents have a responsibility to provide a choice of foods within the framework of the Four Food Groups. When the child is permitted to eat freely from sweets and other empty-calorie foods, he will not obtain sufficient nutrients.

Young children prefer plain, blandly flavored foods that are only lightly seasoned. Mixtures, as in casseroles, are well accepted only as the child becomes older. Some foods that require chewing are essential, but meats that are not chopped or ground may be tough for the preschool child. Lukewarm, rather than hot, foods are preferred. Vegetables are least well liked of all food groups. Strongly flavored vegetables may not be accepted until late school years; some children never learn to like them.

Children sometimes go on food jags; that is, they will eat only certain foods—for example, peanut-butter-and-jelly sandwiches. Usually these diversions of appetite do not last too long if the parents make no particular point of them. If milk is refused as a beverage, it can be given in puddings, or will be accepted if it is occasionally flavored or even colored with vegetable color! American cheese is a good substitute.

Children require snacks to provide for their relatively high energy needs and to avoid excessive hunger at mealtimes. The snacks should be selected largely from the Four Food Groups: fruits and fruit juices; milk; cheese cubes; crackers and peanut butter; raw vegetables; small sandwiches.

By the time a child is ready for school his food likes have increased, but he faces other problems relative to maintaining good nutrition. Mornings in many homes are too often rushed, so that breakfast is a hurried meal or may be skipped entirely. A child who is ill at ease at school may eat poorly at lunch. A short lunch period may be upsetting to the slow eater. Children of this age who are extremely active may become unduly tired before meals.

Observation of the following points will encourage good food habits.

1. Serve meals in a pleasant place and a calm unhurried atmosphere.

2. Provide meals that are colorful, varied in texture and flavor, and attractively served.

3. Don't serve the same food over and over again even if it is a favorite. Even well-liked foods can become tiresome.

4. Provide eating utensils and dishes that are easy for the child to hold and to use. Many vegetables, fruits, meats, and bread may be served as finger foods.

5. Allow sufficient time for meals; breakfast need not be hurried if children are awakened early enough.

6. Don't let the child become too tired before meals. Plan for adequate rest and early bedtime.

7. Plan for snacks as carefully as the meal. Snacks can provide good nutrition. They should not be eaten so close to meals that the appetite is spoiled for the meal.

8. Remember that appetite decreases as the rate of growth slows down during the second, third, and fourth years of life. The toddler may refuse certain foods at this time in trying to assert his independence; don't make too much of this.

CHILD NUTRITION PROGRAMS

The U.S. Department of Agriculture provides substantial assistance through cash and through distribution of commodities to programs designed to improve the nutrition of children. The largest of these programs is the School Lunch which is now available in most of the elementary and secondary schools. The Type A lunch consists of ½ pint milk; 2 ounces of meat, fish, poultry, cheese, or alternate of egg, cooked beans or peas, or peanut butter; 2 servings (at least ¾ cup) of vegetables and fruit; and 1 slice whole-grain or enriched bread or rolls, muffins, corn bread, or biscuits. This lunch furnishes about one third of the recommended allowances.

The Breakfast Program is expanding especially in schools located in low-income areas since it has been shown that many children come to school without breakfast. A breakfast includes milk; fruit or fruit or vegetable juice; bread, biscuits, or muffins; and cereal. In some situations eggs, cheese, meat, fish, or poultry may be included.

Child-care centers, summer school programs, and camps are also aided by cash and commodity distribution. (See Fig. 14–4.) The Special Milk Program provides reimbursement to defray the cost of milk. Children in schools may purchase the milk below cost, or without cost if they are from families with low income.

The WIC Program provides food supplements for women, infants, and

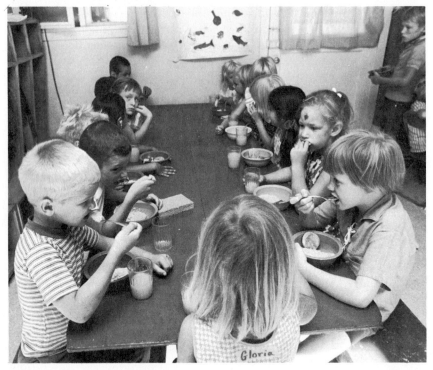

FIGURE 14–4 Child feeding programs of the U.S. Department of Agriculture enable these children of migrant farm workers to eat a nutritious breakfast and other meals at a day-care center. (Mr. Jack Schneider and U.S. Department of Agriculture, Washington, D.C.)

children under 4 years who are at high risk and who have limited incomes. Vouchers are issued for the purchase of foods to supplement their otherwise inadequate diets.

Preadolescent and Adolescent Youth

NUTRITIONAL NEEDS

The caloric needs of boys and girls are somewhat higher than those for men and women, with corresponding higher allowances for thiamin, riboflavin, and niacin. The protein allowances do not differ significantly from those for adults, but the calcium allowance is 1200 mg, which is 50 per cent greater than that for adults. Boys should have an intake of 18 mg iron through 18 years of age, while girls should continue this level of intake throughout the childbearing years. Iodized salt will meet the increased requirement for iodine.

An allowance of 1000 R.E. (5000 I.U.) vitamin A is recommended for boys and of 800 R.E. (4000 I.U.) for girls. Up to 19 years, 10 mcg (400 I.U.) vitamin D should be included daily. The recommended allowance for ascorbic acid is 50 mg at 11–14 years and 60 mg at 15 years and thereafter. See Table 4–1 for other recommended allowances.

The teenage girl frequently becomes pregnant at a time when her own body is still maturing. The mother-to-be needs to increase her already high nutritive allowances by the amounts of nutrients needed for successful pregnancy. (See Chapter 13.)

FOOD SELECTION AND HABITS

The impression is sometimes gained that all teenagers are poorly nourished and always eat great quantities of empty-calorie snacks. In fact, many teenagers have good food habits, are well nourished, and might serve as good examples for others in their age group who need to improve their food habits. Perhaps we have not sufficiently appealed to the teenager himself in terms of his needs for better nutrition. Girls express a particular need for a good figure, a healthy skin, and beautiful hair. They need to understand the patterns of normal maturing of the body so that they do not indulge in bizarre reducing diets. Although a good diet is essential to a healthy skin, they also need to understand that skin problems arise when rapid changes in hormone production are taking place.

Boys are more likely to be interested in tall stature, muscular development, and athletic vigor and stamina. They too have skin problems about which they are concerned. The large appetite of boys helps to ensure an increased intake of needed nutrients along with the foods that are supplying calories.

The diets of boys and girls most frequently fail to meet the recommended allowances for calcium, vitamin A, and ascorbic acid. In addition, girls often do not get enough iron.

Of the food groups, milk requires special emphasis because of the great calcium need. If dark green leafy and deep yellow vegetables and citrus fruits were more adequately consumed, the vitamin A and ascorbic acid intakes would be substantially improved.

Among the particular problems during adolescence are these:

1. Skipped meals. Many high school students keep late hours, get up too late in the morning to eat breakfast, eat a hurried lunch at school, and never quite make up during the rest of the day for their nutritional requirements.

2. Overweight. The pattern of overweight is often set in earlier childhood through a continuing excessive food intake. Active participation in sports rather than watching others engage in sports is important. Weight control should begin in childhood and during adolescence and not be delayed to middle age.

3. Snacks. Boys and girls, as a rule, need some snacks, but their selection should be substantially from the Four Food Groups. A correlation has been established between the excessive intake of sweets, especially those that are sticky, and the amount of tooth decay. This is not to say that any foods are altogether forbidden. Rather, if there is an adequate intake of foods from the Four Food Groups the amounts of empty-calorie foods to satisfy the appetite will be correspondingly reduced.

REVIEW QUESTIONS AND PROBLEMS

1. Visit a food market to determine the kinds of formulas available for infant feeding. Read the labels to see what kind of information is provided.

2. Compare the recommended allowances for calories, protein, calcium, iron, vitamin A, ascorbic acid, and thiamin for the infant at 12 months, the child of two years, the school child of eight years. List the conclusions you can make from these comparisons.

3. Write a schedule for a day for a seven-month-old infant, indicating the kinds and approximate amounts of foods to include at this time.

4. A baby eats one third of the contents of a can of strained fruit. What would you do with the rest of it?

5. Why is egg white not given until toward the end of the first year?

6. What is meant by a Type A lunch? Why is the school lunch program of such importance for the child? Plan a packed lunch for a 12-year-old boy who attends a school where there is no lunch program.

7. Develop suggestions for helping teenagers to improve their food habits.

8. What nutrients require special emphasis during adolescence? What foods will meet these needs?

9. Write a menu for one day for adults. Modify this menu so that it is suitable for a 3-year-old, an 8-year-old, and a 15-year-old boy. Include plans for snacks.

REFERENCES

"Current Concepts in Infant Nutrition," *Dairy Council Digest*, March/April 1976.

Caghan, S. B.: "The Adolescent Process and the Problem of Nutrition," *Am. J. Nurs.*, 75:1728–31, 1975.

Dansky, K. H.: "Assessing Children's Nutrition," *Am. J. Nurs.*, 77:1610–11, 1977.

Ishida, M. C., *et al.:* "Introducing Solid Foods to Infants: An Outline for Instructing Mothers," *Nurs. Digest*, 2:78–83, Summer 1974.

Mayer, J.: "Charting a Course to Good Nutrition with Your Children," *Family Health*, 8:30–32, August 1976.

Mayer, J.: "Baby Foods Grow Up," *Family Health*, 9:36, October 1977.

"Nutrition and Athletic Performance," *Dairy Council Digest*, March/April 1975.

Pipes, P. L.: "When Should Semisolid Foods Be Fed to Infants," *J. Nutr. Educ.*, 9:57–59, 1977.

Safran, C.: "Parents: Experts Tell You What to Do About Balky Vegetable Eaters," *Today's Health*, 51:54, November 1973.

Smiciklas-Wright, H., and D'Augelli, A. R.: "Primary Prevention for Overweight: Preschool Eating Patterns Program," *J. Am. Dietet. A.*, 72:626–29, 1978.

FOOD ACCEPTANCE, CULTURAL FOOD PATTERNS, AND FOOD HABITS

Hunger is the urge to eat and is accompanied by a number of unpleasant sensations. It follows a period when one has been deprived of food, and is generally associated with contraction of the stomach. The individual begins to feel irritable, uneasy, and tired. If a blood sample is taken at this time, the blood sugar level is somewhat low. When food is taken, the individual begins to feel better almost immediately.

Appetite is the anticipation of and the desire to eat palatable food.

People eat not only to satisfy hunger, but also because food has many meanings for them. Good or bad food habits result from the interaction of social, emotional, and cultural factors. In order to help improve your own food habits and to help other people improve theirs, you need to appreciate and understand the variations people have in their likes and dislikes and their attitudes toward food.

Some people have good food habits because they have been fortunate in their early home and school environment. Other people through education have seen the need for change and have been willing to work to modify their habits. Are you one of these?

Factors Affecting Food Acceptance

PHYSIOLOGIC VARIATIONS

Young children have many more taste buds on the tongue and in the cheek, and therefore they have a keener sense of taste, than older individuals. Babies and young children prefer bland foods, whereas teenagers begin to like foods that are more spicy and highly flavored. The number of taste buds diminishes later in life, and old people often lose a sense of taste for certain foods.

The sense of taste varies widely from one individual to another. Some people notice slight differences in taste, and others do not. Some persons like much salt, others only a little; some like very sweet foods, others do not; some like spicy foods, and others prefer bland foods. From day to day, the senses of taste and smell also vary. Smelling food too long at a time, or having a steady diet of certain foods, reduces the response of the sense organs.

The feel of foods is also important. A baby learns about food by feeling it as well as tasting it. We all react favorably to velvety ice cream, crisp rolls, fluffy mashed potatoes, but we are likely to object to sugary fudge, greasy meat, lumpy mashed potatoes, and stringy string beans. Young children don't like very hot or cold foods, but adults usually demand that their foods be piping hot or well chilled.

FAMILY CUSTOMS AND SOCIAL PATTERNS

The family environment has much influence on food habits. Food is more likely to be well accepted when the entire family is together for meals in a happy, relaxed atmosphere. If the homemaker prepares only a few well-liked dishes over and over again, the family members will encounter some difficulty in adapting to other situations. Within the family some allowances may be made for individual likes and dislikes without preparing many separate dishes. If the homemaker selects a variety of foods and prepares them in different ways from time to time, the individual's food experiences are enriched.

Negative attitudes to food may be developed in the home. Children are quick to imitate their parents, who do not eat certain foods. They rapidly note signs of worry, dislike, or anger on the part of the parents and develop antagonisms toward particular foods. They dawdle when they learn it is a way to gain attention. Parents sometimes punish by refusing to give dessert to a child who hasn't finished his meal or bribe and reward with a favorite food like candy if a meal is finished.

Foods are often classed as being for babies, young children, or adults. Milk, cut-up food, peanut-butter-and-jelly sandwiches are looked upon as children's foods; hamburgers, pizza, and large sandwiches are teenage fare; tea and coffee are for adults.

Meat, potatoes, and pie are typical of masculine meals, whereas soufflés, salads, and light desserts are more characteristic of feminine foods.

Some foods have more prestige value than others, and we use them as company foods to honor or impress our friends. They cost more, are hard to get, take a lot of time to prepare, or are unusual. Examples of such status foods are filet mignon, wild rice, baked Alaska, and a fine imported wine. Other foods are sometimes considered to be only for those with low incomes; ground meat, margarine, dry skim milk, dry beans, and fish, for example. Yet any of the latter foods are just as nutritious and can be prepared in as many delicious ways as more expensive foods.

FOOD AND THE EMOTIONS

Did you ever go to a soda fountain for a fancy sundae after taking an examination? Or have you sometimes rewarded yourself for finishing a difficult job with an especially good meal in a restaurant? Do you recall with pleasure certain meals at birthday parties or holidays? Food is often used in one way or another to express or to cover up our feelings of happiness, love, security, worry, grief, loneliness, and so on.

The baby who is held when he is fed associates his food with warmth and security. But a child who is scolded for being messy may associate certain foods with unhappiness. Some teenagers overeat to compensate for a poor record in school or unpopularity with their classmates. Elderly persons living alone often eat far too little, because they are lonely and unhappy. People who are grieving or who can't face the problems that beset them are known to gain excessive weight in some instances, because they find relief in eating excessive quantities of food.

RELIGION AND DIETARY PATTERNS

Various foods have symbolic meanings in religion. Likewise, most religions place certain restrictions upon the use of food. Although the regulations for fasting placed upon Roman Catholics have been liberalized, many Catholics still abstain from meat on fast days; to them fish and cheese may be associated with denial and penitence. Muslims abstain from eating pork, whereas Buddhists are vegetarians and will not eat the flesh of any animal. Seventh Day Adventists are lacto-ovo-vegetarians; that is, they do not eat meat but they use eggs, milk, nuts, and legumes as sources of protein.

Orthodox Jews adhere to dietary laws based upon tradition and the Bible. Animals and poultry are slaughtered according to ritual, and the meat is soaked in water, salted to remove the blood, and washed. This is known as *koshering*. Pork and shellfish are prohibited.

Milk, sour cream, cottage cheese, and cream cheese are widely used, but no dairy foods are served at a meal with meat. Usually two meals each day are dairy meals, and one meal is a meat meal. Separate utensils are used for the cookery of meat and dairy products. Fish, eggs, vegetables, fruits, cereals, and bread may be used at all meals; however, no milk or butter may be used with these foods if they are included in the meat meal.

No food preparation takes place on the Sabbath. Religious festivals are celebrated with special dishes, and much symbolism is attached to food. For example, only unleavened bread is eaten during the Passover. Separate sets of dishes are used during the Passover week. On Yom Kippur (Day of Atonement), the most solemn day of the religious year, no food or drink is taken for 24 hours.

Among the foods widely used by Jewish people are *borsch* (a soup), *gefullte fish*, *blintzes* (thin rolled pancakes filled with cottage cheese or ground beef), *knishes* (pastry with ground meat), *lox* (salted, smoked salmon), *challah* (a braided white bread), *matzo* (flat unleavened bread), *bagel* (doughnut-shaped hard yeast roll), *kuchen* (coffee cake), *leckach* (honey cake served especially at Rosh Hashana, the New Year), and *strudel* (fruit-filled pastry).

REGIONAL PATTERNS IN THE UNITED STATES

Food habits result from the foods that have been available in the various parts of the world. People everywhere tend to like the foods with which they are familiar. Even before tasting a food they will look with suspicion and dislike on something that is unfamiliar. The ease with which people travel from one part of the world to another is doing much to widen our food experiences and to make us more appreciative of other cultures.

Some regional differences still exist in the United States, but for the most part, these are exceptions rather than major departures from the diet. One is likely to associate New England with clam chowder, codfish cakes, Boston baked beans, and lobster; Pennsylvania Dutch, with seven sweets and sours, scrapple, German-type sausage, and shoofly pie; the South, with corn bread, hominy, fried chicken, hot biscuits, turnip and other greens, and sweet potatoes; Louisiana, with French and Creole cookery; the Southwest, with Mexican dishes; the Midwest, with its abundance of dairy products, eggs, and meat and the traditions of Scandinavian, Polish, and German cookery; the Far West, with its luscious fruits and vegetables, salmon, and the influences of the Orient.

VEGETARIAN DIETS

Levels of vegetarianism. A vegetarian diet is one that eliminates one or more of these food groups: meat, poultry, fish, eggs, milk. *Lacto-ovo-vegetarian diets*, used by Trappists, Seventh Day Adventists and others, include milk, milk products, and eggs, but no meat, fish, or poultry. These diets are planned to be nutritionally adequate without difficulty. *Lacto-vegetarian diets* include milk and milk products but no eggs, meat, fish, or poultry. These diets can also be planned to be nutritionally adequate. *Strict vegetarian diets* (also known as *vegans*) include only plant foods. There are many variations of the strict vegetarian diet, some of which are nutritionally adequate when appropriately planned, while others are seriously lacking in nutrients. The *Zen macrobiotic diet* is a diet progressing through several stages, the last of which consists principally of brown rice. This diet, lacking in some essential amino acids, minerals, and vitamins, has resulted in severe malnutrition in persons who have adhered to it for a long period of time. *Fruitarians* consume diets consisting of raw and dried fruits, nuts, honey, and oil. Such diets are deficient in many nutrients.

Reasons for vegetarianism. Probably the most important reason for a vegetarian diet is that a given people adopts a diet of foods that are readily available. In many parts of the world plant foods are abundant, while animal foods are scarce or expensive. In the United States vegetarianism has been adopted by many people because (1) they are concerned about the most efficient use of available land for food production, (2) they believe a vegetarian diet to be more healthful, and (3) their religious or ethical beliefs include such a diet.

The protein problem. Proteins from single plant foods do not furnish sufficient amounts of the essential amino acids to meet the needs for tissue proteins. This is especially true during periods of growth. However, plant foods differ from each other in the kinds and amounts of essential amino acids that they furnish. For example, grains are good sources of methionine but do not have sufficient lysine. Legumes are good sources of lysine, but somewhat deficient in methionine. A general rule, then, is to combine legumes in the same meal with a cereal grain. Thus, beans and corn, as used in Mexican diets, are a good meal combination that compares favorably with meat.

Other nutritional problems. Vitamin B_{12} occurs only in animal foods. Children raised on strict vegetarian diets will not grow properly unless their diets are supplemented with vitamin B_{12}. When no milk is used in the diet, an adequate supply of calcium can be assured if soy milk fortified with calcium is used. Some of the green leafy vegetables are also a good source of calcium. Although an appreciable amount of iron is furnished by an abundant intake of green, leafy vegetables and whole-grain cereals, some of this iron may be poorly absorbed. The absorption of iron from these foods is improved if each meal contains a good source of ascorbic acid.

Cultural Food Patterns

Although people of the United States come from nationality backgrounds from all over the world, the differences in their diets are evident primarily on holidays and family celebrations. Those who adhere more closely to national patterns can readily adapt to the varied supplies of foods in our markets when taught how to do so. A few of the more outstanding examples of some dietary patterns are described briefly.

BLACK AMERICAN

The dietary pattern for black Americans is often described in terms of foods used in the South. However, the foods that are selected by black Americans, as with any group of people, are modified by the geographic location of the community, the neighborhoods in which people live—that is, integrated or largely made up of a single group, the availability of foods in the local markets, and changes in income. For example, some black families living in the North use dietary patterns that differ little if at all from those used by white families who have always lived in the North; other black families have retained the food patterns brought from the South and use them with pride.

"Soul food" is a term recently used to denote foods of the black culture, with particular reference to foods of the black South. Many of these foods originated with the slaves of pre-Civil War days, and continued to be used by poor people in the South, both black and white. At one time such foods lacked status; now they have become fashionable in many places. Some of the typical foods are these:

Meat from every part of the pig: pork chops, ham hocks, bacon, salt pork, spareribs (often barbecued), chitterlings (lining of pig stomach, usually boiled and then fried), and pig's feet, tail, and ears
Fried chicken, fried fish, catfish stew
Wild game when available: coon, possum, beaver, rabbit, squirrel
Greens—turnip, mustard, collard, dandelion, kale—boiled in salt water with ham hocks, bacon, or bits of salt pork; "pot likker" is consumed as well as the greens
Stewed okra, corn, tomatoes
Cornbread in many ways: hoecakes, crackling bread, spoon bread, hush puppies; baking powder biscuits, served hot
Black-eyed peas with molasses and bacon or salt pork
Grits, rice, sweet potatoes, sweet potato pie

Black people do not consume much milk. Recently this has been explained by the fact that a high percentage of adult blacks have an intolerance to lactose, the carbohydrate in milk. The intolerance is probably a hereditary defect in which there is a deficiency or a lack of lactase, the enzyme in intestinal juice that splits up lactose. Milk should not be excluded from the diet of black children, but an awareness of intolerance should be considered. (See p. 65.)

PUERTO RICAN

Many Puerto Ricans have come recently to the large cities of the eastern United States. They are frequently poor, lack employment skills, and live in crowded, often unsanitary, quarters. Because of difficulty in speaking and understanding English, they are likely to patronize small food stores that are owned by Spanish-speaking people. They usually pay much more for the foods they purchase than they would in a supermarket. These and other factors account for a high level of malnutrition, especially among children.

Their staple foods include rice, chick peas, kidney beans, and other legumes, and a variety of *viandas* or starchy vegetables, such as plantain, green bananas, white sweet potato, and others. Dried codfish is often used. Although milk, chicken, and pork are well liked, they are infrequently used because of cost.

Fruits and vegetables have always been available to them in abundance, but they have made limited use of them.

Rice *(arroz)* is eaten once or twice a day and may be combined with a little codfish, legumes, and occasionally chicken *(arroz con pollo)* or pork. The legumes are usually cooked and dressed with a highly seasoned tomato sauce *(sofrito)*. The starchy vegetables are boiled and served with oil, oil and vinegar, or some dried codfish.

MEXICAN

The staple foods of Mexicans include corn, pinto or calico beans, and chili peppers; wheat is now replacing some of the corn. Milk is seldom used, and meat and eggs appear on the menu only two or three times a week. Mexican dishes are seasoned liberally with red chili powder, garlic, onion, and spices.

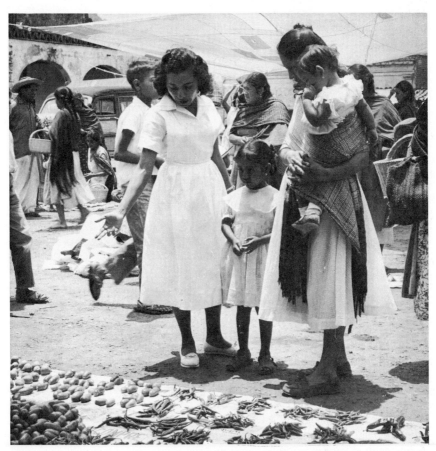

FIGURE 15–1 A community nurse in Mexico points out the importance of selecting fruits and vegetables to supplement the tortilla and black bean diet. *(UNICEF.)*

Dried corn is heated and soaked in lime water, washed, and pounded to a puttylike dough called *masa*. Thin cakes rolled from the masa and baked on a hot griddle are known as *tortillas*. Cheese and ground meat with onion and lettuce may be used to fill tortillas in preparations known as *enchiladas*. *Tamales* consist of highly seasoned ground meat and masa wrapped in corn husks, steamed, and served with chili sauce. *Chile con carne* is a favorite meat and bean dish. (See Fig. 15–1.)

ITALIAN

Pastas such as spaghetti, macaroni, and noodles in many sizes and shapes are characteristic of the Italian diet. Crusty Italian bread is widely used. Chicken, lamb, pork, and veal and a variety of cold cuts are popular but eaten less frequently than in typical American diets. Milk is not used much, but many varieties of Italian cheeses are favored. Vegetables boiled and dressed with oil or oil and vinegar are well liked. Salads and fruits are important parts of the day's meals.

Noodle doughs may be filled with meat, cheese, and vegetable mixtures for such dishes, as *lasagne, ravioli,* and *pizza*. Chick peas, split peas, kidney beans, and lentils are used in such substantial soups as *minestrone*. *Polenta* is a thick cornmeal mush often served plain or with tomato sauce and cheese.

MIDDLE EAST

Round, fat loaves of bread are the staff of life at every meal. Cracked parboiled whole wheat (bulgur) and rice are staple foods eaten as such or with vegetables and meat. Fermented milk (yogurt, matzoon, leben) is preferred to plain milk. Fresh fruits are widely used. Eggplant, zucchini, onions, peppers, okra, cabbage, and cauliflower are favorite vegetables.

Lamb and mutton are preferred, although other meats and poultry are also eaten. Meat is often ground or cut and cooked with wheat, rice, or vegetables. For example, ground meat may be baked in cabbage leaves, and pieces of cut lamb may be placed on skewers with tomato and onion slices for *shashlik*.

ORIENTAL

Rice, wheat, and millet are staple cereals providing most of the calories and protein for people of the Orient. The Chinese use soybeans and soybean sprouts in many dishes. Finely sliced vegetables are cooked by the Chinese for a short time in a little oil (stir-frying) and retain their color and crispness. Chicken, pork, eggs, fish, and shellfish serve as the foundation for many delicious dishes, such as shrimp egg rolls, sweet and sour pork, and chow mein, an American adaptation. Milk, cheese, and beef are not widely used. Sesame oil, peanut oil, and lard are much used. Soy sauce at almost every meal contributes to a high salt intake. Almonds, sesame seeds, and ginger are popular seasonings.

Some Techniques for Changing Food Habits

Good food habits are easily acquired in youth, and it is more difficult to change the habits of people later in life. (See Fig. 15–2.) Perhaps you have found some of your food habits should be improved, or maybe you can help someone in your family or a friend to improve his. The following suggestions may be helpful.

1. A change in food habits is indicated only if the present habits lead to poor nutrition. Remember that persons who have good food habits need not

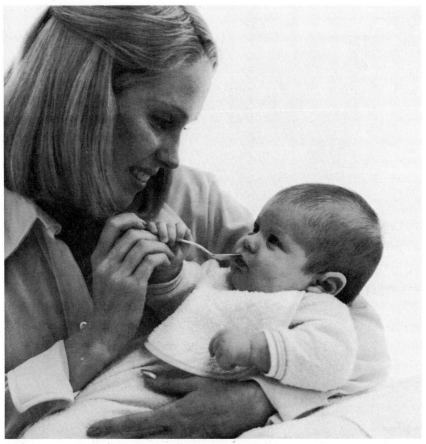

FIGURE 15–2 Good food habits are established during infancy. The environment should be pleasant, secure, and relaxed. *(Gerber Products Company, Fremont, Michigan.)*

like every nutritious food. Also, it is not necessary to omit all foods that are poor sources of the nutrients.

2. Find out what reasons are most likely to appeal to the individual. Boys are often motivated on the basis of growth in stature, physical vigor, and ability in sports. The teenage girl, on the other hand, desires a slim figure to be in the latest fashion, or a clear skin and glossy hair. Neither boys nor girls are likely to be interested in the promise of health or of a good old age, but they might like to impress their friends with their cosmopolitan tastes in food. Older people, on the other hand, are interested in weight control from the standpoint of health or for diet control of some disease problems.

3. Look at the whole diet pattern—not just at one meal pattern or the snacks. List the good points of the diet as well as the weaknesses. Start with the good points for building a better pattern.

4. Be realistic in what can be accomplished. Expect only small changes at the time. Make allowances for strong likes and dislikes. Don't suggest foods that are too expensive, hard to get, or contrary to one's beliefs.

5. Encourage the individual to become adventurous in trying new foods at home or when eating out.

6. Provide practical suggestions for preparing foods in attractive ways.

Specific techniques for the development of good food habits in infants and children are listed in Chapter 14.

REVIEW QUESTIONS AND PROBLEMS

1. A young man away from home for the first time writes that the food he is getting is not to his liking. List as many reasons as you can that affect his food acceptance.

2. What nationality food patterns are found in your community? Write a menu for one day that would be well liked by one nationality group.

3. If possible, visit a food market that caters to a particular nationality group. What foods do you find that are not often seen in supermarkets?

4. A 14-year-old girl is 15 lb overweight. She skips breakfast and drinks little milk, eats no bread, and does not like vegetables. In what ways could you approach her to improve her food habits?

REFERENCES

Berkowitz, P., and Berkowitz, N. S.: "The Jewish Patient in the Hospital," *Am. J. Nurs.*, 67:2335, 1967.

Goldberg, J.: "Vegetarianism," *Family Health*, 10:30–31, April 1978.

Kight, M., *et al.*: "Nutritional Influences of Mexican-American Foods in Arizona," *J. Am. Dietet. A.*, 55:557–61, 1969.

Mayer, J.: "A Matter of Taste," *Family Health*, 8:26–31, April 1976.

Mills, E. R.: "Psychosocial Aspects of Food Habits," *J. Nutr. Educ.*, 9:67–68, 1977.

Register, U. D., and Sonnenberg, L. M.: "The Vegetarian Diet. Scientific and Practical Considerations," *J. Am. Dietet. A.*, 62:253–61, 1973.

Sakr, A. H.: "Dietary Regulations and Food Habits of Muslims," *J. Am. Dietet. A.*, 58:123–26, 1971.

Soulsby, T.: "Russian-American Food Habits," *J. Nutr. Educ.*, 4:170–72, 1972.

Yohai, F.: "Dietary Patterns of Spanish-Speaking People Living in the Boston Area," *J. Am. Dietet. A.*, 71:273–77, 1977.

16

Illness Caused by Food | BACTERIAL AND VIRAL INFECTIONS | BACTERIAL
INTOXICATIONS | PARASITE INFESTATIONS | NATURAL TOXICANTS | CHEMICAL
POISONING | RADIOACTIVE FALLOUT • Preservation of Foods | CAUSES OF
FOOD SPOILAGE | METHODS OF FOOD PRESERVATION | NUTRITIVE VALUES OF
PROCESSED FOODS • Additives | INTENTIONAL ADDITIVES | INCIDENTAL
ADDITIVES

SAFEGUARDING THE FOOD SUPPLY

Food is the nation's biggest business. Each American consumes about 1400 pounds of food in a year. Considering the number of people involved in growing, processing, and selling this large amount of food, the record of safety is excellent. In fact, the food supply is as safe, wholesome, and nutritious as any in the world. This is so because of many interrelated factors: (1) an agriculture dependent upon scientific methods and controls; (2) a system of rapid transport to market under controlled conditions of temperature and sanitation; (3) a highly developed food technology that enables processing of food under high standards of quality control; (4) a rapid turnover in the market place; and (5) intelligent handling by the consumer whether in the home or institution. Each step in the chain from farm to consumer is protected by legislation to ensure compliance to high standards (see Chapter 17).

Although the overall record is excellent, there is no room for careless handling of the food supply. Death from botulin poisoning is rare, but its dramatic occurrence provides headlines in the news. Milder illness from food poisoning occurs to millions every year, but for the most part such illness goes unnoticed and unreported. Only when such illness strikes infants or an institution where many elderly people are living is there concern; these people may, in fact, die from the infections that would be only mild to healthy adults.

Illness Caused by Food

BACTERIAL AND VIRAL INFECTIONS

Large numbers of organisms in food may cause bacterial infection. The bacteria grow rapidly in the moist warm intestinal environment and in 12 to

36 hours produce symptoms such as fever, vomiting, distention, cramping, and diarrhea. The illness is usually mild, lasts for two or three days, and is not usually reported to public health authorities. The dehydration and electrolyte imbalance that sometimes occur are poorly withstood by infants and elderly people.

Salmonella account for a high incidence of bacterial infections. Meat, poultry, fish, eggs, and dairy products that are eaten raw or inadequately heated are frequently the source of infection. For example, raw egg in an eggnog may be the source; or a butcher block, kitchen counter, or utensil that has been in contact with raw meat or poultry could contaminate another food placed upon it.

Typhoid fever is caused by a species of Salmonella. It was a major public health problem at the beginning of this century, but the illness is now uncommon because of the greater safety of water and milk supplies.

Clostridium perfringens, also known as the gas gangrene organism, appears normally in the soil, in sewage, and in the intestinal tract of man. The bacteria are readily destroyed by heat, but the spores survive even after five or six hours of heating. If a cooked food such as meat or gravy is allowed to stand at room temperature for several hours, the spores germinate and produce tremendous numbers of bacteria. If the food so grossly contaminated is eaten, it produces the typical gastrointestinal upsets. Such infections do not occur when food is eaten immediately after cooking. Nor do they occur if food is refrigerated promptly after cooking so that the spores do not germinate. However, if large masses of foods are refrigerated, considerable growth of bacteria can occur before the center of the food mass is adequately chilled; therefore, such foods should be spread out in thin pans for rapid cooling.

Other bacterial infections that may be food borne are *shigellosis* (bacillary dysentery), *brucellosis* (undulant fever) from raw milk from infected animals, *tularemia* (rabbit fever), and *streptococcal* infections, such as strep throat and scarlet fever.

Viral infections include the common cold and infectious hepatitis. The infections are transmitted by direct contact or by contamination of food or water supplies.

BACTERIAL INTOXICATIONS

Some bacteria produce a toxin that causes the illness. The symptoms, which are mild to severe, appear much more rapidly than in bacterial infections—usually in one to six hours after the meal.

Staphylococcal poisoning occurs after eating food that has been contaminated with staphylococci and kept at temperatures ranging between 10° and 60° C (50° and 140° F) for three or four hours. Custards, cream fillings in pastries, cream puffs, cream sauces, chicken salad, croquettes, potato salad, poultry dressing, ice cream, ground meat, and stews are some of the foods that provide the ideal medium for rapid growth of the bacteria. During growth the bacteria produce the toxin that leads to the illness.

The staphylococci are present in infected cuts of the skin, in pimples, and in the nose and throat of persons handling food. Failure to wash hands or bringing a cut finger in contact with food is sufficient to contaminate the food. High heat destroys the bacteria, but does not destroy the toxin that has already been produced. The foods that are most frequently contaminated are not heated sufficiently to destroy the bacteria and are subsequently not refrigerated promptly.

Botulism. *Clostridium botulinum* is an organism found in soils all over the world, and therefore infects vegetables grown on them. The bacteria produce spores that germinate under anaerobic (without air) conditions. As the bacteria grow, they produce the deadly poison *botulin.*

Botulism is rare but about two thirds of all cases are fatal. The toxin affects the nervous system, leading to dizziness, headache, double vision, and paralysis of the muscles leading to respiratory and cardiac failure.

Botulism is traced to canned products, especially home-canned foods, that have been insufficiently sterilized. The spores germinate in the can, and the bacteria in turn produce the toxin. Nonacid foods such as meat, corn, peas, green beans, asparagus, mushrooms, and beets are good media for growth. Acid foods such as tomatoes and certain fruits are not favorable for growth. Boiling a food for at least 10 minutes destroys the toxin. The contents of any can with bulging ends should be discarded without even tasting the food.

PARASITE INFESTATIONS

Trichinella spiralis is a worm that becomes embedded in the muscle tissue of pork. Trichinosis in humans results when infected pork that has been insufficiently cooked is eaten. The larvae develop in the intestinal tract and grow to adult size in a few days. They invade the blood and lymph circulation and involve the muscles of the abdominal wall, the diaphragm, the thorax, the biceps, and the tongue. Muscular pain, chills, and fever result.

Trichinella are destroyed by cooking pork until no trace of pink is present. The organisms are killed at about 60° C (140° F) but the recommended temperature for cooking pork is 77° C (170° F). Trichinella are also destroyed by freezing at −18° C (0° F). Trichinella infestation is now uncommon because all states require that only cooked garbage be fed to pigs.

Tapeworms. Beef or pork tapeworm infestation occurs when cattle graze on sewage-polluted pastures or hogs eat polluted garbage. When man eats infected meat that is raw or rare, the tapeworm continues its reproductive cycle in the intestinal tract. The best controls are to prevent pollution of pastures, to feed only cooked garbage to pigs, and to avoid eating raw or rare meat.

Endamoeba histolytica is a protozoa that is transmitted by food handlers who are carriers of the organism, or by contaminated water supplies. The illness, amebic dysentery, is acute, chronic, or intermittent. The diarrhea may be profuse and bloody with erosion of the intestinal mucosa. Abscesses of the liver, lung, brain, and other tissues sometimes occur. The infestation is more common in tropical areas.

NATURAL TOXICANTS

Many natural constituents of foods produce intoxication when those foods are eaten. Some examples of these are

Rhubarb leaves, extremely high in oxalic acid
Green part of sprouting potatoes: solanine, an alkaloid, causes pain, vomiting, jaundice, diarrhea; when peeling potatoes the green part should be completely removed
Certain species of mushrooms and toadstools contain deadly poisons
Monkshood, foxglove, deadly nightshade, wild parsnip, and hemlock contain poisonous alkaloids
Raw soybeans contain a factor that inhibits the activity of the digestive enzyme trypsin; cooking destroys the trypsin inhibitor
Cottonseed contains the toxic pigment gossypol; processing removes this pigment
Mycotoxins are toxins produced by molds growing on grains and nuts. Aflatoxins are produced by a mold growth on Brazil nuts and peanuts. The problem is important especially in African countries where peanuts often mold on the ground. Discarding nuts with broken shells and discolored, shriveled nut kernels removes the danger.

CHEMICAL POISONING

Food may be accidentally contaminated by poisonous chemicals. Lead poisoning can occur if food is exposed to dust containing lead or if food is kept in containers made with solders, alloys, or enamel containing lead.

Zinc, an essential mineral element, is toxic in excessive amounts. Illness was reported in a group of people who drank lemonade made in a galvanized can. The acid of the lemon juice had dissolved out zinc from the can. The discharge of mercury into rivers and oceans can lead to fish contaminated with greater than tolerable limits; poisoning from this source was recently reported in Japan.

Pesticides have sometimes been accidentally mistaken for a food ingredient, or have been ingested by children who had access to them. Pesticides used in excess of regulations are a potential hazard to fruits and vegetables. Careful washing of foods before their use reduces this hazard.

RADIOACTIVE FALLOUT

Nuclear testing has increased the amount of strontium 90 and iodine 131 in the atmosphere and consequently in the soil. Cattle may transmit strontium 90 from the grasses they eat to their milk, and plants grown on such soils may also contain radioactive elements. The absorption of large quantities of iodine 131 by the body increases the possibility of thyroid cancer. About four fifths of the strontium 90 is excreted in the urine, but some is deposited in the bones and gonads. A liberal intake of calcium appears to be protective against excessive deposit of strontium 90. The Atomic Energy Commission and the U.S. Public Health Service measure the amounts of radioactive fallout in food supplies from time to time. Presently, the amounts are well below any danger levels.

Preservation of Foods

CAUSES OF FOOD SPOILAGE

Bacteria and parasites in food are a frequent cause of illness; yeasts produce fermentation, as in fruit juices and cider; molds attack berries, citrus fruits, breads, jellies and jams, and other foods. Enzymes, normally present in food, cause chemical changes that lead to softening of the food, development of off flavors, loss of some nutrients such as vitamin C, darkening of peeled fruit, or rancidity of fats. Physical factors also cause undesirable changes in food: milk in clear glass bottles exposed to a few hours sunlight loses much of its riboflavin and takes on a tallowy flavor; ice cream held too long in a freezer may become grainy or gummy. Animals or insects may contaminate food with hairs, droppings, or insect fragments.

Foods are contaminated by any of the following ways:

1. Preparation by persons whose hands have not been washed after each use of the handkerchief or toilet, or contact with other source of dirt and filth.

2. Exposure to dust, flies, insects, and nasal sprays of persons who cough or sneeze.

3. Use of equipment and dishes that are poorly cleaned and rinsed.

4. Failure to refrigerate fresh or cooked food promptly, thus speeding up the action of bacteria, molds, yeasts, and enzymes.

METHODS OF FOOD PRESERVATION

Food preservation aims (1) to destroy microorganisms as by heat, or (2) to retard their growth by removal of moisture or the use of cold temperatures. Chemical changes are minimized by avoiding exposure to air and light, by reducing the environmental temperature, and by destroying enzymes.

Dehydration, one of the oldest methods of preservation, eliminates the moist environment that microorganisms need for their growth.

Freezing inactivates bacteria and enzymes. Foods stored in the home freezer at −18° C (0° F) may be left for several weeks or months (depending on the product) with minimum loss of texture, color, flavor, or nutritive value. Once foods are thawed, bacteria and enzymes are reactivated and the foods should be used promptly before spoilage can occur.

Freeze-drying consists in rapidly freezing the product and then removing the moisture in a vacuum.

Cookery. The cooking or baking of food leads to destruction of microorganisms and enzymes. Lower temperatures, such as those attained in a double boiler, are not sufficient to destroy some organisms, such as *Salmonella* in eggs. Some spores of bacteria and some toxins are not destroyed by the heat used in ordinary cooking methods.

Pasteurization is the application of heat to destroy pathogenic bacteria, but it does not sterilize the product. In the high-temperature, short-time process now widely used, milk is held at 160° F for at least 15 seconds. Milk and cream for the manufacture of cheese, ice cream, and butter is usually pasteurized.

Canning is still the primary means used to preserve foods for long periods of time. Home canning is far less frequent than at one time. Meat, poultry, and nonacid vegetables, such as corn, peas, and green beans, should be canned only with a pressure cooker for specified times in order to ensure destruction of the spores of *Cl. botulinum.*

Chemical preservation. Sugar has some preservative effect when used in high concentrations for jams, jellies, and preserves, but molds will grow on the surfaces unless they are protected from air. Brine is used for pickles, sauerkraut, and pickled fish. Sodium benzoate may be used in a limited number of products, including margarine. Sulfur dioxide prevents the darkening of apples and apricots during dehydration. Calcium propionate in bread, and sorbic acid in cheese wrappings retard mold growth.

NUTRITIVE VALUES OF PROCESSED FOODS

Many people have the mistaken notion that processed foods have been "robbed of their nutrients." Commercial processing techniques today ensure maximum retention of nutrients. In fact, fruits and vegetables that have been frozen or canned at the peak of their quality may be higher in nutritive value than those sold as fresh in markets where the temperatures were too high or the products were held for too long a period.

In canned foods the water-soluble vitamins and minerals distribute evenly between the solid and liquid. Suppose one fourth of the contents were liquid, then up to one fourth of the water-soluble nutrients would be lost if the liquid were discarded. Thus, the general rule: use liquids in which foods have been canned or cooked.

Additives

The words "additive" or "chemical" strike fear in people who do not understand that all foods, and all living things, are composed of chemicals, and that there are safe and legitimate uses for additives in foods. Our present system of processing and marketing would be impossible if no additives could be used, and food spoilage would greatly increase. The additives permitted in foods are normally metabolized in the body or excreted so that no harm results. Their use is carefully controlled by the Food and Drug Administration. (See Chapter 17.)

INTENTIONAL ADDITIVES

An intentional additive is any substance of known composition that is added to food to serve some useful purpose. Additives are used to (1) improve nutritional values: thiamin, riboflavin, niacin, and iron in the enrichment of flours and cereals; vitamin D in milk; iodine in salt; and vitamin A in margarine; (2) improve keeping qualities: tocopherol (vitamin E) or other antioxidants to prevent rancidity in fats or in cereal products (see also Chemical Preservation, p. 171); and (3) improve esthetic qualities of foods: emulsifiers to give smooth texture to ice cream, cheese, peanut butter, and other foods; leavening agents such as yeast, baking powder, baking soda in breads, cakes; artificial sweeteners to reduce caloric content; flavoring; and coloring. It is unlawful to use additives to mask faulty processing or handling, or to cover up inferior ingredients, or to deceive the consumer in any way.

INCIDENTAL ADDITIVES

Some chemicals gain entrance to foods from contact during growing or processing, or from the package itself. Since such incidental additives cannot be completely eliminated, it is essential that safe pesticides be used within the allowed levels; that all processing be carried on under the strictest controls of safety and sanitation; and that packaging be rigidly tested for its safety. Federal and state laws determine the maximum levels of such incidental additives that will be tolerated in a product.

REVIEW QUESTIONS AND PROBLEMS

1. Visit a local market or restaurant to observe the practices in the handling of food. List the good practices and any that require improvement.

2. What would you do if you opened a can of food that appeared to be spoiled?

3. Following a picnic many people became ill from eating chicken salad. What organism probably caused the illness? How did it probably gain entrance to the food? Give several rules for avoiding such illness.

4. What is meant by botulism? Trichinosis? How can they be avoided?

5. Read the labels on the following packaged foods and list the additives contained in them: hydrogenated fat, breakfast cereal, bread, gelatin dessert powder, cake mix,

process cheese, and canned soup. List the reasons for as many of these additives as you can.

REFERENCES

Food Additives: What They Are. How They Are Used. Manufacturing Chemists Association, 1825 Connecticut Ave., N.W., Washington, D.C., 1972.

Heenan, J.: *Can Your Kitchen Pass the Food Storage Test,* HEW Pub. No. (FDA)74–2052, Consumer Information Center, Pueblo, CO 81009.

Keeping Food Safe to Eat, Home and Garden No. 162, U.S. Department of Agriculture, Washington, D.C.

Olcott, H. S.: "Mercury, DDT, and PCBs in Aquatic Food Resources," *J. Nutr. Educ.,* 4:156–57, Fall 1972.

Rensberger, B., and Roueché, B.: "When Americans Are a Swallow Away from Death," *Today's Health,* **49**:41, September 1971.

Taylor, A., Jr.: "Botulism and Its Control," *Am. J. Nurs.,* **73**:1380–82, 1973.

Tschirley, F. H.: "Pesticides: Relation to Environmental Quality," *JAMA,* **224**:1157, 1973.

Werrin, M., and Kronick, D.: "Salmonella Control in Hospitals," *Am. J. Nurs.,* **66**:528–31, 1966.

17

CONSUMER CHALLENGES • Food Protection Through Legislation | FOOD, DRUG, AND COSMETIC ACT | MEAT AND POULTRY INSPECTION | FEDERAL TRADE COMMISSION | STATE AND LOCAL LEGISLATION • Read the Label | SOME DEFINITIONS | FOOD LABELING | NUTRITIONAL LABELING | LABELING FOR SPECIAL DIETARY USES • Selection by Food Groups | GENERAL RULES FOR ECONOMY | MILK GROUP | MEAT GROUP | VEGETABLE-FRUIT GROUP | BREAD-CEREAL GROUP | FATS | SWEETS AND CONDIMENTS

FOOD LEGISLATION, LABELING, AND SELECTION

CONSUMER CHALLENGES

Many persons spend more money for food than for any other item. Today's consumer faces great challenges in selecting food from the thousands of items available in any supermarket. Dietitians and nurses in their daily work and also in their neighborly contacts within their own communities are constantly asked about the comparative values of foods.

The tremendous rise in food costs in recent years means that the homemaker tries to be much more selective in her food marketing. She is anxious to know how one product compares with another not only in quantity per unit price but also in nutritive values. Many people are concerned about the additives in foods and want to know what protection they have that these additives are indeed safe and serve a useful purpose. Other individuals require modified diets. For example, someone who is allergic to wheat and eggs needs to be able to identify the products that are wheat-free and egg-free. Another person whose physician has prescribed a cholesterol-restricted fat-controlled diet (see Chapter 24) is interested in the cholesterol and fat content of foods.

These and many other consumer problems are answered through knowledge of legislation that protects the quality of the food supply as well as the honesty of claims made for the product. The regulations for labeling will help consumers to make wise choices for nutritional values as well as ingredients. Finally, consumers need information concerning good choices within the several food groups.

174

Food Protection Through Legislation

FOOD, DRUG, AND COSMETIC ACT

The first federal food and drug law was passed in 1906 and was replaced in 1938 by a more comprehensive Federal Food, Drug, and Cosmetic Act— also known as the "Pure Food and Drug Law." This law pertains to food, other than meat and poultry products, sold in interstate commerce and imported and exported foods. It requires that foods be pure, wholesome, and honestly labeled.

Amendments. Several amendments to the law have been enacted. The Miller Pesticide Amendment of 1954 enables the establishment of safe tolerances of pesticides that may remain in foods after they have been harvested. The Additives Amendment of 1958 provides that an additive may be used in a food product only if it can be shown to improve the nutritive quality, appearance, or keeping properties of a food and not to cover up the use of an inferior food. The amendment requires the manufacturer to submit evidence from experimental work on animals that an additive is safe before it may be included in a food product for sale. The Food and Drug Administration examines the evidence, seeks further proof if necessary, and then issues or refuses a permit for the use of the additive, depending upon its findings. The Color Additive Amendment of 1960 provides for the establishment of safe tolerance levels for all colors used in foods. The Fair Packaging and Labeling Act passed by Congress in 1966 authorizes the FDA to set up regulations for packaging and labeling that avoids deceptive practices.

GRAS list. In 1958 when the Food Additives Amendment was enacted about 600 substances were excluded from testing. They had been used for long periods of time without any known harm to consumers, and were "generally recognized as safe" (GRAS). The list included salt, baking powder, baking soda, spices, and minerals and vitamins added to food for enrichment, as well as other substances.

In 1968 the public as well as some scientists became concerned when cyclamates (one of the artificial sweeteners on the GRAS list) were found to produce bladder cancer in animals. The amount of cyclamate required to produce the cancer was so large, that a human being would find it impossible to consume an equivalent amount. Nonetheless, the Delaney clause of the additives amendment specifies that no substance may be added to food if it produces cancer at any level whatsoever. As a result the entire GRAS list is being tested to determine whether any of the substances will produce cancer at any level of feeding.

Enforcement. The food and drug law, together with its amendments, is enforced by the Food and Drug Administration of the Department of Health, Education, and Welfare. Under the law, factories and warehouses may be in-

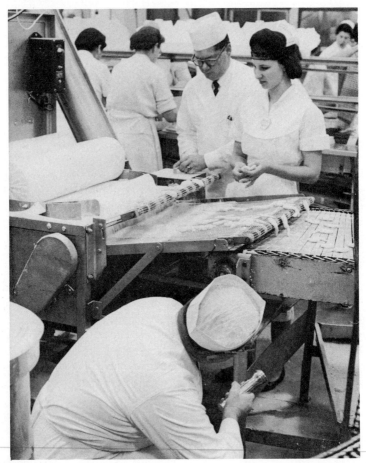

FIGURE 17–1 Plant inspection is one of the activities of the Food and Drug Administration authorized by federal legislation. *(FDA photo.)*

spected to ascertain that the raw materials together with processing, packaging, and storage facilities are sanitary. (See Fig. 17–1.) Adulterated and misbranded products may be seized by inspectors and destroyed or relabeled, depending upon the nature of the offense. Flagrant violations may result in the imposition of fines or imprisonment by the courts.

Interpretation of the law. A food is *adulterated* if it contains dirt, filth, or decomposed material or any substance harmful to health; if it is prepared, packaged, or stored under unsanitary conditions; if it is made from diseased animals; if it contains additives that conceal the poor quality of the food; if it contains unsafe additives, uncertified food colors, or pesticide residues in excess of tolerances; if the packaging material contains substances harmful to health.

Misbranded food is that which has a false, misleading label; a package that fails to specify the weight, measure, or count of the food; a package that is of misleading size, so that the consumer thinks he is getting more than he actually is; a label that does not clearly state the use of imitations, including artificial color, flavorings, and preservatives; a label that fails to list the name of the manufacturer, packer, or distributor; a label that does not list the amounts of nutrients in products for which a nutritional claim is made.

The Food and Drug Administration also establishes what a product actually is by setting standards of *identity, quality,* and *fill.* Foods for which an official standard has been set must contain amounts of ingredients not below the prescribed minimum nor above the legal maximum. This regulation applies also to the addition of required amounts of nutrients for enrichment and fortification. For nonstandardized products the ingredients are listed in order from the greatest amount to the least. Standards of quality for canned vegetables, fruits, and meats, and other products pertain to the color, flavor, and freedom from defects. Standards of fill specify how full a container must be.

MEAT AND POULTRY INSPECTION

The Meat Inspection Act of 1906 and its amendments of 1967 and the Poultry Inspection Act of 1957 accomplish the objectives of the pure food law for meat and poultry. The Bureau of Animal Husbandry of the U.S. Department of Agriculture is charged with the enforcement of these acts. The acts provide for the inspection of premises for processing animals and poultry, the live animals, and the carcasses. Meat that is inspected and is fit for consumption is labeled "U.S. Inspected and Passed," and that which is unfit for human consumption is labeled "Inspected and Condemned." (See Fig. 17–2.) The Act also applies to manufactured meat products and provides for the proper use of additives, the correct labeling of the product, and the maintenance of standards of identity.

FEDERAL TRADE COMMISSION

Advertising for products that are involved in interstate commerce is regulated by the Federal Trade Commission. In recent years some of the food supplements

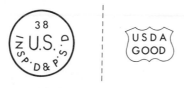

FIGURE 17–2 The round inspection stamp on meat indicates that the meat is wholesome. The shield indicates the grade of meat; grading of meat is not required by law. *(U.S. Department of Agriculture, Washington, D.C.)*

such as vitamins and so-called health foods were seized because false claims were made for nutritive values or for cures for disease.

STATE AND LOCAL LEGISLATION

Because federal legislation applies only to foods sold in interstate commerce, the individual states have passed laws that are similar to the federal laws. The state and local ordinances for the protection and pasteurization of milk, and the regulations for public eating establishments, have usually been patterned after the codes set up by the U.S. Public Health Service.

The U.S. Department of Agriculture maintains a voluntary grading service for the quality of livestock, poultry, dairy products, fruits, and vegetables. Many state departments of agriculture cooperate with the federal government in the training of state inspectors and in setting up comparable standards for intrastate products.

Read the Label

SOME DEFINITIONS

In order to interpret labels consumers need to have a clear understanding of several descriptions of foods.

Restored applies to the addition of nutrients to a processed food so that it has the same value as the original food. For example, suppose the original food contained 5.0 mg iron per pound, and lost 1.0 mg in processing; the addition of 1.0 mg iron restores it to the original value.

Fortification is the addition of one or more nutrients that may or may not have been present in the original food; for example, the addition of vitamin D to milk, vitamin A to margarine, and iodine to salt.

Enrichment is the addition of thiamin, riboflavin, niacin, and iron to flours and cereals according to specified standards set by the Food and Drug Administration. This constitutes a restoration of nutrients removed in the processing of grain, and, in the case of iron, fortification as well.

A *dietary supplement* is a product specially formulated to furnish additional nutrients to a regular diet. It includes vitamins, minerals, and/or protein in the form of foods, capsules, tablets, pills, powders, or liquids.

Engineered, formulated, or *fabricated* foods are products developed by manufacturers from one or more ingredients. They are termed *analogs* when they simulate another food; for example, textured vegetable protein made from soybeans may simulate a pork chop or sausage or other meat product. Several breakfast drinks have been developed for use in place of orange juice, and are similar in color, flavor, and nutrient content. One of the important points to be aware of in choosing a fabricated food is that it furnishes the same amount and variety of nutrients that are contained in the food it replaces.

FOOD LABELING

The principal display panel for a packaged or canned food product must include (1) the common name of the product, (2) the net weight in ounces, including the liquids used for packing as well as the solids, and (3) the name and address of the manufacturer, packer, or distributor. A description of the product is also given; for example, "condensed" for soups that are to be diluted when used; "cream style" for corn; whole, halves, pieces, etc., for fruits.

The ingredients for nonstandardized products must be listed in the order of their predominance; that is, the ingredient in the largest amount listed first, the second largest next, and so on. This listing includes the common names of ingredients. The common names of additives are chemical terms that have little meaning to most consumers. Nevertheless, their listing represents a protection to the consumer.

More than 300 products are manufactured under a standard of identity. Manufacturers are not required to list the ingredients for these products, since they are formulated according to standard recipes set by the Food and Drug Administration. However, manufacturers are now being urged to list ingredients in these products so that consumers can be better informed.

NUTRITIONAL LABELING

The Food and Drug Administration has adopted regulations pertaining to the labeling of processed foods for nutritional information. This labeling will permit consumers to compare the nutritive values of one product with another; to count calories; to learn which foods contribute substantial amounts of nutrients and which foods contain few nutrients; to compare new food products with familiar ones; and to select appropriate foods for modified diets.

Nutritional labeling is voluntary on the part of manufacturers for most foods, but it is hoped that food processors will generally provide such information. Full nutritional labeling is required for (1) any product for which a claim of nutritional value is made in labeling or advertising, and (2) any product that contains one or more added nutrients, such as foods that are restored, fortified, or enriched.

Labeling standard. The U.S. Recommended Dietary Allowances (U.S. RDA) replaces the Minimum Daily Requirements (MDR) which is now outdated. Although the standard is based upon the Recommended Dietary Allowances (Table 4–1, p. 32), the two tables must not be confused and used interchangeably. For example the RDA has 17 categories for age, sex, pregnancy, and lactation, while the U.S. RDA applies generally to all persons over 4 years

TABLE 17–1   U.S. RECOMMENDED DIETARY ALLOWANCES (U.S. RDA) FOR ADULTS
AND CHILDREN OVER 4 YEARS

Required		Optional	
Protein	65 gm *	Vitamin D	400 I.U.
Vitamin A	5000 I.U.	Vitamin E	30 I.U.
Vitamin C	60 mg	Vitamin B_6	2.0 mg
Thiamin	1.5 mg	Folacin	0.4 mg
Riboflavin	1.7 mg	Vitamin B_{12}	6 mcg
Niacin	20 mg	Phosphorus	1.0 gm
Calcium	1.0 gm	Iodine	150 mcg
Iron	18 mg	Magnesium	400 mg
		Zinc	15 mg
		Copper	2 mg
		Biotin	0.3 mg
		Pantothenic Acid	10 mg

* If the protein efficiency ratio of protein is equal to or better than that of casein, U.S. RDA is 45 gm.

except pregnant and lactating women. The allowances in the U.S. RDAs, in most cases, include the highest levels specified in the recommended allowances within this age category. Thus, they exceed the needs of most people. Compare, for example, the U.S. RDA with the recommended dietary allowance for a child of 10 years, a boy of 16 years, and a woman of 35 years. Three U.S. RDA standards have also been proposed for infants under 12 months, children up to 4 years, and pregnant and lactating women. Such standards apply to products intended especially for these groups.

Nutrition information on any label must follow the format and order set by the Food and Drug Administration. The percentage of the U.S. RDA are required for protein and seven vitamins and minerals; the manufacturer may list percentages for twelve additional vitamins and minerals. (See Table 17–1 and Fig. 17–3.)

LABELING FOR SPECIAL DIETARY USES

Any product sold for a special dietary use must contain full nutritional labeling and use the appropriate U.S. RDA. Six prohibitions apply to the labeling of products. No claim can be made (1) that the product in itself prevents, treats, or cures disease; (2) that a diet of ordinary foods cannot furnish adequate nutrients; (3) that inadequate diet is due to the soil on which the foods are grown; (4) that transportation, storage, or cooking of foods may result in an inadequate diet; (5) that nonnutritive ingredients such as inositol, paraminobenzoic acid, or bioflavinoids have nutritional value; and (6) that a natural vitamin is superior to a synthetic vitamin.

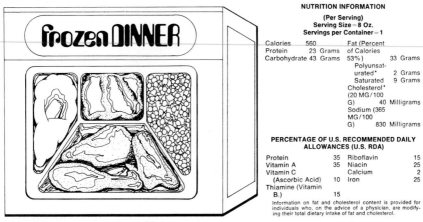

NUTRITION INFORMATION

(Per Serving)
Serving Size = 8 Oz.
Servings per Container = 1

Calories	560	Fat (Percent		
Protein	23 Grams	of Calories		
Carbohydrate	43 Grams	53%)	33 Grams	
		Polyunsat-		
		urated*	2 Grams	
		Saturated	9 Grams	
		Cholesterol*		
		(20 MG/100		
		G)	40	Milligrams
		Sodium (365		
		MG/100		
		G)	830	Milligrams

PERCENTAGE OF U.S. RECOMMENDED DAILY
ALLOWANCES (U.S. RDA)

Protein	35	Riboflavin	15
Vitamin A	35	Niacin	25
Vitamin C		Calcium	2
(Ascorbic Acid)	10	Iron	25
Thiamine (Vitamin			
B.)	15		

Information on fat and cholesterol content is provided for
individuals who, on the advice of a physician, are modifying their total dietary intake of fat and cholesterol.

FIGURE 17–3   Nutrition information such as that provided by this product will help consumers to compare food products and also to determine whether a product is appropriate for a given modified diet. *(Food and Drug Administration, Rockville, Maryland.)*

Cholesterol and fat.   Any product that is labeled for cholesterol must state the amount of cholesterol in milligrams per serving and per 100 grams of food. The fatty acid content of food may be stated if the total fat content is more than 2 gm per serving. It should include the grams of total fat, grams of fat from saturated fatty acids, grams of fat from polyunsaturated fatty acids, and per cent of calories from fat. When information on cholesterol and fatty acids is included in labeling, the following statement must also appear on the label: "Information on fat (and/or cholesterol) content is provided for individuals who, on the advice of a physician, are modifying their total dietary intake of fat (and/or cholesterol)."

Selection by Food Groups

GENERAL RULES FOR ECONOMY

1. Eat meals at home most of the time. Carry lunches to work whenever practical.

2. Read food columns in newspapers to learn which foods are plentiful and lower in cost. Take advantage of advertised specials in newspapers.

3. Plan menus in advance and prepare a market order. Be prepared to modify your plans if when you get to the market you find that some foods are too expensive or are not available.

4. Avoid buying foods on impulse.

5. Read labels and compare prices, weights, grades, and nutritional values of different brands.

6. Buy fresh foods in season. Fresh foods out of season are usually more costly than canned or frozen foods.

7. Compare cost of convenience and home-prepared foods. Many canned and dried products and some frozen products are about as low in cost as home-prepared foods and save considerable time for the homemaker. Highly perishable convenience foods, such as salad mixes of fruits or vegetables and bakery foods, are likely to be much more expensive.

8. Consider the nutritive value of the snack foods—popcorn, candy, pretzels, soft drinks, and others. Is too much of your food budget spent for these?

9. Purchase only the amounts that are likely to be used by the family. Use leftovers promptly. (See Fig. 17–4.)

10. Store foods properly. Use leftovers within 24 hours.

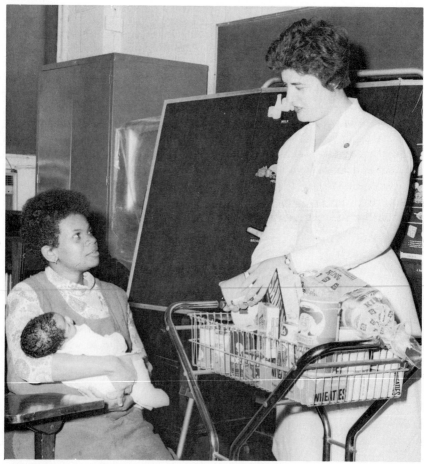

FIGURE 17–4 A market basket is used to illustrate the nutritive and economic values of foods. *(School of Nursing, Thomas Jefferson University, Philadelphia.)*

MILK GROUP

Of fluid milks, fresh milk costs the most, evaporated milk is intermediate in cost, and skim milk made from nonfat dry milk costs the least. Almost all fresh pasteurized milk is fortified with vitamin D. Skim milk, nonfat dry milk, and skim evaporated milks are fortified with vitamins A and D. Purchasing fresh milk in a supermarket is less expensive than having it delivered to the home. For families that require large amounts of milk the half-gallon and gallon containers are economical.

Nonfat dry milk makes a palatable beverage when it is mixed according to directions and thoroughly chilled before serving. For people who have been accustomed to drinking whole milk it usually takes a week or so to adjust to the flavor of skim milk. Many people are now drinking milk with lower fat content in order to reduce their intake of saturated fat, cholesterol, and calories. A good compromise is to mix one part whole milk with one part nonfat milk made from dry milk. This reduces fat, cholesterol, and caloric content as well as cost.

Evaporated milk has the same nutritive value as fresh milk when it is mixed with an equal amount of water. It may be used in any cooked dishes that require milk. Evaporated milk may be whipped for desserts and may be used on cereals and as whitener for coffee.

Cream, yogurt, cream cheese, and ice cream are more expensive dairy products, and should be used infrequently when the budget is limited. Half-and-half contains 12 per cent fat, coffee and cultured sour cream about 18 per cent fat, and whipping cream 30 to 40 per cent fat. Many people now prepare yogurt in the home at low cost.

Cottage cheese, American cheddar and Swiss cheese, and process cheeses are relatively inexpensive sources of protein, and provide good occasional substitutes for a meat meal. Imported cheeses such as Roquefort, Gouda, Camembert, Edam, Gorgonzola, and many others are more expensive.

MEAT GROUP

Although the meat group is important for protein, iron and other minerals, as well as some B-complex vitamins, many people spend more money than necessary for this group. They buy larger amounts than are needed for good nutrition and they select expensive cuts. With limited budgets this expenditure often restricts the amount spent for the other food groups, especially fruits and vegetables. Acceptable daily meat allowances for adults are 4–5 ounces. At this level, the saturated fat and cholesterol intakes are moderate, and the cost of this group can be kept within reasonable limits. Frequent substitution of poultry and legumes for meat reduces not only the cost but also the fat and cholesterol intake.

Meat that bears the round purple stamp of the Meat Inspection Board is safe and wholesome, but this stamp is no indicator of quality. The cost of meat depends upon the grade, with U.S. Choice, Good, Standard, and Commercial grades being most common. Prime grade is seldom seen on the retail market. Choice grades of meat come from younger animals and are more tender than the cuts from older animals. The lean of Choice grade is well marbled with streaks of fat. Such meat will give the most tender steaks, chops, and oven roasts. Meats graded as Good are leaner than choice or prime cuts and lower in cost and in saturated fat and calories.

Rib and loin cuts of meat, such as steaks, chops, and rib roasts, are tender and usually more expensive than cuts from the more exercised parts of the animal, such as the flank, the shoulder used for pot roasts, Swiss steak, and meat loaf. Less tender cuts are very flavorful if properly cooked. Beef, lamb, and pork liver are much less expensive than calves' liver and just as nutritious.

When comparing the costs of meat, one should note the amount of fat, bone, and gristle in relation to the lean. Some lower-priced cuts of meat are sometimes more expensive because there is so little lean. One pound of lean meat, such as ground beef or round steak, will serve three to four persons. Steak and chops, because of the amount of bone and fat, will usually require 1 lb for two persons. Meat with much fat and bone, such as brisket and short ribs, will serve only one to two persons per pound.

Chicken and turkey have been good buys in recent times. The relative proportion of bone and skin to lean meat is somewhat higher than in the meat of larger animals.

Fish, whether fresh, canned, or frozen, is likely to be less expensive than meat. Shellfish, such as oysters, lobsters, shrimp, and crabs, are luxury items except where locally available.

Eggs. Eggs are priced according to quality and size. Top-quality eggs, grade AA and A, have a thick, gelatinous white and a round, high yolk that does not break easily. Such eggs are good for poaching, cooking in the shell, and frying. Grade B eggs have thinner whites and flatter yolks. They are suitable for cooking and baking, but they have a somewhat less delicate flavor for table use.

Eggs are sorted according to size, based on weight per dozen: extra large, 27 oz; large, 24 oz; medium, 21 oz; and small, 18 oz. Medium and small eggs are usually a good buy in the fall, whereas large eggs may be a good buy in the spring. Medium eggs are a better buy if their cost is at least one eighth less per dozen. White and brown eggs are equally good. Always buy eggs that have been kept under refrigeration.

Legumes. Legumes are a good protein source when the budget is limited, and they lend themselves to a variety of uses. Split peas, navy beans, Lima beans, kidney beans, lentils, soybeans, chick peas, and peanuts are among the varieties available. Peanut butter is a good buy. Dried legumes require soaking and a longer cooking time.

Textured vegetable protein (TVP) is sold under a variety of names. It is prepared from soybeans and is an excellent extender for meats such as hamburgers and meat loaf. When combined with meat the quality and amount of protein is as good as though the dish had been prepared from meat alone.

VEGETABLE-FRUIT GROUP

Fresh, frozen, dehydrated, and canned fruits and vegetables may be purchased. Fresh fruits and vegetables, especially those locally grown, are often less expensive in season. Canned or frozen fruits and vegetables are likely to be better buys at other times of the year. Frozen orange juice is less expensive than freshly squeezed juice, but usually costs a little more than canned juice. Frozen vegetables prepared with butter or cream sauces are appreciably higher in cost than plain vegetables that would be seasoned at the time of cooking.

Fruits should be ripe, firm, free from decay spots, and not soft or with mold spots. Vegetables should be firm, crisp, and clean—not wilted or bruised. Overripe fruits or too mature vegetables are not good economy even though the price may be somewhat lower.

A canned product should be selected for its use; for example, whole fruit may be desired when it is to be served as a dessert, but fruit pieces are just as good for a mixed salad or for pastries. Likewise, grade A peas may be preferred for buttered peas, but grade B peas would be suitable for a casserole dish.

BREAD-CEREAL GROUP

Enriched or whole-grain breads, cereals, pastas, and flours should be purchased. Enriched white bread is the least expensive way to purchase bread. Day-old bread, when available, is somewhat reduced in price. Many specialty breads that contain butter, stone-ground flour, honey, raisins, or other flavor ingredients and sweet breads and rolls are considerably more expensive. Many homemakers today find much satisfaction in baking their own breads and rolls.

Cooked breakfast cereals are usually less expensive than dry breakfast cereals. For variety, some of each should be used. When selecting cereals compare the nutritive values of one serving of one kind or brand of cereal with another. Some cereals contain appreciably more iron and B-complex vitamins than do others. Also compare the cost per unit price. Unit prices are posted directly below the display of each brand of cereals. For cereals the unit price is expressed as cost per pound. Finally, compare the list of ingredients. Some sugar-coated cereals are not only more costly than plain cereals, but a significant percentage of the calories are derived from sugar that supplies no minerals or vitamins.

FATS

Butter and margarine are of equal nutritive value and are comparable in flavor. Regular margarines are much less costly than butter, but special margarines that are high in polyunsaturated fat are only slightly lower in cost than butter. Consumers today are using more oils—corn, cottonseed, soybean, safflower, and less hydrogenated shortenings or lard because of the differences in polyunsaturated fat content.

SWEETS AND CONDIMENTS

Cane and beet sugars cost less than raw, brown, and confectioners' sugars. Molasses is a good buy, because it contains iron as well as carbohydrates. It can be used for many dishes, such as baked beans, gingerbread, cookies, puddings, and sometimes in a glass of milk for children. Honey, maple sugar and syrup, and candies represent expensive ways to buy sweets.

Spices, flavoring extracts, and herbs are important additions, because they enhance the flavors of food so much. Flavors are rapidly lost to the air, and only small containers of infrequently used seasonings should be purchased. Coffee, tea, catsup, meat sauces, pickles, and relishes add interest to meals. Depending upon the choices made, these food adjuncts may increase the food expenditure appreciably.

REVIEW QUESTIONS AND PROBLEMS

1. Visit a supermarket and examine carefully the labeling for a can of fruit, a package of cereal, a package of biscuit mix, a frozen dinner, a brand of soft margarine, a loaf of bread, and a package of some dietetic food. What information do you find on the label of each? How would you evaluate this information for the nutritional importance of the product?

2. What national laws protect the food supply?

3. When is labeling for nutritional information required for a food product?

4. List four practices that would lead a product to be adulterated.

5. List four ways in which a product would be seized because it was misbranded.

6. Examine the labeling for two brands of instant potatoes. Are they fortified with vitamin C? How much per serving? How does this compare with the vitamin C content of one serving of fresh potatoes?

7. Compare the cost of a pound of round steak, short ribs, chuck roast, and rib roast. How many servings per pound of each?

8. A homemaker tells you that she cannot afford to buy enough milk for her family including herself, her husband, and four children ages 6, 8, 11, and 14. How much milk should she include each day? Show how much money she could save by using half of the day's allowance as whole milk and half as nonfat dry milk, as compared with all fresh milk.

REFERENCES

Bauman, H. E.: "What Does the Consumer Know About Nutrition?" *JAMA*, 225:61–62, 1973.

Council on Foods and Nutrition: "Improvement of the Nutritive Quality of Foods," *JAMA,* **225**:116–18, 1973.

Day, H. G.: "Food Safety—Then and Now," *J. Am. Dietet. A.,* **69**:229–34, 1976.

Deutsch, R.: "Where You Should Be Shopping for Your Family," *Today's Health,* **50**:16, April 1972.

Food Shopper Language, U.S. Department of Agriculture, Consumer Information Center, Pueblo, CO 81009

Food for Thrifty Families, Revised 1977. U.S. Department of Agriculture, Consumer Information Center, Pueblo, CO 81009

McGill, M.: "Nutrition Labeling," *Family Health,* **6**:35–37, November 1974.

Moore, J. L., and Wendt, P. F.: "Nutrition Labeling—A Summary and Evaluation," *J. Nutr. Educ.,* **5**:121–25, April 1973.

Stephenson, M.: "Making Food Labels Informative," *FDA Consumer,* **9**(8):13–17, 1975.

UNIT **IV**

DIET THERAPY

18 ILLNESS AND FOOD ACCEPTANCE | ILLNESS AND NUTRITION | MEDICATIONS AND DIET | DIET THERAPY | THE DIETARY PRESCRIPTION | THE NURSE'S ROLE IN NUTRITIONAL CARE | GOOD TRAY SERVICE | THE PATIENT AND HIS MEALS | FEEDING THE PATIENT

NUTRITION AND DIET FOR THE PATIENT

ILLNESS AND FOOD ACCEPTANCE

The many physiologic, cultural, economic, and emotional factors affecting food acceptance have been discussed in Chapter 15. The person who is ill must face added problems related to his meals. Diet is related to both the comfort and the treatment of the patient, but sometimes it is necessary to take therapeutic measures that may distress rather than provide immediate comfort. The nurse plays an essential role in helping to bridge this gap. (See Fig. 18–1.)

Illness itself often reduces interest in food because of anorexia, gastrointestinal distention, or discomfort following meals. Inactivity and some drugs also reduce the desire for food.

The patient in a hospital may be away from home for the first time. He probably misses his family and the sociability of family meals. He finds that the food pattern in the hospital and the time for meals differ, more or less, from his usual pattern. He finds it difficult to manage a tray in bed. His food intake is affected by his worries about mounting hospital bills, about return to work, or about the extent of his return to full health.

If the diet is modified, the patient may be getting less or more food than he normally eats. The change in flavor or texture of some diets is not appealing. Often he is unwilling to accept any change, worried about how he will get the new foods for his diet at home, or bothered about the inconvenience of sticking to a diet that is different from that of his family or friends. Some modified diets make him feel that he is deprived and punished.

191

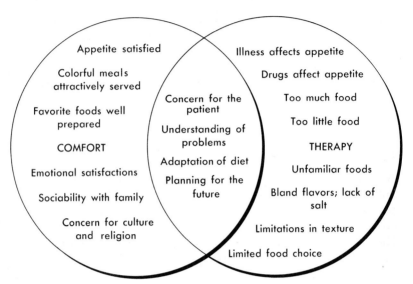

FIGURE 18–1   Patients seek comfort through food. Modified diets may present many problems. The nurse must help the patient to solve these problems.

In his illness the patient becomes more self-centered, and he reacts by being irritable or even angry. He complains incessantly about his food in order to get more attention, or he is quite indifferent to his diet, eats poorly, and ignores the suggestions made by doctors, nurses, or dietitians.

ILLNESS AND NUTRITION

Illness has many effects on the body's ability to use nutrients and upon the specific requirements. Lack of appetite, vomiting, and pain often prevent the intake of a sufficient amount of food. In severe diarrhea the absorption of all nutrients is poor, so that loss of weight, dehydration, and signs of malnutrition may be found. A fever increases the rate of metabolism, thus increasing the need for calories, protein, and vitamins. In metabolic diseases nutrients are not utilized fully; for example, the untreated diabetic patient will not make adequate use of carbohydrate. The patient who must remain in bed or in a wheelchair for a long time usually loses increased amounts of nitrogen and calcium from his body. As the student becomes more experienced in the care of patients, she will undoubtedly find numerous examples of the effects of illness upon nutrition.

MEDICATIONS AND DIET

Some drugs interfere with food intake because they produce nausea and vomiting. Others reduce the absorption of nutrients because they interfere with enzyme activity, block the absorption of some vitamins, or lead to diarrhea. On the other hand, food can also interact with the medications so that absorption is reduced. Thus, the peak of effectiveness of the drug may never be reached. The nurse, dietitian, and pharmacist must take these factors into account to assure maximum effectiveness of the drug as well as optimum food intake and utilization. Table A-6 outlines the interaction of some commonly used drugs and diet.

DIET THERAPY

An appropriate diet is essential in the total-care plan developed for each patient. The normal diet is the basis on which all *therapeutic* or *modified* diets are planned. Usually the diet supplements medical and surgical care; sometimes it is the specific treatment for the disease.

Diet therapy accomplishes one or more of these aims: (1) maintains normal nutrition; (2) corrects nutritional deficiency, for example, high-protein diet; (3) changes body weight, as with low- or high-calorie diets; (4) adjusts to the body's ability to use one or more nutrients, for example, diabetic diet; (5) permits maximum rest to the body or an organ, as with a soft, low-calorie diet in six feedings.

The normal diet may be modified for (1) consistency and texture; (2) flavor; (3) energy value; (4) nutrient levels such as fat, protein, carbohydrate, sodium, and others; or (5) food categories such as types of fats or elimination diets for allergies.

THE DIETARY PRESCRIPTION

The physician orders the appropriate diet for each patient, just as he orders medications and other therapy. Each prescription is the result of an evaluation of the patient's symptoms, laboratory tests if they have been done, and his nutritional needs. In some instances priority must be given to one aspect of diet, while other requirements are deferred for a later time. For example, a very low-residue diet is lacking in some vitamins, but such a diet might be essential for an acute gastrointestinal disorder or prior to surgery. The nutritional lack can be correlated by means of a vitamin supplement until a more liberal diet can be taken.

Diets should be described exactly in terms of the changes to be made in consistency, flavor, and level of nutrients; for example, 1800-kcal, 500-mg sodium, soft diet. The use of the term "special diet" should be discouraged for it has little meaning. Likewise, the terms "high" and "low" have meaning only when they are used with reference to the normal diet or when a given diet manual specifies the nutritive value. For example, a low-calorie diet might mean 800 kcal to one individual, 1200 kcal to another, and 1800 kcal to a man whose normal requirement is 2600 kcal per day. Diets should not be named for persons or diseases; the latter practice is likely to be a continual reminder to the patient of his condition.

A correct, nutritious, attractive, and well-prepared meal for a patient requires the teamwork of the medical, nursing, and dietary services. In the hospital the dietitian translates the diet prescription into a menu and supervises the food preparation and service to the patient. If a selective menu is used, the dietary technician or nurse may help the patient to select his meals according to the diet prescription.

The nurse has the most continual direct contact with the patient and makes certain that he receives and consumes his meals under the best circumstances. As a nurse you would expect to prepare the patient for his meals so that his tray can be served as soon as it arrives. Perhaps you may need to feed him. Helping the patient to accept his diet by giving encouragement and praise is a decided contribution. This also means that you avoid criticism if he is not eating well, or pity because the diet is one you would not like very much.

Observing, listening, and reporting are three important functions performed by the nurse in nutritional care. How well the patient eats his food, what kinds and amounts of food are refused, and the patient's attitude toward his food are readily determined. You are more likely than anyone else to observe problems such as these: poorly fitting dentures and inability to chew; a sore mouth and pain when acid juices are taken; arthritic fingers that make it difficult to cut up food; portions that are too large for some elderly persons or too small for teen-agers; difficulty in breathing so that eating a large meal at one time is not possible; between-meal feedings interfering with the appetite for the meals; fatigue and poor appetite at the end of the day; and many others.

By listening you show your general interest in and your understanding of the patient, and help him to express his feelings and perhaps to "blow off steam." You begin to learn that some foods are favorites, others are thoroughly disliked, and still others cannot be eaten because of religious beliefs. You become aware of what food means to the patient, and what concerns the patient may have about the diet he will have when at home.

Acting upon your information is essential to the best care of the patient. Sometimes it is direct action on your part. More often it involves reporting to the nursing supervisor, dietitian, or physician, depending upon the circumstances.

GOOD TRAY SERVICE

Meals are often the high point of the day for patients. An attractive tray of well-prepared food presented cheerfully to a patient who is ready for his meal goes a long way toward ensuring acceptance. The essentials of good tray service are

1. A tray of sufficient size for uncrowded arrangement of dishes.
2. An immaculately clean, unwrinkled tray cover and napkin.
3. An attractive pattern of spotless china, sparkling glassware, and shining silverware.
4. Convenient orderly arrangement of all items on the tray so that the patient can easily reach everything.
5. Portions of food suitable for the patient's appetite.
6. Food attractively arranged with appropriate garnishes.
7. Hot foods served on warm plates and kept warm with a food cover; cold foods served on chilled dishes.
8. Trays promptly served to the patient so that food is at its best.

THE PATIENT AND HIS MEALS

A pleasant cheerful environment is essential to the greatest enjoyment of food. Before the tray is served the nurse should make every effort to provide surroundings that are clean, orderly, and well ventilated. Activities not associated with meal service should be avoided as far as possible while patients are eating. If an interruption in a meal is unavoidable because of a doctor's visit, or if there is a delay because of a laboratory test, arrangements should be made to keep food hot (or chilled, as the case may be) in a nearby kitchen.

Before the trays arrive the patient's hands should be washed, and if the patient is in bed, he should be positioned so that he is comfortable and able to feed himself. The tray should be checked as soon as it reaches the patient's room to be certain that everything needed is there and is convenient for the patient. Sometimes it is necessary to butter the bread, open food containers, or cut the meat. The patient should be encouraged to eat, but should not be made to feel that he must hurry. Trays should be removed promptly when the patient has finished his meal.

FEEDING THE PATIENT

Acutely ill, handicapped and elderly infirm patients often must be fed. Feeding a patient requires patience and understanding, especially if the patient eats slowly. (See. Fig. 18–2.) If you can imagine how you would want someone fed who is very dear to you, you could probably set up a good guide. Here are some suggestions:

Before starting to feed the patient, make certain that you have everything you need. If the patient eats very slowly, make some arrangement to keep the food hot (or cold). Sit, rather than stand, so that you and the patient will be more comfortable and relaxed. If the patient is blind, give an attractive description of the food you are about to feed him. Offer small amounts of

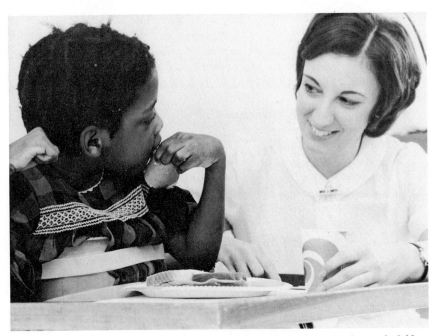

FIGURE 18-2 A nurse provides assistance and encouragement to a handicapped child at mealtime. *(Handicapped Children's Unit, St. Christopher's Hospital for Children, Philadelphia.)*

food at a time, and encourage the patient to chew his food well. Alternate one food with another, as the individual would normally do if he were feeding himself. Offer a beverage as seems indicated or as the patient requests it.

Focus upon the patient, rather than on the feeding process. Avoid giving the impression that the feeding is a bother to you and that you must hurry. Talk to the patient about pleasant things, and also give him a chance to talk. Listen thoughtfully and with interest to what he has to say. Explain the reasons for any change in his diet, and give encouragement when he makes progress.

REVIEW QUESTIONS AND PROBLEMS

1. List some changes that occur in illness and that affect the nutrition of the patient.

2. Keep a record for a few days of the things that annoy you about food service. Also list the comments about food made by your friends and by patients. What reasons can you assign for these complaints? How would you as a nurse help the patient to better acceptance of his diet?

3. What is meant by *diet therapy?* What purposes can be served by diet therapy?

4. Why are the following names for diet undesirable: cardiac diet, Meulengracht diet, ulcer discharge diet, low-salt diet?

5. Prepare a detailed list of ways in which you, as a nurse, can assist the patient with his nutrition.

6. Observe the meals served to patients for whom a house diet has been prescribed. How do they differ from normal diets with which you are familiar? Explain any differences you have noted.

REFERENCES

American Hospital Association: "Statement on a Patient's Bill of Rights," *Hospitals*, 47:41, February 16, 1973.
Butterworth, C. E., and Blackburn, G. L.: "Hospital Malnutrition," *Nutr. Today*, 10:8, March/April 1975.
Chappelle, M. L.: "The Language of Food," *Am. J. Nurs.*, 72:1294–95, 1972.
Dolan, P. O., *et al.:* "Patients' Coffee Hour," *Am. J. Nurs.*, 74:479–80, 1974.
Etzwiler, D. D.: "The Patient Is a Member of the Medical Team," *J. Am. Dietet. A.*, 61:421–23, 1972.
Johnson, C. A.: "The Needs for Better Nutritional Care: Who's Responsible," *J. Am. Dietet. A.*, 67:219–21, 1975.
Luckmann, J., and Sorensen, K. C.: "What Patient's Actions Tell You About Their Feelings, Fears, and Needs," *Nursing 75*, 5:54–61, 1975.
Robinson, C. H.: "Updating Clinical Dietetics: Terminology," *J. Am. Dietet. A.*, 62:645–48, 1973.

NUTRITION EDUCATION AND DIETARY COUNSELING

The focus in this chapter is on the role of the nurse and dietetic technician in dietary counseling as it might take place in the hospital, clinic, or nursing home, usually under the supervision of a dietitian or as an assistant to the dietitian.

Dietary counseling refers to the process whereby an individual is led to modify his diet according to a specific problem presented at a given point in time. The problem might relate to the need to improve a normal diet in order to correct or prevent a dietary deficiency; to modify a diet for a specific disease condition; or to modify a diet to eliminate certain excesses that could increase the risk of some chronic disease.

Nutrition education denotes a body of knowledge that enables the individual to select and maintain a dietary pattern based on principles of nutrition science. In addition to knowledge of nutrition science it takes into consideration the practical applications in terms of food for nutritive adequacy, food costs and preparation, as well as attitudes, beliefs, cultural factors, and emotional meanings the individual holds regarding food.

OPPORTUNITIES FOR NUTRITION EDUCATION

Nutrition education should be available to the healthy and the ill; the school child and teenager, mature adults, and the older person. It can be realized through individual or group discussion on an informal basis; by participation in classroom settings; and through books, magazines, radio, and television. (See Fig. 19–1.)

198

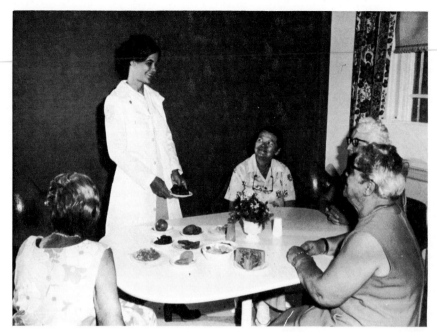

FIGURE 19-1 Dietitians and nurses provide dietary counseling on the essentials of normal nutrition to persons who do not require a modified diet. *(Veterans Administration Medical Center, Bay Pines, Florida.)*

The nurse and dietetic technician share a responsibility with dietitians, physicians, teachers, and others for educating people concerning the essentials of a good diet. For modified diets the dietitian is the person best qualified to give dietary counseling, but she may call upon the nurse or dietetic technician to amplify or to reinforce the counseling. In addition, there are frequent opportunities for informal education while working with patients. Here are a few situations in which information might be given:

Answering questions regarding specific foods on the tray; reasons for the method of preparation, portions, choice

Answering questions about a diet list that the patient has been given; helping the patient to select correct foods from a menu

Helping a patient plan his own menus using a diet list such as the exchange lists

Answering general questions about nutrition that the patient might ask during the day.

There are also opportunities for participation in group discussions; for example:

Discussion-demonstration of the food groups: what they are; what foods are found in each group; what nutrients are contributed by each group

Exchange lists: what foods are included in each group; exercises in planning menus using these lists (low-calorie diet, Chapter 22; calculated diet for diabetic patients, Chapter 23; modified fat diet, Chapter 25). See also Table A-2.
Demonstration on home preparation of baby foods
Exercises in label interpretation
Menu planning in a weight-control program
Preparation of posters and exhibits for group education.

WHAT SHOULD THE CONSUMER KNOW?

To be fully informed regarding the selection of a good diet, the consumer should have knowledge concerning:

The body's use of food: digestion; absorption; functions; interrelationships of nutrients in the body; elimination of wastes
The effect of activity and physical state (growth, pregnancy, ill health) on nutritional needs
Recommended Dietary Allowances; U.S. RDA
The ways in which psychology, emotions, cultural patterns affect food acceptance and intake
The caloric and nutritive value of foods; use of food tables
Food groupings suitable for meal patterns that are nutritionally satisfactory
Food selection for economy and quality; interpretation of labels
Storage and preparation of foods for maximum nutritive values
Sources of information to aid in analysis of published statements on nutrition

SOURCES OF INFORMATION

Your study of nutrition and this text provide you with a background of information that you can use in answering many questions or in discussing nutrition problems. If you are not certain that your information is reliable, don't hesitate to say "I don't know, but I will find out for you" or "I don't know, but I will ask the dietitian to talk with you." Other sources of information that you might also consult are

Books on diet and nutrition in your nursing and medical library
Community or state public health nutritionists
County or state food and nutrition specialists in the Cooperative Extension Service
College teachers of food and nutrition
Home economists in food industry; for example, local dairy council

Essentials of Dietary Counseling

Counseling may take place at the bedside of a patient, in a clinic, or in the home. Regardless of the setting it is essential that privacy be maintained, that interruptions be avoided, and that there be no distracting noise. A patient is more likely to be attentive some time following a meal than he would be when he is hungry or when he has just finished his meal.

Effective counseling takes time. An initial session during which the diet history is obtained requires one-half to one hour. Later sessions might require as little as 15 minutes. For patients in the hospital it is often advantageous to break up the initial counseling into several shorter sessions. In this way the patient is more alert, and also has opportunity to think about the content between sessions and to raise questions.

COUNSELOR-PATIENT RELATIONSHIP

Dietary counseling requires constant interaction between patient and counselor. It is not a one-sided lecture by the counselor telling the patient what to do.

The dietary counselor must be able to interpret the principles of dietary change into practical terms that the patient can understand. She believes that the individual can change his dietary habits, but also realizes that change is likely to occur gradually. She understands the patient's needs and values. She is able to communicate at the level of the person being counseled. She respects the individual's dignity and maintains confidentiality.

The patient is an active participant in the counseling process. He provides the information pertaining to his diet history and food intake; listens to the counselor's evaluation of his food patterns and the reasons why changes are recommended; sets his own goals for what he can realistically accomplish; studies the materials that he is given; and makes notations of questions he needs to ask.

SOME INTERVIEWING TECHNIQUES

Listening thoughtfully to the patient is an important aspect of counseling. As a counselor you should permit the patient to give as much information as possible without too many interruptions. Be aware of his attitudes as well as what he says.

A record of food intake is more reliable if the patient can have some visual reminders of size of portions: measuring spoons, several sizes of glasses and cups, measuring cup, and ruler.

After the patient has had opportunity to describe his food intake, it is usually necessary to follow up with more questions. You should avoid questions that suggest a right answer; for example, "What did you have for breakfast?" and "Did you eat cereal?" suggest that the patient should have eaten breakfast that included cereal. Better: "When did you first eat yesterday?" and "What did you eat at that time?" Usually you will need to obtain specific details concerning kinds of foods, methods of preparation, and amounts; for example,

"What kind of bread?" "How many slices?" "What did you put on the bread?" "How was the meat cooked?" "How much gravy did you use?"

The diet history. An adequate diet history tells the counselor about the patient's food habits and provides the basis for all counseling that follows. The patient's chart gives much information that is pertinent to the diet, and these items should be identified before the initial counseling session:

Age
Weight, height, changes in weight status; desirable weight
Present illness: symptoms, diagnosis, important laboratory findings
Digestion: appetite, chewing, swallowing, nausea, vomiting, distention, cramping
Elimination: normal, constipation, diarrhea
Physical handicaps: lack of teeth, mouth soreness, need for self-help devices
Social relationships: occupation, family, residence, ethnic background, religion
Income: adequacy, need for financial assistance

The aspects of diet that you will need to question the patient about include:

Meal and snacking patterns: when, where, with whom, when skipped; away from home: how often, type of facility
Food preparation: by whom, facilities for shopping, cooking
Previous modified diets: self-prescribed or by physician; how long; why; results
Mineral-vitamin supplements: prescribed by whom; kind
Food likes and dislikes; food allergies
24-hour recall of food intake

When the diet history has been completed the counselor makes an evaluation with the patient. For example, the good characteristics of the present pattern as well as the deficiencies might be compared with the Four Food Groups.

Motivation and goal setting. Without the patient's interest, motivation, and decision making, any efforts by the dietetic-nursing team in counseling will be wasted. Fear of ill health is an important motivating factor for some people; for example, the patient recovering from a heart attack is more likely to stick to a low-calorie modified-fat diet than is a person who appears to be healthy. The pregnant woman is motivated to accept a better diet as something she is doing for the well-being of her baby. The adolescent girl is motivated in terms of her figure, and the boy in terms of vigor for athletics, and so on.

Realistic goals are necessary if diet behavior is to be changed. Losing 50 pounds in 8 months might seem like an endless task, but a goal of "six pounds this month" seems easier to achieve. A child who thoroughly dislikes a food cannot be expected immediately to consume a recommended quantity of that food; a better goal might be one or two bites of the food. The diabetic patient who has not been eating breakfast may have goals related to time of getting up in the morning, or development of menus that have appeal at breakfast time, or others.

Instruction. The patient requires information on a diet plan that has been individualized according to his circumstances; food lists that apply to his diet; how to use the food lists; food selection in the market; reading labels; and details concerning food preparation.

At each point in the instruction the patient should be encouraged to ask questions. Following the counseling session the patient will strengthen his understanding of his diet by writing out menus from food lists; keeping a record of what he eats during the day; reading labels to determine whether a food can be used on a given diet. Such activities should be checked by the counselor for any errors or misunderstanding.

Behavior modification is a process now widely used to change the individual's habits to those that are more desirable. With respect to diet it consists of keeping a detailed record of all behavior related to food and then identifying the changes that must take place. The program requires skilled therapists such as psychologists, dietitians, and nurses; it would not be initiated by dietetic technicians or nurses not trained in these skills.

Follow-up. Successful dietary change almost always requires some follow-up to the initial counseling. Patients should have access by telephone to the dietitian, dietetic technician, or nurse to answer simple questions or to allay fears. Visits to the clinic as necessary help to assure the patient that he is following his diet correctly, to encourage continued adherence to the diet, and to provide opportunity for additional information. Many hospitals provide classes for patients on a given dietary regimen; for example, diabetic patients, or pregnant women, or patients on renal dialysis. Such classes provide a common bond of understanding between patients, as well as furnishing information concerning the dietary regimen.

REVIEW QUESTIONS AND PROBLEMS

1. Develop a form for a diet history. Complete the diet history by interviewing one of your classmates. Evaluate the nutritional adequacy of the diet record.
2. Plan a lesson that you might use in demonstrating how to prepare baby foods in the home.
3. Prepare a poster that shows the food groups for a lacto-ovo-vegetarian diet.
4. How would you respond to these questions or comments of patients:
   a. I am allergic to citrus fruits. What foods could I depend on to get enough vitamin C?
   b. Should I take vitamin pills when I go home?
   c. They forgot to put a salt shaker on my tray.
   d. I've been drinking raw milk because pasteurized milk has lost most of its nutrition.

REFERENCES

American Dietetic Association: "Position Paper on Nutrition Education for the Public," *J. Am. Dietet. A.*, **62:**429–30, 1973.

American Dietetic Association: "Position Paper on the Scope and Thrust of Nutrition Education," *J. Am. Dietet. A.*, **72:**302–305, 1978.

Danish, S. J.: "Developing Helping Relationships in Dietary Counseling," *J. Am. Dietet. A.*, **67:**107–10, 1975.

Myers, M., *et al.:* "Guidelines for Diet Counseling," *J. Am. Dietet. A.*, **66:**571–75, 1975.

Storie, F.: "A Philosophy of Patient Teaching," *Nurs. Outlook*, **19:**378, 1971.

MODIFICATIONS OF THE NORMAL DIET FOR TEXTURE

Normal, Fluid, and Soft Fiber-Restricted Diets

NORMAL DIET AND ITS MODIFICATIONS

The normal, regular, general, or house diet is the most frequently used of all diets. A normal diet, like a modified diet, is of great importance in a therapeutic sense. With satisfactory food intake the body's tissues are continuously maintained, and there is opportunity for repair from the effects of illness. On the other hand, the patient's failure to eat a normal diet could lead to loss of body tissue and a prolonged convalescence.

The normal diet in hospital usage follows the principles outlined in the preceding units, and is planned to provide the Recommended Dietary Allowances. The Four Food Groups offer a convenient basis for menu planning, and diets in this section will be arranged according to these groups. The normal diet in the hospital requires no restrictions upon food choice. Strongly flavored vegetables, fried foods, cakes, pies, pastries, spicy foods, and relishes all have a place on the menu, but they should be used with discretion.

Liquid Diets

CLEAR-FLUID DIET

This is an allowance of tea, coffee or coffee substitute, and fat-free broth. Ginger ale, fruit juices, flavored gelatin, fruit ices, and water gruels are sometimes given. Small amounts of fluid are offered every hour or two to the patient.

205

The diet is used for 24 to 48 hours following acute vomiting, diarrhea, or surgery.

The primary purpose of this diet is to relieve thirst and to help maintain water balance. Broth provides some sodium, and fruit juices contribute potassium. Carbonated beverages, sugar, and fruit juices, when used, furnish a small amount of carbohydrate.

FULL-FLUID DIET

This diet consists of liquids and foods that liquefy at body temperature. It is used for acute infections of short duration and for patients who are too ill to chew. It may be ordered as the first progression from the clear-fluid diet following surgery or in the treatment of acute gastrointestinal upsets.

The diet is offered in six feedings or more. Initially, amounts smaller than those represented by the plan below are given. To increase the caloric intake,

FULL-FLUID DIET

Food Allowance for One Day

6 cups milk
2 eggs (in custards or pasteurized eggnog)
1–2 oz strained meat
1 cup strained citrus juice
½ cup tomato juice
½ cup vegetable purée
½ cup strained cereal
2 servings dessert: soft custard,
    Junket, plain ice cream, sherbert, or
    plain gelatin
2 tablespoons sugar
1 tablespoon butter
Broth, bouillon
Tea, coffee, carbonated beverages
Flavoring extracts, salt

Protein: 85 gm
Calories: 1950

Sample Menu

Breakfast
Grapefruit juice
Strained oatmeal with butter, hot milk, and
    sugar
Milk
Coffee with cream and sugar

Midmorning
Orange juice
Soft custard

Luncheon
Broth with strained beef
Tomato juice
Vanilla ice cream
Milk

Midafternoon
Milk

Dinner
Cream of asparagus soup
Eggnog, commercial, pasteurized
Strawberry gelatin with whipped cream
Tea with lemon and sugar

Bedtime
Chocolate malted milk

TABLE 20–1   FOOD ALLOWANCES AND SAMPLE MENU
FOR SOFT FIBER-RESTRICTED DIET

Food Allowances	Sample Menu *
Beverages—coffee, tea, carbonated	*Breakfast*
Bread—white, fine whole-wheat, rye without seeds; white crackers	Orange sections Oatmeal Milk
Cereal foods—dry (except bran) and well-cooked breakfast cereals; hominy grits, macaroni, noodles, rice, spaghetti	Sugar Whole-wheat toast Butter or margarine
Cheese—mild, soft, such as cottage and cream; Cheddar; Swiss	Coffee with cream, sugar
Desserts—plain cake, cookies; custards; plain gelatin or with allowed fruit; Junket; plain ice cream, ices, sherbets; plain puddings, such as bread, cornstarch, rice, tapioca	*Luncheon* Tomato bouillon Melba toast Salmon loaf Egg sauce
Eggs—all except fried	Asparagus tips Soft roll
Fats—butter, cream, margarine, vegetable oils and fats in cooking	Butter or margarine Golden cake with fluffy white icing
Fruits—raw: ripe avocado, banana, grapefruit or orange sections without membrane; canned or cooked: apples, apricots, fruit cocktail, peaches, pears, plums—all without skins; Royal Anne cherries; strained prunes and other fruits with skins; all juices	Milk; tea, if desired *Dinner* Grapefruit juice Small club steak
Meat—very tender, minced, or ground; baked, broiled, creamed, roast, or stewed: beef, lamb, veal, poultry, fish, bacon, liver, sweetbreads	Baked potato without skin, butter Buttered julienne green beans
Milk—in any form	Dinner roll with butter or margarine
Soups—broth, strained cream or vegetable	Apple crisp Milk
Sweets—all sugars, syrup, jelly, honey, plain sugar candy without fruit or nuts, molasses Use in moderation	Tea or coffee, if desired
Vegetables—white or sweet potato without skin, any way except fried; young and tender asparagus, beets, carrots, peas, pumpkin, squash without seeds; tender chopped greens; strained cooked vegetables if not tender; tomato juice	
Miscellaneous—salt, seasonings and spices in moderation, gravy, cream sauces	

* May be given in six feedings by saving part of the food from the preceding meal.

1 pt light cream may be substituted for 1 pt milk. The protein level of the full-fluid diet may be increased by adding nonfat dry milk to fresh milk, cream soups, cereal gruels, or custards. Strained meats may be added to broth or to hot tomato juice.

Soft Diets

MECHANICAL SOFT DIET

The Mechanical Soft Diet differs from the normal diet only in that it is limited to soft foods for those who have difficulty in chewing because of no teeth or poorly fitting dentures. No restriction is made upon the diet for seasonings or method of food preparation.

The normal diet is modified in the following ways:

1. Meat and poultry are minced or ground; fish usually is sufficiently tender without further treatment.

2. Vegetables are cooked. They may be cooked a little longer than usual to be sure they are soft, and may be diced or chopped.

3. Chopped raw tomatoes and chopped lettuce are sometimes used.

4. Soft raw fruits: banana, citrus sections, berries, grapes, diced soft pear, peach, apple, apricots, melons. All canned and frozen fruits.

5. Soft rolls, bread, and biscuits instead of crisp rolls, crusty breads.

6. All desserts on a normal diet that are soft, including pies with tender crusts, cakes, puddings. Finely chopped nuts and dried fruits.

SOFT FIBER-RESTRICTED DIET

The Soft Fiber-Restricted Diet is a nutritionally adequate diet that differs from the normal diet in being reduced in fiber content and soft in consistency. It is used intermediately between the Full-Fluid Diet and the normal diet following surgery, in acute infections and fevers, and in gastrointestinal disturbances. The food allowances and a sample menu for the Soft Fiber-Restricted Diet is shown in Table 20–1.

REVIEW QUESTIONS AND PROBLEMS

1. What foods are usually allowed on a clear-fluid diet? What nutrients are supplied by this diet? When is it used?

2. Keep a record of the normal diet served to a patient for one day. What changes would you make in this menu so that it would be suitable for a patient who has no teeth?

3. Modify the normal diet recorded for question 2 so that it is suitable for a patient who has an infection, with an order for a soft diet.

4. List four situations when a soft diet might be used.

DIETARY CALCULATIONS WITH

EXCHANGE LISTS

NEED FOR CACULATED DIET

A number of conditions require control of the quantities of one or more constituents of the diet; for example, obesity, diabetes mellitus, hyperlipidemias, and others. A daily calculation for the specific foods of the menu would be extremely time consuming and impractical. As a matter of fact, even the detailed calculation would give only an approximate value for the actual intake because no two samples of the same kind of food are completely identical in their composition. Furthermore, people vary considerably in their metabolism from day to day.

EXCHANGE LISTS

This chapter describes a practical, rapid method for planning diets by using average values for groups of foods. The Exchange Lists for Meal Planning, revised 1976 (Table A-2, p. 345) were prepared by a joint committee of The American Dietetic Association, The American Diabetes Association, and the National Institutes of Health.

An *exchange list* is a grouping of foods in which the carbohydrate, protein, and fat values are about equal for the items listed. The six exchange lists include:

List 1. Nonfat milk is the basis for the milk exchanges. If low-fat or whole milk is used, the adjustment is made by (1) using the fat value stated in the table for the calculation of the diet, or (2) subtracting the designated fat exchanges from the day's total for fat.

List 2. All vegetables except starchy vegetables are included here. Starchy vegetables appear on List 4, Bread Exchanges.

List 3. Fruit exchanges are based on the amounts of fruits or fruit juice that will supply 10 gm carbohydrate. Thus, one may choose for an exchange 1 small apple, or ½ small banana, or ½ cup orange juice, or 2 prunes, etc. (See Fig. 21–1.)

List 4. Bread exchanges include breads, rolls; dry and cooked cereals; starchy vegetables; and some prepared foods. When prepared foods are used, fat exchanges as specified must be subtracted from the day's total. For example, if 2 pancakes are used for 2 bread exchanges, the day's fat allowance would be reduced by 2 exchanges. (See Fig. 21–2.)

List 5. Lean meat is the basis for the meat exchanges. When medium-fat or high-fat meats are used the adjustment is made by (1) calculating for the values of these meats in the development of the diet plan, or (2) subtracting the designated fat exchanges from the day's total for fat. The meat list also includes dried peas and beans and peanut butter. (See Fig. 21–3.)

List 6. Fats high in polyunsaturated fat are listed separately from those high in saturated fat. (See Fig. 21–4.)

METHOD FOR DIETARY CALCULATIONS

The physician, and in some situations the dietitian, prescribes the amounts of carbohydrate, protein, and fat that are to be used in measured diets. Using

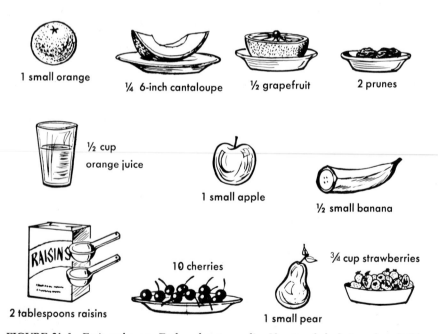

1 small orange

¼ 6-inch cantaloupe   ½ grapefruit   2 prunes

½ cup orange juice

1 small apple

½ small banana

2 tablespoons raisins

10 cherries

1 small pear

¾ cup strawberries

FIGURE 21–1 Fruit exchanges. Each exchange supplies 10 gm carbohydrate and negligible protein and fat. See List 3 in Table A-2 (p. 346) for additional choices.

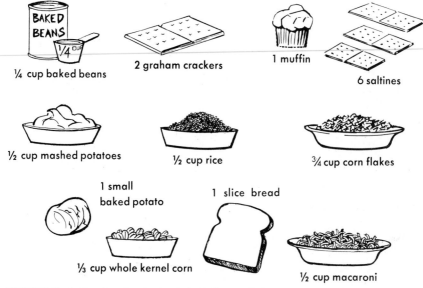

FIGURE 21–2   Bread exchanges. Each food illustrated above yields approximately 15 gm carbohydrate, and 2 gm protein. See List 4 of Table A-2 (p. 347) for additional choices.

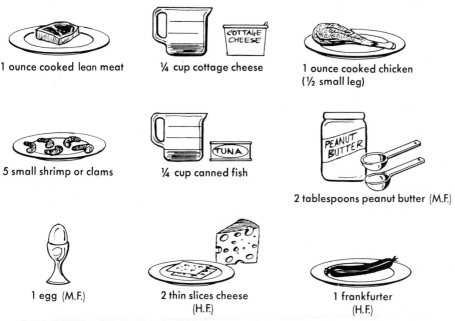

FIGURE 21–3   Meat exchanges. Each exchange provides 7 gm protein. Low-fat exchanges furnish 3 gm fat; medium-fat (M.F.) exchanges 5.5 gm fat, and high-fat (H.F.) exchanges 8 gm fat. About 3 exchanges are used for an average dinner serving of cooked meat; use 4 oz raw, lean meat to equal 3 oz cooked. See List 5 in Table A-2 (p. 348) for additional choices.

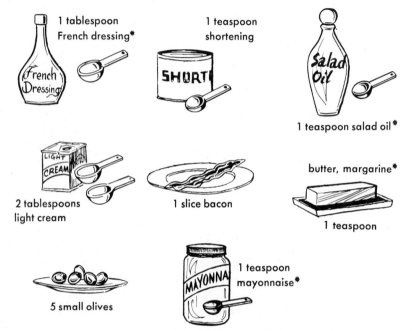

FIGURE 21–4 Fat exchanges. Each of the foods illustrated above provides approximately 5 gm fat per exchange. See List 6 in Table A-2 (p. 350) for additional choices.

*When safflower, corn, cottonseed, or soy oils are used, these are high in polyunsaturated fatty acids. Soft tub or stick margarines made with these oils are also high in polyunsaturated fatty acids.

the values for the exchange lists, the dietitian, dietetic technician, or nurse calculates the number of exchanges to be furnished by the diet.

The steps in diet planning are listed below. A sample calculation in Table 21–1 illustrates the procedure.

1. Become familiar with the patient's usual pattern of meals, the food likes and dislikes, and so on. Whether the patient eats at home, carries lunches, or eats in a restaurant will affect the planning. The amount of money that can be spent, the preparation facilities, and the cultural patterns must be considered.

2. Include basic foods to ensure adequate levels of minerals and vitamins: 2 cups milk (3 or more for children and pregnant or lactating women); two servings vegetables; two servings fruit, including a good source of ascorbic acid; four to five exchanges meat; wholegrain or enriched bread and cereal.

3. List the carbohydrate, protein, and fat values for the milk, vegetables, and fruit.

4. Subtract the carbohydrate value of these foods (74 in the example) from the carbohydrate level prescribed (150 gm). Divide the difference by 15 to determine the number of bread exchanges (5 in the example).

TABLE 21–1   SAMPLE CALCULATION OF DIET
CARBOHYDRATE: 150 GM; PROTEIN: 70 GM; FAT: 70 GM

Exchange List	Number of Exchanges	Carbohydrate gm	Protein gm	Fat gm
Milk, nonfat	2	24	16	—
Vegetables	2	10	4	—
Fruit	4	40	—	—
		(74 *)		
Bread	5	75	10	—
			(30 †)	
Meat, lean	6	—	42	18
				(18 ‡)
Fat	10	—	—	50
Totals for the day		149	72	68

* 150 − 74 = 76 gm carbohydrate to be supplied from bread exchanges
  1 bread exchange = 15 gm carbohydrate
  76 ÷ 15 = 5 bread exchanges
† 70 − 30 = 40 gm protein to be supplied from meat exchanges
  1 meat exchange = 7 gm protein
  40 ÷ 7 = 6 meat exchanges
‡ 70 − 18 = 52 gm fat to be supplied by fat exchanges
  1 fat exchange = 5 gm fat
  52 ÷ 5 = 10 fat exchanges

5. Total the protein values of the milk, vegetables, and bread exchanges (30 in the example). Subtract from the protein prescribed (70). Divide the difference by 7 to determine the number of meat exchanges (6 in the example).

6. Total the fat values for milk and meat (18 in the example) and subtract from the total fat prescribed (70). Divide the difference by 5 to determine the number of fat exchanges (10 in the example).

7. Check the calculations to be certain that they are correct. It is not a good idea to split the bread, fruit, and meat exchanges into half.

8. Divide the total exchanges for the day into meal patterns according to the physician's diet order and the patient's preference. Two sample menus illustrate differing applications of the diet calculated in Table 21–1.

REVIEW QUESTIONS AND PROBLEMS

1. List the foods in the vegetable group that are especially rich in vitamin A and ascorbic acid.

2. Why are some vegetables included in the bread list? List five of them.

3. Plan a breakfast that includes the following exchanges: nonfat milk, 1; fruit, 1; bread, 2; fat, 3.

4. Calculate the carbohydrate, protein, and fat value of the following day's allowance: milk, 2; vegetables, 3; fruit, 3; bread, 4; lean meat, 5; medium-fat meat, 2; fat, 5.

5. Arrange a day's allowance from question 4 into three meals. Write a sample menu for the pattern you have set up.

Two Sample Menus Based on Calculations in Table 21–1

Breakfast
Cantaloupe—¼ small
Wheat flakes—¾ cup
Milk—1 cup skim
Enriched toast—1 slice
Margarine—2 teaspoons

Lunch
Sandwich
 Whole-wheat bread—2 slices
 Sliced chicken—2 ounces
 Mayonnaise—2 teaspoons
 Margarine—2 teaspoons
 Lettuce
Apple—1 small
Milk—1 cup skim

Dinner
Roast lamb, lean—4 ounces
Potato, baked—1 small
Broccoli—1 medium stalk or ½ cup cut
Carrots—½ cup
Margarine—4 teaspoons for potato and vegetables
Pears, water packed—2 halves
Coffee or tea

Snack
Orange—1 small

Breakfast
Prunes—4 medium
Egg, poached—1 *
Toast—2 slices
Margarine—1 teaspoon

Lunch
Salad:
 Tuna fish—½ cup
 Celery—¼ cup
 French dressing—1 tablespoon
 Lettuce
Carrot sticks—½ medium carrot
Plain roll—1
Margarine—1 teaspoon
Strawberries—¾ cup
Milk, 2 per cent—1 cup *

Dinner
Roast loin of pork—3 ounces *
Beets—½ cup
Peas—½ cup
Corn muffin—1 *
Margarine—2 teaspoons for muffin and vegetables
Grapes—12
Coffee or tea

Snack
Milk, 2 per cent—1 cup *

* 1 egg: subtract ½ fat exchange
3 ounces pork loin: subtract 1½ fat exchanges
2 cups 2 per cent milk: subtract 2 fat exchanges
1 corn muffin: subtract 1 fat exchange
Day's fat allowance: 10 exchanges
10–5 = 5 exchanges from fat list

PROBLEMS OF WEIGHT CONTROL

Low- and High-Calorie Diets

HAZARDS OF OVERWEIGHT AND UNDERWEIGHT

Obesity or excessive fatness of the body is a hazard to health. Imagine your reaction if you were told to carry a 25-lb package with you wherever you went! That is exactly what the overweight person must do—10, 25, 50 lb or whatever the excess may be. It goes with him whether he walks upstairs, or ties a shoelace, or tries to hurry for a train. The extra weight makes demands upon his heart, his blood circulation, his back, his feet, and so on. It is no surprise that obese people more often have heart disease and hypertension; they also have gallbladder disease, diabetes, and other chronic diseases more frequently. They face an extra risk if they require surgery. The obese pregnant woman is more likely to have complications than the woman of normal weight.

Underweight, though less emphasized, also presents dangers to health. Underweight persons are more likely to have infections and disturbances of the gastrointestinal tract. Tuberculosis is more frequent among young, underweight people.

FATNESS AND BODY TYPES

Obesity refers to excessive fatness. *Overweight* implies weight above normal that might be explained by increased muscular development, as in the athlete; or it could mean excessive fatness. The terms are often arbitrarily applied as follows: overweight is a condition in which the body weight is 10 to 19 per cent above desirable weight, and obesity is present when the body weight is

215

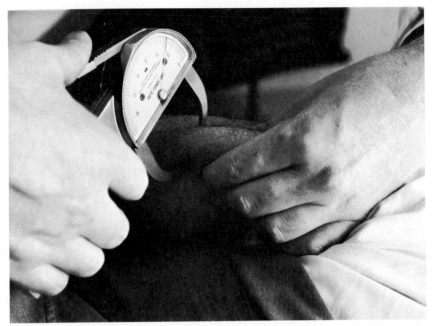

FIGURE 22–1 The degree of body fatness is determined by measuring the thickness of a skinfold with a caliper. *(Roche Medical Image, Hoffman-LaRoche, Inc.)*

20 per cent or more above desirable weight. People who are 15 per cent or more below desirable weight are *underweight.* (See Table A-3, p. 351).

The degree of body fatness may also be determined by measuring the thickness of skin folds of the upper arm or abdomen with a caliper. (See Fig. 22–1.)

Body type seems to be related to obesity. Persons who have the *ectomorphic* body type (thin, angular) seldom become obese, while those who are *endomorphic* (round, soft) are more likely to become obese. Body type is an inherited characteristic, and obesity seems to "run in families." (See Fig. 22–2.)

BALANCING ONE'S WEIGHT

Gaining or losing weight is simply a question of balancing food calories with the body's need for calories. One kilogram of fat is equal to about 7500 kcal. Thus, if you have 500 kcal every day above what your body needs, you will gain about ½ kg (1 lb) in a week. If your intake is 500 kcal below your needs, you will lose about ½ kg in a week.

Let us take another example. Suppose you need 2000 kcal a day, but your daily diet averages 2100 kcal. In 30 days this excess adds up to 3000 kcal. You would gain about 0.4 kg or 0.9 lb in that month (3000 ÷ 7500 = 0.4).

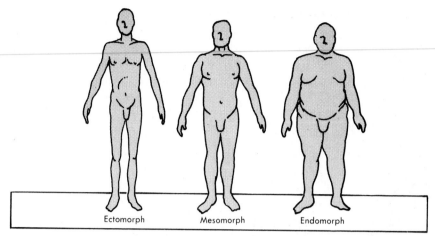

Ectomorph   Mesomorph   Endomorph

FIGURE 22–2   Types of body build.

Perhaps this does not seem like very much gain, but in one year it amounts to 5 kg (11 lb).

To keep in balance you would need to eliminate the surplus calories from your diet. You could also avoid gaining weight by increasing your activity. By walking a mile a day the average adult uses about 100 to 125 calories; so this increase in exercise would help to avoid weight gain.

CAUSES OF OVEREATING AND UNDEREATING

Too often we assume that obese people simply eat tremendous amounts of food. In fact, however, obesity more often results because of the little extras day by day; perhaps an extra pat of butter, a second roll, a snack, a second piece of candy, or a rich dessert each day rather than a low-calorie dessert.

Not all obese people eat more than normal-weight people. Several recent studies have shown that many obese boys and girls actually eat less than normal-weight boys and girls. However, they were found to be much less active. Failure to get enough exercise meant that their diets, which seemed quite normal, furnished too many calories for them. Likewise, many adults probably do not eat large amounts of food, but they are so inactive that their intakes are excessive for them.

The list on page 218 presents some of the factors that might be responsible for failing to balance one's calories with body weight.

PREVENTION OF OBESITY

To avoid obesity one must first understand fully the reasons for excessive calorie intake as described in the preceding section. But there must also be the will to take prompt measures when the first few extra pounds appear. It

Some Reasons for Calorie Intake in Excess of Needs	*Some Reasons for Inadequate Calorie Intake*
1. Family patterns of rich, high-calorie foods; mother often has reputation of being a good cook	1. Family pattern places emphasis upon low-calorie foods; few rich desserts, for example
2. Good appetite; likes to eat; likes many rich foods; may dislike fruits and vegetables	2. Small appetite; has little interest in eating; has many dislikes; unpalatable therapeutic diets
3. Ignorance of calorie value of foods	3. Ignorance of essentials of an adequate diet
4. Skips breakfast; is a frequent nibbler; coffee breaks with high-calorie snacks	4. Skips meals; seldom makes up for skipped meals; rarely nibbles

5. Pattern of living
  a. Sedentary occupation; idleness
  b. Riding to work or school
  c. Little exercise during leisure
  d. Often sleeps more as he becomes older.
	5. Pattern of living
	  a. Often tense
	  b. Overactive
	  c. Not enough sleep and rest

6. Emotional outlet: eats to overcome worry, boredom, loneliness, grief	6. Emotional outlet: unhappy, worried, grieving, but refuses to eat
7. Many social events with rich foods; frequent eating in restaurants	7. Often lives alone; misses sociability; doesn't like to eat alone
8. Lower metabolism with increasing age, but failure to reduce intake	8. Illness and infection; fever, diarrhea; hyperthyroidism
9. Influenced by pressures of advertising for many high-calorie foods	9. Affected by claims for fad diets; may get inadequate diet

is much easier to prevent obesity than to treat it. Prevention is most effective when patterns of diet and exercise are established early in life. Mothers need to know that the fat baby is not necessarily the healthiest baby, and that they should not force the infant to eat every last bit of food. The early introduction of cereal and other baby foods before the baby really needs them could contribute to overweight babies. Preschool children should not be bribed or rewarded with food; they should have a variety of activities so that they do not depend too much upon food for pleasure.

In families where one or both parents are obese, children are very likely to become obese and remain so throughout life. This can be prevented by changing the eating patterns so that fewer calorie-rich foods are eaten. Use fruits for desserts often and cakes, pies, or pastries seldom; broil, stew, or roast meats instead of frying; put less butter and cream on vegetables and learn to use other flavorings.

Children should be urged to get more exercise and should be expected to perform some chores requiring daily physical activity. Family recreation needs to include more participation in physical activity and somewhat less of the quiet pastimes such as watching television and riding about in automobiles.

Diets for Obesity

PLANNING FOR WEIGHT LOSS

Any program of weight loss of more than a few pounds should be directed by a physician. If a weight-losing program is to be successful, the individual must be convinced of the rewards that will come: better health, a slimmer figure, more pep, and perhaps a longer life. Although a low-calorie diet is used only so long as weight needs to be lost, each obese person must be convinced that he needs to modify his lifetime eating habits. If he fails to do this, he will gain back all the pounds he has lost.

It is important to set a reasonable goal. A weekly weight loss of ½ to 1 kg (1 to 2 lb) is better than a crash program that leaves one tired and unwilling to continue. If one needs to lose 25 kg (55 lb), six to nine months is not an unreasonable time allowance.

Keeping a weekly weight chart is a good idea. The person should weigh at the same time every week on the same scale and with the same amount of clothing. He needs to know that the scales might not show any weight loss for the first week or two because, in some instances, water is temporarily held in the tissues when people are placed on reducing diets. After a while this water will be released from the tissues, and the weight loss will show up.

Exercise has its place in a weight-reduction program. Walking is one of the best exercises. People can walk a few extra blocks to work or make it a practice to see a little more of the outdoors on foot rather than from an automobile window. Moderate exercise does not increase the appetite as some claim. For very obese persons, or those who have been ill, the recommendation for exercise by the physician should be followed closely. It is never a good idea for a person who has been sedentary to suddenly engage in violent exercise.

THE LOW-CALORIE DIET

Women usually lose satisfactorily on diets restricted to 1000 to 1500 kcal, whereas men lose satisfactorily on diets furnishing 1200 to 1800 kcal. Bed patients, such as those with heart disease, are often placed on diets restricted to 800 to 1000 kcal, and sometimes less.

The daily food allowances for the 1000-, 1200-, and 1500-kcal diets are somewhat higher in protein. (See Table 22–1.) This is desirable, because it provides most people with a feeling of satisfaction. Also, it helps to correct the greater losses of muscle tissue that occur during reducing. No matter how

TABLE 22–1   LOW-CALORIE DIETS BASED ON FOOD EXCHANGE LISTS *

	1000 kcal	1200 kcal	1500 kcal
		number of exchanges	
Milk, nonfat	2	2	3
Vegetables	2	2	2
Fruit	3	3	4
Bread	2	3	4
Meat, lean	8	9	9
Fat	2	4	4
Protein, gm	80	89	99
Fat, gm	34	47	57
Carbohydrate, gm	94	109	146
Energy, kcal	1002	1215	1493

* Choices from the Exchange Lists are given in Table A-2 (p. 345)

carefully they are planned, diets that provide less than 2000 kcal daily may not meet the recommended allowances for iron, zinc, magnesium, and for vitamin E and folacin. This does not mean that nutritional deficiency will necessarily occur in the individual. It is not a problem except where a diet is to be used for several months. Then a multivitamin-mineral supplement may be prescribed.

The exchange lists are used for planning the daily food choices for low-calorie diets. Usually the food allowances are divided into three approximately equal meals. Skipping breakfast is not a good idea. Some people prefer to have a midafternoon or bedtime snack, and these may be included by saving some milk or fruit from the meal. Of course, tea or coffee without cream or sugar, and bouillon may also be used.

Meals on a low-calorie diet should be attractive and palatable. Herbs and spices may be used to lend variety to vegetables and meat preparation. Meats, fish, and poultry should be lean, and prepared by broiling, roasting, or stewing. Fresh fruits or canned unsweetened fruits are used. Vegetables may be used in salads for variety in texture and flavor, and add bulk to the diet. Low-calorie salad dressings are available commercially or may be prepared at home. Labels must be read to determine the fat and caloric equivalent. Mineral oil should never be used in salad dressings or other food preparation since the oil will reduce the absorption of fat-soluble vitamins.

Low-calorie diets do not include sweetened carbonated beverages, cakes, cookies, candy, fried foods, sweetened fruits, pastries, pies, potato chips, pretzels, puddings, and so on. Occasionally the physician may permit an alcoholic beverage in limited amounts in place of a bread exchange. Persons on low-calorie diets need to be especially conscious of the little extras often added to the diet, such as a teaspoon of butter, a tablespoon of cream, or a little gravy. Of course,

TABLE 22–2 SAMPLE MENUS FOR LOW- AND HIGH-CALORIE DIETS

1200-kcal Diet	High-Calorie Diet (3000–3200 kcal)
Breakfast	
Half grapefruit	Half grapefruit
Poached egg—1	Dry cereal—1 cup
Rye toast—1 slice	Milk, whole—1 cup
Margarine or butter—1 teaspoon	Poached egg—1
Coffee—no cream or sugar	Rye toast—1 slice
	Margarine or butter—2 teaspoons
	Sugar for cereal and coffee—2 teaspoons
	Cream for coffee—2 tablespoons
Luncheon	
Salad plate:	Cream of mushroom soup—1 cup
Whole tomato stuffed with	Saltines—2
Salmon—3 ounces	Salad plate:
Diced celery—2 tablespoons	Whole stuffed tomato with
French dressing—1 tablespoon	Salmon—3 ounces
Lettuce	Diced celery
Roll, plain—1	French dressing—1 tablespoon
Milk, skim—1 cup	Lettuce
Plums, unsweetened—2	Roll, plain—1
	Margarine or butter—2 teaspoons
	Jelly—1 tablespoon
	Milk, whole—1 cup
	Plums in syrup—2
	Sugar cookie—1
Dinner	
Sautéed veal cutlet with thyme and lemon (use 2 fat exchanges for sautéeing)—4 ounces	Sautéed veal cutlet with thyme and lemon
Corn—⅓ cup	Mashed potato—½ cup
Asparagus spears—3	Asparagus spears
Milk, skim—1 cup	Dinner roll—1 plain
Tea with lemon	Margarine or butter—3 teaspoons for vegetables and roll
	Milk, whole—1 cup
	Cherry pie
Evening snack	
Cherries—10 large	Chicken sandwich:
Cheese, low fat—1 ounce	Bread—2 slices
	Mayonnaise—2 teaspoons
	Chicken—1½ to 2 ounces
	Milk, whole—1 cup

even occasionally eating a piece of pie or cake will wreck the efforts that may have been made toward dieting all day!

A sample menu for a 1200-kcal diet is shown in Table 22–2.

BEHAVIORAL MODIFICATION

Behavioral modification is a technique in which learned eating behaviors are changed. Physicians, dietitians, nurses, or psychologists trained in the technique of behavioral modification provide the guidance for individuals or groups. To begin such a program the individual keeps a daily record of when he eats, where he eats, the social situation while eating (alone, with family, with friends, etc.), the activities associated with eating (studying, watching TV, picnic, etc.), the mood at the time of eating, the kinds and amounts of foods eaten, and so on.

The completed records are analyzed by the counselor to see what behaviors require modification. For example, to the person who eats when he is bored some suggestions for activity are given to take the place of eating. The person who eats too rapidly may be told to put his fork down with each bite, to chew each mouthful more completely, and to swallow the food before taking the next bite. The individual who eats in front of TV or while reading in the living room might change his behavior by always eating only when he sits down at the table. None of these changes can be imposed on the individual. Rather, the person must see the possibilities and then act upon them.

Reinforcement is important. This is brought about by scheduled appointments with the counselor. Sometimes one can set up a contract, that is, the individual earns "points" for observing changes in behavior. The points are then exchanged for something the person very much desires.

SURGERY

In persons who are massively obese (350 lb or so) and in whom the obesity is life-threatening, surgery is sometimes performed in which the jejunum is attached to about 10 cm of terminal ileum, thus "bypassing" most of the ileum. As a result, far fewer calories and nutrients are absorbed and weight is lost. There are many problems associated with such surgery: severe diarrhea, decreased absorption of vitamins, and imbalances of potassium, magnesium, and other mineral elements in the blood circulation.

FAD DIETS

People who are overweight do not always remember that they did not become so in just a few days, and yet they often expect to return to normal weight in a short time. They are frequently misled by advertising as well as articles in magazines or newspapers that promise spectacular losses in a few days; for example, "Lose 9 pounds in 9 days." Some fad diets do not supply the protein, minerals, and vitamins needed by the person who is reducing. As a result, such diets lead to weakness and ill health if they are used for a long time. Other fad diets are based upon bizarre food combinations or unusual proportions of carbohydrate, fat, and protein. No specific food or combination of foods has any special ability to increase the rate of weight loss, nor does the proportion of carbohydrate to fat or protein make any difference. Among the fad diets that come and go, and that are *not* recommended, are the nine-day diet; the grapefruit diet; the meat and fat diet, also known as the high-protein, high-fat, low-carbohydrate diet; liquid protein diet; powdered protein diet; the "Air Force" diet (the U.S. Air Force did *not* recommend this diet); the "Mayo" or egg diet (the Mayo Clinic did *not* subscribe to this diet); the grape juice diet; banana-skim milk diet, and many others.

Formula diets as liquids or as diet bars are widely used and people often ask about their value. Usually they include the nutritional essentials for which recommended allowances have been established; they are convenient to use; and they take away the problems of dietary planning. An important disadvantage is that they do not retrain the individual to a new pattern of eating once the weight has been lost. If used exclusively, the formula diets provide little bulk, and constipation may be a problem. Formula diets are probably most useful for individuals who substitute them for one meal a day and who need to lose only a few pounds.

Reducing candies and pills of various kinds have no place in the reducing program. They are a waste of money and may be dangerous. Some pills cause diarrhea and increased excretion of water by the kidney—a temporary weight loss that is soon replaced; it is fat, not water, that one should lose. Other pills lead to overactivity of the thyroid, increase in metabolism, and increase in heart rate; the results could be disastrous. Obesity is rarely caused by endocrine disturbances.

Diet for Underweight

INDICATIONS FOR HIGH-CALORIE DIET

Long illness not infrequently leads to much weight loss because of nausea, lack of appetite, and inability to eat. In some individuals vomiting and diarrhea lead to failure to absorb all nutrients, so that weight loss and undernutrition become severe. Moreover, the individual with an upset gastrointestinal tract is often so uncomfortable that he is reluctant to eat.

Other patients with a high fever lose much weight, because each degree Fahrenheit rise in body temperature increases the rate of metabolism by about 7 per cent. Thus a temperature of 102° or 103° would considerably increase the calorie needs. Occasionally, an individual has a very high metabolic rate because of an overactive thyroid. Although hyperthyroidism is usually treated by drugs or surgery, many individuals have lost much weight before they sought medical advice.

THE HIGH-CALORIE DIET

About 500 kcal daily above the normal caloric requirements are needed in order to gain 0.4 kg (1 lb) per week. Ordinarily, a 3000- to 3500-kilocalorie diet is considered to be high in calories for the adult. In some cases of marked weight loss and greatly increased metabolism, 4000 to 4500 kcal are indicated. A sample menu for a high-calorie diet is shown in Table 22–2. Note that the menu items used in the low- and high-calorie diets were, for the most part, the same. The increase in calories was brought about by substituting a high-calorie dessert and adding butter, sugar, jelly, bread, soup, and so on.

Weight loss is often accompanied by loss of protein tissue as well as fat tissue. Therefore it is necessary to provide a liberal protein allowance—usually 100 gm per day. When the undernutrition is severe, the physician may prescribe supplements to correct vitamin and mineral deficiencies.

Weight gain for some people is just as difficult as weight loss is for others. Usually the person who requires 3000 kcal will be found to be consuming only half as many calories. To suddenly place before him a tray loaded with food can only result in further loss of appetite and reluctance to eat. The high-calorie diet, then, must begin with the patient's present intake. Perhaps some changes are first made to a menu selection that is somewhat higher in calories but that does not contain much extra bulk. The increase in the amount of food is usually achieved gradually.

All the following foods rapidly increase the calorie content of the diet: light or coffee cream on fruit or on cereal, sour cream for baked potato or in salad dressings, whipping cream, half milk and half cream, ice cream; butter, margarine, mayonnaise, and other salad dressings; jelly, jam, marmalade, honey, sugar, candy; cake, cookies, puddings, pie, and pastry.

Many persons find an excess of fats or sugars to be nauseating, so it is important that the above foods be used with care. On the other hand, one should avoid filling up the patient on too many bulky low-calorie foods, such as vegetables and fruits.

Three meals a day plus a bedtime snack are, as a rule, preferable to three meals plus midmorning and midafternoon feedings. Often the between-meal feedings take the edge off the appetite, so that the meals are less well eaten. However, such quickly digested and absorbed foods as fruit juice with crackers and cookies increase the calorie intake without interfering with the appetite. Three examples of calorie-rich bedtime snacks follow.

Chicken salad sandwich	Chocolate milk shake	Strawberry ice cream
Milk	Oatmeal raisin cookies	Angel food cake

REVIEW QUESTIONS AND PROBLEMS

1. What are the effects of obesity on health?

2. A patient is 12 kg (26 lb) overweight. If he needs 1800 kcal a day but eats a diet that provides 1200 kcal a day, how long would it take him to lose this weight?

3. List eight factors in the American way of life that make it easy to gain weight.

4. Plan menus for three days for a man on a 1500-kilocalorie diet, using the food allowances in Table 22–1.

5. Visit a supermarket and make a list of five products that are claimed to be low in calories. Read the label information. What conclusions do you reach?

6. If a person eats all his meals in a restaurant, what are some suggestions you could give him so that he does not gain weight?

7. Plan five bedtime snacks for a person who is trying to gain weight. Be certain these snacks also provide a good supply of nutrients.

8. Discuss ways by which you might improve the food intake of a patient who has a very poor appetite and for whom a high-calorie diet has been ordered.

REFERENCES

American Dietetic Association: "Statement on Diet Protein Products," *J. Am. Dietet. A.,* 73:547–48, 1978.

D'Augelli, A. R., and Smiciklas-Wright, H.: "The Case for Primary Prevention of Overweight through the Family," *J. Nutr. Educ.,* 10:76–78, 1978.

Evans, R. I., and Hall, Y.: "Social-Psychologic Perspective in Motivating Changes in Eating Behavior," *J. Am. Dietet. A.,* 72:378–83, 1978.

Felig, P.: "Four Questions about Protein Diets," *N. Engl. J. Med.,* 298:1025–26, 1978.

Heydman, A. H.: "Intestinal Bypass for Obesity," *Am. J. Nurs.,* 74:1102–1104, 1974.

Mahoney, M. J., and Caggiula, A. W.: "Applying Behavioral Methods to Nutritional Counseling," *J. Am. Dietet. A.,* 72:372–77, 1978.

Mayer, J.: "Should You Starve Yourself Thin?" *Family Health,* 9:24–26, February 1977.

Michiel, R. R., *et al.:* "Sudden Death in a Patient on a Liquid Protein Diet," *N. Engl. J. Med.,* 298:1005–1007, 1978.

Schanche, D. A.: "Diet Books That Poison Your Mind . . . and Harm Your Body," *Today's Health,* 52:56–61, 1974.

VanItallie, T. B., and Yang, M-U.: "Current Concepts in Nutrition. Diet and Weight Loss," *N. Engl. J. Med.,* 297:1158–61, 1977.

Winckler, I.: "Nutrition Today. This Slimming Business," *Nurs. Times,* 72:1968–69, 1976.

23

DIABETES MELLITUS

Diet Controlled for Carbohydrate, Protein, and Fat

Diabetes mellitus is a metabolic disease that affects the endocrine system of the body and the use of carbohydrate, fat, and protein. Specifically, there is not enough insulin available for the body's needs. In some patients the islands of Langerhans of the pancreas do not produce enough insulin; in others the pancreas requires some stimulation to manufacture enough insulin; and in still others the insulin that is produced cannot, for some reason, be used by the tissues.

INCIDENCE

About 10 million persons in the United States have diabetes, although almost half of them are unaware that they are diabetic. Persons who have a family history of diabetes and who are overweight are more likely to have diabetes. It has been estimated that there are as many as 50 million persons who are diabetic carriers. Obviously, the campaigns to detect diabetes in the population should be vigorously supported. Two types of diabetes are recognized.

Non-insulin dependent diabetes, also known as *maturity-onset* or *adult-type* diabetes, accounts for most patients with the disease. About 80 per cent of all diabetics are 40 years of age or over. Of this group at least 90 per cent are obese. The disease is usually mild, stable, and can be regulated by diet alone or by diet and oral compounds. Complications are likely to develop if weight is not lost or hyperglycemia persists. These patients seldom have ketosis.

Insulin-dependent diabetes, also referred to as *juvenile diabetes,* accounts for about 20 per cent of all known cases of diabetes. The onset is sudden in children or young adults. The disease is also seen in adults of any age who are of normal weight or underweight. This type of diabetes is often severe, requires insulin and diet regulation to sustain life. There may be wide fluctuations between hypoglycemia and ketosis. Vascular changes are present in most patients and life expectancy is shortened.

SYMPTOMS AND LABORATORY FINDINGS

Diabetes in adults is often so mild that it is detected only by blood and urine tests. Children and adults with insulin-dependent diabetes show many of the symptoms described below.

Because the blood glucose cannot be used by the tissues, the level of sugar in the blood rises (hyperglycemia). After a night's fast the blood sugar remains above the normal level (70 to 120 mg per 100 ml). If a *glucose tolerance test* is made the diabetic patient shows a curve that begins at a higher level and stays higher than the curve for a normal person. The curve comes down slowly for the diabetic person, but sharply for the normal person. (See Fig. 23–1.)

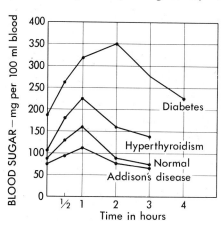

FIGURE 23–1 **The glucose tolerance test shows differences in various disorders of carbohydrate metabolism.**

When the blood sugar exceeds the renal threshold (180 mg per 100 ml), some sugar is excreted in the urine (glycosuria). To excrete the sugar, water is taken from the tissues. Thus, the patient complains of frequent urination (polyuria) and increased thirst (polydipsia). The appetite is often increased (polyphagia) because the patient is not fully utilizing the food he normally eats.

When the body is unable to use carbohydrate, it oxidizes more and more fat to supply energy. The liver breaks down the fatty acids to ketones (acetone, beta-hydroxybutyric acid, acetoacetic acid). Normally, the ketones are further broken down to yield energy and the end products carbon dioxide and water. However, in diabetes the breakdown of fatty acids is more rapid than the body can care for. Some of the ketones are excreted in the urine (ketonuria, acetonuria). The ketones are acid products. When they accumulate in the blood the pH of the blood is lowered; the patient then has symptoms of acidosis or diabetic coma.

In addition to the symptoms described above, patients often complain of poor healing of cuts and scratches; boils; itching; cold feet; numbness and tingling of the extremities; and blurring of vision. Cardiovascular disease, renal diseases, and blindness are complications in patients who have had diabetes for many years.

ESSENTIALS OF TREATMENT

The goals of treatment are (1) to relieve symptoms; (2) to enable the patient to lead a normal life; and (3) to prevent or delay the onset of complications. The following are crucial requirements if these goals are to be met: (1) maintenance of normal weight; (2) regular spacing of meals; (3) normal nutritional requirements with normal proportions of carbohydrate, fat, and protein; (4) usually restriction of cholesterol and modification of the type of fat; (5) use of oral compounds or insulin, if not controlled by diet alone; (6) regulation of physical activity; and (7) attention to body hygiene. For children two additional requirements are maintenance of normal rate of growth and emotional well-being.

THE DIET PRESCRIPTION

Energy. Weight control is the single most important objective of dietary management. An overweight patient is initially placed on a diet that permits a loss of ¾ to 1 kg (1½ to 2 lb) each week. From 1000 to 1200 kcal is suitable for obese women and 1200 to 1500 kcal for obese men. The diets described on p. 345 are suitable without further calculations of the diet for protein, fat, and carbohydrate.

Individuals of normal weight are given sufficient calories to maintain weight:

In bed	25 kcal per kg (11 kcal per lb)
Sedentary	30 kcal per kg (14 kcal per lb)
Moderately active	35 kcal per kg (16 kcal per lb)

Protein. About 15 to 20 per cent of total calories are provided by protein. This corresponds to about 1 to 1.5 gm per kg body weight, an allowance that is typical of American diets.

Carbohydrate. Approximately 50 to 55 per cent of calories are furnished by carbohydrate. Severe restriction of carbohydrate is no longer recommended. Diets that provide more liberal intake of carbohydrate do not proportionately increase the hyperglycemia or the need for insulin or oral compounds.

Fat. The remaining calories (30 to 35 per cent) are furnished by fat. Most physicians recommend that saturated fats should be kept at a minimum (about 10 per cent of total calories) and that polyunsaturated fats should be increased to at least 10 per cent of total calories. Cholesterol is preferably restricted to 300 mg daily. These limitations on the kinds and amounts of fat are intended to maintain blood cholesterol levels at a lower level and thus to prevent or delay the onset of cardiovascular complications.

Let us suppose that a diet is being planned for a sedentary individual weighing 60 kg who needs 1800 kcal.

$$0.20 \times 1800 \text{ kcal} = 360 \text{ kcal from protein}$$
$$360 \div 4 = 90 \text{ gm protein}$$

$$0.50 \times 1800 \text{ kcal} = 900 \text{ kcal from carbohydrate}$$
$$900 \text{ kcal} \div 4 = 225 \text{ gm carbohydrate}$$

$$0.30 \times 1800 \text{ kcal} = 540 \text{ kcal from fat}$$
$$540 \div 9 = 60 \text{ gm fat}$$

DIETARY PLANNING

The patient's economic status, time and place for meals, food preparation facilities, and cultural and religious preferences must be considered when planning the daily meals. Since the type of fat is modified, food selection from the exchange lists is restricted to skim milk and skim-milk products, low-fat meat, and fats high in polyunsaturated fatty acids. Most of the carbohydrate is derived from the bread exchanges that furnish complex carbohydrate which are more gradually digested and absorbed. Simple sugars are restricted to those present in milk, vegetables, and fruits; other sugars are avoided since they are digested and absorbed so rapidly that hyperglycemia occurs. One way in which the prescription calculated above might be calculated using the exchange lists is shown in Table 23–1.

TABLE 23–1   SAMPLE CALCULATION FOR DIET: CARBOHYDRATE, 225 GM; PROTEIN, 90 GM; FAT, 60 GM

	Exchanges	Carbohydrate gm	Protein gm	Fat gm
Milk, nonfat	2	24	16	—
Vegetables	2	10	4	—
Fruit	4	40	—	—
		(74)		
Bread	10	150	20	—
			(40)	
Meat, lean	7	—	49	21
Fat	8	—	—	40
Totals		224	89	61

Meal distribution of carbohydrate. The division of carbohydrate at meal-time depends upon whether the patient is taking insulin or not, and the results of tests for sugar in the urine. For example, the 225 gm of carbohydrate in the calculation on p. 229 might be divided as follows:

Breakfast	Lunch	Dinner	Bedtime	
75 (1/3)	75 (1/3)	75 (1/3)		No insulin; without or with oral compounds
45 (2/10)	68 (3/10)	67 (3/10)	45 (2/10)	With insulin

FOOD PREPARATION AND SERVICE

All foods for the diet are measured according to the amounts in the exchange lists. Level measures with standard measuring cups and spoons are used. When purchasing meat, for 3 oz of cooked meat allow:

4 oz raw lean meat or fish, if there is no waste;
5 oz raw meat, fish, or poultry, if there is a small amount of bone or fat to be trimmed off;
6 oz raw meat, fish, or poultry, if there is much waste.

Foods are prepared using only those allowed on the meal pattern. No extra flour, bread crumbs, butter, or other foods may be used. Many recipes are available from diabetic cookbooks and can be adapted to the patient's prescription.

Meats may be broiled, baked, roasted, or stewed. If they are fried, some of the fat allowance must be used.

Water-packed fruits (canned without sugar) are available in most food markets and may be used according to the exchange lists. Frozen or canned fruits packed with sugar must be avoided. It is important to read labels carefully. (See Fig. 23–2.)

Snacks are permitted only if they are calculated in the diet plan. They are necessary with the long-acting insulins. The patient may have coffee, tea, fat-free broth, unsweetened gelatin, chicory, Chinese cabbage, endive, escarole, lettuce, parsley, radishes, and watercress without calculating them.

Each patient's tray is a teaching aid. The patient should be instructed to become visually accustomed to the size of portions. He should learn to relate the specific foods on his tray to the exchange lists.

As a nurse you should consistently check the patient's tray after each meal to know how well he is eating. If he is taking insulin and refuses food, an arrangement is made for a substitution so that he will not go into insulin shock.

```
DIETETIC PEACHES

Nutritional Information per ½ cup serving

Calories                40
Protein                  1    gm
Carbohydrate            14    gm
Fat                      0    gm
Sodium                 3.5    mg
(Less than 2.7 in 100 gm)


Percentage of U.S. Recommended Daily Allowances (U.S.R.D.A.)

Protein                  *
Vitamin A                4
Vitamin C                2
Thiamin                  *
Riboflavin               *
Niacin                   4
Calcium                  *
Iron                     *


*Contains less than 2% of U.S.R.D.A. of these nutrients

        Ingredients: Peaches, Pear, Apple, and
                Grape Juices from Concentrates
```

FIGURE 23–2   Foods intended for use in therapeutic diets must be labeled with information concerning nutritive values.

A typical meal pattern and sample menu for the diet calculated on p. 229 is shown in Table 23–2. Note that the pattern provides three meals of approximately equal carbohydrate value plus a bedtime meal.

INSULIN AND ORAL COMPOUNDS

Patients with insulin-dependent diabetes always require insulin. The kind and amount of insulin are determined by the physician. Intermediate-acting insulin (NPH, globin, lente) is widely used. It reaches peak activity in 9 hours and activity extends over 24 hours. It is often used in combination with a short-acting insulin (regular, crystalline) which has a peak activity in 3 to 4 hours, and a duration of 6 to 8 hours. Long-acting insulins (PZI—protamine zinc, and lente) are used less frequently. Insulin must be given by injection because it would be digested and made inactive if given by mouth. (See Fig. 23–3.)

TABLE 23–2   TYPICAL MEAL PATTERN AND SAMPLE MENU *

Meal Pattern	Exchanges	Carbohydrate gm	Sample Menu
Breakfast			
Fruit	1	10	Sliced orange—1 small
Bread	3	45	Bran flakes—½ cup
			Whole-wheat toast—2 slices
Milk, nonfat	1	12	Nonfat milk—1 cup
Fat	2	—	Soft-type margarine—2 teaspoons
Coffee or tea		—	
		67	
Luncheon			
Meat	3	—	Turkey sandwich:
Bread	3	45	bread—3 slices
			turkey—3 ounces
Fat	3	—	mayonnaise or margarine—3 teaspoons
			lettuce
Fruit	2	20	Banana—1 small
		65	
Dinner			
Meat, lean	4	—	Beef tenderloin—4 ounces
Vegetable	2	10	Tossed green salad
			Broiled tomato; zucchini squash
Bread	3	45	Mashed potato—½ cup
			Plain roll—2
Fruit	1	10	Peach—1 medium
Fat	3	—	French dressing—1 tablespoon
			Margarine—2 teaspoons
		65	
Snack			
Nonfat milk	1	12	Nonfat milk—1 cup
Bread	1	15	Graham crackers—1
		27	

* Carbohydrate distribution for patient not taking insulin who desires an evening snack. Also appropriate for patient with intermediate-acting insulin plus regular insulin before breakfast.

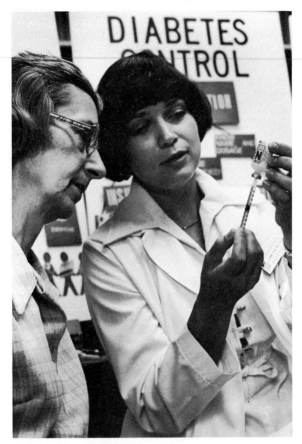

FIGURE 23-3 Patients with diabetes mellitus require counseling regarding (1) techniques of insulin administration or use of oral compounds, (2) diet, (3) general hygiene, and (4) complications of the disease. *(Metropolitan Medical Center, Minneapolis and Jeffrey Grosscup, photojournalist.)*

Patients with insulin-resistant diabetes can almost always be managed successfully with diet alone, or with diet and oral compounds. These compounds are not insulin, but sulfonylureas including tolbutamide (Orinase), tolazamide (Tolinase), chlorpropamide (Diabinese), and acetohexamide (Dymelor). Their action is to stimulate the pancreas to produce insulin.

INSULIN SHOCK

Insulin shock is the effect of too much insulin. It occurs because the patient has failed to eat some of his food; he has increased his activity; or he has a gastrointestinal upset so that the nutrients are not being normally absorbed.

The symptoms of insulin shock result from the marked lowering of the blood glucose. The patient becomes weak, nervous, pale, and hungry. He trembles, perspires, complains of headache, and may become irrational in behavior as if intoxicated. If he is not given carbohydrate promptly he becomes drowsy, disoriented, and eventually unconscious. Prolonged hypoglycemia is damaging to the brain cells because glucose is the only form of energy used by nervous tissue.

Patients who take insulin should always carry some lump sugar or hard candy in case they feel the signs of a reaction. Orange juice or other fruit juice or tea with sugar may be given to the patient who has signs of insulin shock. When the patient is unconscious glucose is given intravenously.

DIABETIC COMA (ACIDOSIS)

Diabetic coma is caused by inadequate insulin to meet body needs. The patient may have failed to follow his diet, or to take the prescribed insulin, or may have an infection.

When the insulin supply to the body is inadequate, the blood sugar rises and glycosuria occurs. A rapid increase of incompletely metabolized fatty acids in the blood leads to a low blood pH. The patient may complain of thirst, headache, frequent urination, fatigue, and drowsiness. His face becomes red, his skin is hot and dry, and his breath has a sweetish (acetone) odor. Nausea and vomiting sometimes occur. The respirations become rapid and the pulse is fast. Finally, the patient lapses into unconsciousness.

Immediate medical attention is required for the patient who goes into diabetic coma. Treatment includes insulin and fluid therapy.

SOME FALLACIES AND FACTS

1. *Fallacy.* A patient who has an infection and who is eating poorly should stop taking his insulin.

Fact. The insulin requirement is usually higher in fevers and infections. The patient should take his insulin and take fluids supplying carbohydrate if he cannot eat solid foods. He should continue to test his urine, and should alert his physician.

2. *Fallacy.* A "free" diet means the patient can eat anything he wants.

Fact. Patients permitted to eat so-called "free" diets must observe regular meal hours and must eat foods that meet their nutritional requirements. They are generally told not to eat concentrated sweets such as sugar, candy, jelly, cake, and cookies. The single and double sugars are rapidly absorbed thus causing the blood sugar to become sharply elevated and making control more difficult.

3. *Fallacy.* Honey can be used in place of cane sugar.

Fact. Honey is about 80 per cent carbohydrate, chiefly fructose. The fructose is eventually used as glucose, thereby requiring insulin. Therefore, the use of honey is not desirable.

4. *Fallacy.* Dietetic foods may be used as desired by diabetic patients.

Fact. Dietetic foods contain some carbohydrate, protein, and fat. Their use is seldom justified, and these foods are relatively expensive. If they are used, the patient should check with the dietitian or physician so that the value can be calculated into the diet.

REVIEW QUESTIONS AND PROBLEMS

1. What is the cause of diabetes mellitus?

2. What symptoms are seen in patients with diabetes?

3. What tests are used to determine whether an individual has diabetes?

4. A diabetic diet is essentially a normal diet. How does the diet differ from the normal pattern?

5. The menu for a family dinner is beef stew with potatoes, carrots, onions; tossed salad with Russian dressing; rolls and butter; lemon meringue pie; milk. Tell exactly how you would adapt this menu for a patient who is allowed the following exchanges: milk, 1; vegetables, 2; fruit, 1; lean meat, 3; fat, 2.

6. Why is a bedtime feeding ordinarily used for patients who are taking insulin?

7. List ten foods that diabetic patients usually should avoid.

8. Why must insulin be given by injection? What is meant by *oral compound?*

9. What symptoms would lead you to suspect that a patient is having an insulin shock? What would you do?

REFERENCES

Brunzell, J. D.: "Use of Fructose, Sorbitol, or Xylitol as a Sweetener in Diabetes Mellitus," *J. Am. Dietet. A.,* **73:**499–506. 1976.

Committee on Food and Nutrition, American Diabetes Association: "Principles of Nutrition and Dietary Recommendations for Patients with Diabetes Mellitus: 1971," *Diabetes,* **20:**633–34, 1971.

Fletcher, H. P.: "The Oral Antidiabetic Drugs: Pro and Con," *Am. J. Nurs.,* **76:**596–99, 1976.

Guthrie, D. W., and Guthrie, R. A.: "Diabetes in Adolescence," *Am. J. Nurs.,* **75:**1740–44, 1975.

Guthrie, D. W.: "Exercise, Diets and Insulin for Children with Diabetes," *Nursing 77,* **7:**48–54, February 1977.

Hayter, J.: "Fine Points in Diabetic Care," *Am. J. Nurs.,* **76:**594–99, 1976.

Jouganatos, D. M., and Gabbe, S. G.: "Diabetes in Pregnancy: Metabolic Changes and Current Environment," *J. Am. Dietet. A.,* **73:**168–71, 1978.

Kaufmann, S. J.: "In Diabetic Diets, Realism Gets Results," *Nursing 76,* **6:**74–77, November 1976.

Salzer, J. E.: "Classes to Improve Diabetic Self-Care," *Am. J. Nurs.,* **75:**1324–25, 1975.

Trayser, L. M.: "A Teaching Program for Diabetics," *Am. J. Nurs.,* **73:**92–93, 1973.

Wolfe, L. W.: "Insulin: Paving the Way to a New Life," *Nursing 77,* **7:**38–41, November 1977.

24

Endocrine Disorders | HYPERTHYROIDISM | HYPOGLYCEMIA | ADDISON'S
DISEASE • **Enzyme Deficiencies** | PHENYLKETONURIA | GALACTOSEMIA
• **Bone and Joint Diseases** | ARTHRITIS | GOUT | OSTEOPOROSIS

VARIOUS METABOLIC DISORDERS

Endocrine Disorders

HYPERTHYROIDISM

Clinical findings. Excessive secretion by the thyroid gland leads to an
increase in the metabolic rate by as much as 50 per cent. Some of the symptoms
are weight loss, nervousness, increased appetite, prominent eyes, and enlarged
thyroid gland. The increased metabolic rate leads to rapid loss of glycogen
from the liver, and some tissue wasting, and in severe cases to signs of cardiac
failure. Calcium and phosphorus excretion is often increased, resulting in osteoporosis (see p. 241). Most patients are treated with antithyroid drugs to bring
the metabolic rate to normal. In some instances surgery is required.

Dietary management. If there has been much weight loss a diet supplying
3000 to 4000 kcal and 100 to 125 gm protein is needed. (See p. 224.) Snacks
are provided between meals and at bedtime. Mineral and vitamin supplements
are often prescribed. Coffee, tea, alcohol, and tobacco are usually eliminated
because of their stimulating properties.

HYPOGLYCEMIA

The incidence of hypoglycemia is greatly exaggerated by faddists who claim
that most fatigue and anxiety can be explained on this basis. The facts are
otherwise, and hypoglycemia can be diagnosed only by determining the fasting
blood sugar and a glucose tolerance test.

Hypoglycemia means low blood sugar, and is a symptom of a number of conditions. It occurs when a patient with diabetes mellitus has taken too much insulin or oral compounds or has failed to eat. Similar symptoms occur in some patients who have had a gastrectomy so that food passes through the intestinal tract rapidly. (See Dumping Syndrome, p. 310.) It also occurs in Addison's disease, and is sometimes a functional disorder.

Functional hypoglycemia (hyperinsulinism).   No organic lesion is present. When the individual eats carbohydrate-rich foods there is increased production of insulin and the blood sugar drops 2 to 4 hours after meals with typical hypoglycemic symptoms: weakness, hunger, nervousness, trembling, increased perspiration, and occasionally loss of consciousness.

Dietary management.   The diet is calculated using meal exchange lists as described in Chapter 21. The diet prescription is planned as follows:

1. The calorie level is sufficient to maintain desirable weight.
2. Carbohydrate is restricted to 75 to 100 gm. This reduces the amount of insulin that is produced. The carbohydrate is supplied by milk, fruit and vegetable exchanges; bread exchanges are usually omitted.
3. The protein intake is increased to 100 to 150 gm; about 50 per cent of protein can be metabolized to glucose for the body's needs but the slower rate of absorption does not stimulate the production of insulin.
4. The remaining calories are provided by fat.
5. The daily food allowance is divided so that each meal provides the same amount of protein, fat, and carbohydrate.

ADDISON'S DISEASE

This is a relatively rare, serious disorder of the adrenal gland in which there is insufficient production of one or more hormones. Deficient production of *aldosterone* leads to excessive excretion of sodium and water in the urine, and increased retention of potassium. These changes lead, in turn, to lowered blood volume, dehydration, and hypotension. Patients may have a craving for salt, thirst, profound weakness, vomiting, diarrhea, and changes in heart rhythm.

Deficient production of other hormones, *glucocorticoids*, leads to rapid depletion of liver glycogen and to hypoglycemia a few hours after meals. If no food has been eaten for 10 to 12 hours hypoglycemia is severe.

Mild insufficiency is often controlled by increasing the salt intake and by giving five to six meals daily. Cortisone may be prescribed to control hypoglycemia. When the deficiency is severe deoxycorticosterone (DOCA) is prescribed to control the mineral metabolism.

A high-protein, low-carbohydrate diet is essential in order to reduce the stimulation by insulin and the subsequent hypoglycemia. Simple sugars are especially avoided. Midmorning, midafternoon, and late evening snacks high in protein and low in carbohydrate are used.

Enzyme Deficiencies

More than a hundred enzyme deficiencies have been identified. These are generally inherited and are sometimes called inborn errors of metabolism. Many of them are evident shortly after birth and others are acquired later in life. Deficiency of the intestinal enzymes leads to malabsorption, discussed further in Chapter 29.

PHENYLKETONURIA

Clinical findings. Phenylketonuria occurs in about 1 infant of every 10,000. The infant is born without the enzyme necessary to use phenylalanine, one of the essential amino acids. As a result the level of the blood phenylalanine is increased and phenylketones are also excreted in the urine—hence the name phenylketonuria (PKU). The deficiency can be diagnosed shortly after birth by blood and urine tests.

High blood levels of phenylalanine are toxic. The infants are usually blond, blue-eyed, fair, and often have eczema. Untreated infants are hyperactive, irritable, and have an unpleasant personality. They have a persistent musty or gamey body odor caused by the production of the phenylketones. If the disease is not diagnosed in the first months of life, mental retardation is usually severe.

Dietary management. Phenylketonuria is successfully treated by a phenylalanine-restricted diet when diagnosis is made in the first months of life. If treatment is delayed, the mental retardation that has occurred cannot be reversed.

The phenylalanine is adjusted to maintain a normal level in the blood. Since this is an essential amino acid, some must be provided to meet normal growth needs. This has been estimated to be 20 to 30 mg per kg. Thus, a 3-month infant weighing 6 kg would need 120 to 180 mg phenylalanine daily.

Proteins contain about 5 per cent phenylalanine. The recommended allowance for protein for a 6 kg infant is about 13 gm. From milk formulas and supplementary foods this would supply 650 mg phenylalanine, which is about 4 to 5 times as much as he should have.

A special formula Lofenalac® is used for these infants.* It supplies just enough phenylalanine for growth and is adequate for all other nutrients. As the infant grows, ordinary foods that are low in phenylalanine are added. Mothers are given detailed food lists for fruits, vegetables, breads, and cereals from which to choose, and careful instructions are needed for measurement. Even low-protein foods such as fruits contain some phenylalanine and must be given in measured amounts. (See Fig. 24–1.)

Successful treatment depends upon dietary adjustment at frequent intervals.

* Mead Johnson & Company, Evansville, Indiana.

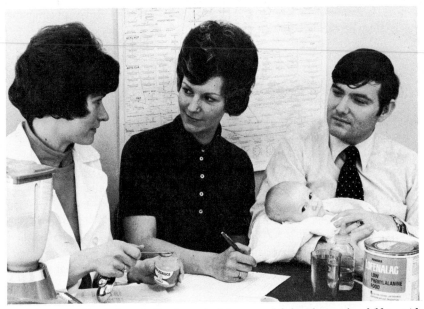

FIGURE 24–1 Detailed counseling is required for successful diet therapy for children with phenylketonuria or other metabolic errors. The dietitian and nurse will provide follow-up from time to time. *(Handicapped Children's Unit, St. Christopher's Hospital for Children, Philadelphia.)*

Based upon the blood levels of phenylalanine the diet is adjusted so that the amount furnished to the body is just sufficient for growth needs. As the child grows the diet is increased to meet all nutritional requirements. The low-phenylalanine diet is continued throughout the early years of childhood. Whether it needs to be continued indefinitely is not yet known.

GALACTOSEMIA

Clinical findings. From birth infants with this condition lack *transferase,* a liver enzyme that converts galactose to glucose. Galactose is one of the simple sugars resulting when lactose is digested. When the enzyme is absent the levels of galactose in the blood reach toxic levels. A few days after birth the infant has vomiting, diarrhea, drowsiness, edema, liver failure, and hemorrhage. If the infant survives, mental retardation is severe.

Dietary management. A galactose-free formula must be started within the first few days of life. Nutramigen®, ProSobee®, Mul-Soy®, and MBF (Meat-Base Formula) are suitable.* Since milk is the only food that supplies

* Nutramigen® and ProSobee®, Mead Johnson & Company, Evansville, Indiana. Mul-Soy®, Syntex Laboratories, Palo Alto, California. MBF (Meat-Base Formula), Gerber Products Company, Fremont, Michigan.

lactose, other foods are added to the infant's diet as he grows. All milk-containing foods must be rigidly excluded. A list of such foods is given on p. 287.

Bone and Joint Diseases

ARTHRITIS

Some 20 million Americans are afflicted with arthritis; of these at least 3 million are limited in their activity. The chronic, painful, and often disabling nature of the disease leads arthritic patients each year to spend some 435 million dollars on phony diets, drugs, and devices.

No diet will cure arthritis or modify its course. Patients are well advised to eat a normal diet selected from the four food groups. Young patients who have rheumatoid arthritis and who are underweight may need to increase their caloric intake. On the other hand, the older patient with osteoarthritis is sometimes obese and should lose weight to reduce the burden on weight-bearing joints.

Steroids or aspirin should be taken with meals to reduce gastric irritation. Salt restriction is required when steroids cause retention of fluids and sodium. Patients with severe deformities often need the advice of physical and occupational therapists in the use of devices to aid in normal activities; for example, special utensils for feedings, and methods for food preparation adapted to physical limitations.

GOUT

Gout is an inherited condition of abnormal purine metabolism. Purines are nitrogen-containing compounds that are broken down in the body to uric acid. Normally uric acid is eliminated in the urine. In gout the blood uric acid is elevated and some of the uric acid is deposited as an insoluble salt in the metatarsal, knee, and toe joints, often causing severe pain.

Medications are effective in relieving pain and in increasing the excretion of uric acid. A high-fluid intake is desirable. A purine-restricted diet, by itself, is of little value but is recommended by some physicians together with medications. Patients are usually advised to avoid foods that are high in purines: liver, kidney, brains, sweetbreads, heart, sardines, anchovies, broth, meat soups, and meat gravies.

During an acute attack some physicians recommend the omission of meat, fish, and poultry which are moderate sources of purines. When the acute attack has subsided, small servings of meat, fish, and poultry are again introduced. Milk, cheese, eggs, and legumes are good protein sources in the low-purine diet.

Many patients with gout are obese. Weight loss increases the blood level of uric acid and may bring about an acute attack. If recommended, weight loss should be gradual and never rapid. A low-calorie diet should not be initiated during an acute attack because this could further aggravate the symptoms. Starvation regimens are prohibited.

OSTEOPOROSIS

Osteoporosis is extremely common in older women. The bones contain less bone substance than usual and are more porous. Weight-bearing bones break easily and are hard to repair. Low back pain is frequent, there is gradual loss in height, and the appearance of the "dowager's hump." Osteoporosis occurs in many persons who are immobilized, in diseases of malabsorption such as sprue (see Chapter 29), and is often associated with decreased estrogen production after the menopause. Hormone therapy and mineral supplements are generally recommended.

Osteoporosis occurs less frequently in geographic areas where the water supply is high in fluoride. The disease is less common in persons who have had an adequate intake of calcium throughout life. A high-calcium diet—that is, one containing a quart of milk a day—is often prescribed; it may be of some help in preventing further damage.

REVIEW QUESTIONS AND PROBLEMS

1. What diet modification is sometimes ordered for a patient with hyperthyroidism? Why?

2. What are some conditions in which hypoglycemia is present?

3. Why is a low-carbohydrate diet recommended for functional hypoglycemia?

4. What is meant by phenylketonuria? Why is early treatment with diet essential?

5. What foods contain large amounts of phenylalanine? Why is some phenylalanine included in the diet for patients with phenylketonuria?

6. A patient with arthritis says he has heard that a low-carbohydrate diet is useful in treating his condition. How would you respond to this?

7. What is meant by a low-purine diet? When is it used? What foods are restricted?

8. Why is weight loss by patients with gout introduced cautiously?

REFERENCES

Acosta, P. B., et al.: "Methods of Dietary Inception in Infants with PKU," J. Am. Dietet. A., 72:164–69, 1978.

Eliott, D. D.: "Adrenocortical Insufficiency: A Self-Instruction Unit," Am. J. Nurs., 74:1115–30, 1974.

Hernandez, L. A.: "Gout," Nurs. Times, 72:898–900, 1976.

Hudson, F. P.: "Phenylketonuria," *Nurs. Times,* **71:**687–89, 1975.

MacRae, I.: "Arthritis, Its Nature and Management," *Nurs. Clin. North Am.,* 8:643–52, 1973.

Reyzer, N.: "PKU," *Am. J. Nurs.,* 78:1895–98, 1978.

Soika, C. V.: "Combatting Osteoporosis," *Am. J. Nurs.,* **73:**1193–97, 1973.

"Statement on Hypoglycemia," *J.A.M.A.,* **223:**682, 1973.

HYPERLIPIDEMIAS AND

ATHEROSCLEROSIS

Cholesterol-Restricted, Modified-Fat Diets

Each year more than one million persons in this country die of heart attack, stroke, and other diseases of the heart and blood vessels. Coronary heart disease alone accounts for over 600,000 deaths; about one fourth of these coronary deaths occur under 65 years.

ATHEROSCLEROSIS

Atherosclerosis, the most common form of hardening of the arteries, refers to the thickening of the inner walls (intima) of the blood vessel. It is the most frequent cause of heart attacks and strokes. It can lead to aneurysm (dilation) of the abdominal aorta or gangrene of the leg.

Atherosclerosis develops gradually throughout life. In childhood fatty streaks appear in the inner lining of the blood vessel. These streaks do not lead to any clinical symptoms. In early adult years fatty materials and cholesterol continue to be deposited and are covered with thick fibrous layers of connective tissue. These deposits are known as *atheroma*, or *plaques*. The channel through which the blood flows becomes narrower, and it is increasingly difficult to supply enough blood to the tissues. In later years angina pectoris is a manifestation of this deficiency of blood (ischemia). (See Fig. 25–1.)

The plaques sometimes ulcerate and hemorrhage, or the rough surfaces can initiate blood clotting. If the vessel is blocked by a clot, the tissue served by that vessel dies. Blocking of a coronary vessel, also known as a coronary occlusion, results in myocardial infarction; sudden death occurs if a principal

243

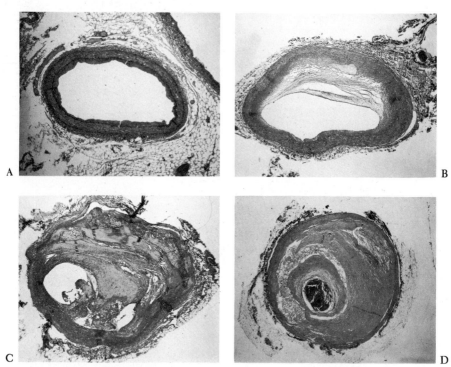

FIGURE 25–1   Gradual development of atherosclerosis in a coronary artery, leading to a heart attack. (A) normal artery; (B) deposits formed in inner lining of the artery; (C) deposits harden; (D) normal channel is blocked by a blood clot. *(American Heart Association.)*

vessel is affected. Occlusion of a vessel to the brain is a stroke (cerebral thrombosis), while blockage of a blood vessel in the leg leads to gangrene.

RISK FACTORS

The three major factors that increase the risk of atherosclerosis and coronary heart disease are elevated blood lipids, hypertension, and cigarette smoking. Dietary factors, especially saturated fat and cholesterol, are associated with elevated blood lipids, while a high salt intake may be a factor in hypertension. Many other factors also increase the risks: (1) males between the ages of 45 and 64 years are highly susceptible; (2) a family history of heart and blood vessel disease; (3) tension, frustration, emotional stress, meeting deadlines, and drive to achieve; (4) sedentary occupation and lack of exercise; (5) obesity; and (6) diabetes mellitus. Even the relative softness of drinking water in some geographic areas has been listed by some research workers as a risk factor. There is considerable lack of agreement on the excessive consumption of coffee (more than 5 cups daily) as a risk factor.

HYPERLIPIDEMIAS

Hyperlipidemia refers to an elevation of the blood lipids, and includes cholesterol, triglycerides, or elevation of specific lipoproteins.

Hypercholesterolemia refers to an elevation in the serum level of cholesterol, while *hypertriglyceridemia* is an elevation of serum triglycerides.

Hyperlipoproteinemia refers to the elevation in the serum level of one or more of the lipoproteins. The lipoproteins are the means by which insoluble fats are carried in the blood stream. They fall into four groups:

1. *Chylomicrons:* the form carried in the lymph and blood 1 to 8 hours after a meal; contain triglycerides attached to a very small amount of protein; they give a milky appearance to the blood serum.

2. *Very low-density lipoproteins* (VLDL) or *prebeta-lipoproteins:* consist chiefly of triglycerides synthesized in the body and attached to some protein; carry a small amount of cholesterol.

3. *Low-density lipoproteins* (LDL) or *beta-lipoproteins:* derived chiefly from the prebeta-lipoproteins; account for most of the cholesterol in the circulation.

4. *High-density lipoproteins* (HDL) or *alpha-lipoproteins:* contain the largest percentage of protein, and about one fourth of the cholesterol in the circulation.

The level of the first three groups in the blood is affected by the amount and kinds of fat in the diet, while that of the high-density lipoproteins remains relatively constant. Based upon the amounts of triglycerides, cholesterol, and specific lipoproteins, Fredrickson and his associates have classified hyperlipoproteinemias into five types. A physician makes a diagnosis and prescribes appropriate diet and other therapy depending upon the medical history, the physical examination, and the laboratory findings. Some of the characteristics of each type are included in the following outline.*

TYPE I
> Inability to clear chylomicrons from plasma because of deficiency of enzyme *lipoprotein lipase;* triglycerides very high; cholesterol normal or elevated
> Rare; usually familial; children or young adults
> Abdominal pain with fat ingestion; pancreatitis; xanthomas; enlarged spleen and liver

TYPE IIa
> Elevated betalipoproteins; elevated cholesterol; normal triglycerides. Must differentiate between cholesterol present in low and high density lipoproteins; excess cholesterol in low density lipoproteins is harmful while that in high density lipoproteins may be protective
> Common at all ages; often familial (probably autosomal dominant); may be secondary to excessive cholesterol intake, nephrosis, liver disease, myxedema, myeloma

---

* Data from D. S. Fredrickson *et al.: Dietary Management of Hyperlipoproteinemia. A Handbook for Physicians.* National Heart and Lung Institute, Bethesda, Md., revised 1974.

Xanthomas and vascular disease often in early adulthood; corneal arcus; early incidence of ischemic heart disease

TYPE IIb

Elevated betalipoproteins, cholesterol, and triglycerides

Common; may be familial

Sensitive to caloric intake

TYPE III

Abnormal form of betalipoproteins determined by laboratory analysis; elevated cholesterol and triglycerides

Relatively uncommon; usually familial (recessive)

Tuboeruptive lesions of elbows, knees, buttocks; palmar xanthomas; increased incidence of coronary and peripheral vessel disease at an early age

TYPE IV

Increase in endogenous triglycerides (prebeta or very low density lipoproteins); cholesterol normal or slightly high; about half have abnormal glucose tolerance; some have elevated uric acid

Very common; usually found after second decade; may be familial; often secondary to diabetes mellitus

Few external signs; xanthomas if triglycerides very high; associated with early atherosclerosis and vascular disease; exacerbated by obesity

TYPE V

Extremely high triglyceride levels originating from chylomicrons (exogenous triglycerides) and prebetalipoproteins (endogenous triglycerides); cholesterol level somewhat elevated; abnormal glucose tolerance and hyperuricemia often found

May be familial; often secondary to diabetic acidosis, nephrosis, pancreatitis, alcoholism

Intolerance to fat from the diet (exogenous) and also fat synthesized in the body (endogenous); symptoms similar to Type I, usually after age 20; abdominal pain with fat ingestion; enlargement of spleen and liver

DIETARY MODIFICATION

Diet is the primary therapy for all types of hyperlipidemia. Medications are ordered only when diet alone does not bring about the necessary lowering of the blood lipids. A summary of the characteristics of the diets for each type are shown in Table 25–1. Several characteristics apply to all diets.

1. All diets furnish recommended allowances for protein, minerals, and vitamins to maintain satisfactory nutrition for indefinite periods of time. For women during the childbearing years the iron level of the diet is below recommended allowances.

2. Obesity is a frequent problem. When it is present, any nutritionally balanced low-calorie diet can be used. (See Chapter 22.) Weight loss should approximate ½ to 1 kg (1 to 2 lb) per week. With loss of weight the blood lipid levels are usually lowered and may even reach normal levels. When desired weight is achieved, the maintenance diet is adjusted according to the type of hyperlipoproteinemia.

TABLE 25-1 SUMMARY OF DIETS FOR TYPES I–V HYPERLIPOPROTEINEMIA

	Type I	Type IIa	Type IIb and Type III	Type IV	Type V
Diet prescription	Low Fat 25–35 gms.	Low Cholesterol Polyunsaturated fat increased	Low Cholesterol Approximately: 20% cal. Pro. 40% cal. Fat 40% ca. CHO	Controlled CHO Approximately 45% of calories Moderately restricted cholesterol	Restricted Fat 30% of calories Controlled CHO 50% of calories Moderately restricted cholesterol
Calories	Not restricted	Not restricted	Achieve and maintain "ideal" weight, i.e. reduction diet if necessary	Achieve and maintain "ideal" weight, i.e. reduction diet if necessary	Achieve and maintain "ideal" weight, i.e. reduction diet if necessary
Protein	Total protein intake is not limited	Total protein intake is not limited	High protein	Not limited other than control of patient's weight	High Protein
Fat	Restricted to 25–35 gms. Kind of fat not important.	Saturated fat intake limited Polyunsaturated fat intake increased	Controlled to 40% calories (polyunsaturated fats recommended in preference to saturated fats)	Not limited other than control of patient's weight (polyunsaturated fats recommended in preference to saturated fats)	Restricted to 30% of calories (polyunsaturated fats recommended in preference to saturated fats)
Cholesterol	Not restricted	As low as possible; the only source of cholesterol is the meat in the diet	Less than 300 mg.—the only source of cholesterol is the meat in the diet	Moderately restricted to 300–500 mg	Moderately restricted to 300–500 mg.
Carbohydrate	Not limited	Not limited	Controlled—concentrated sweets are restricted	Controlled—concentrated sweets are restricted	Controlled—concentrated sweets are restricted
Alcohol	Not recommended	May be used with discretion	Limited to 2 servings (substituted for carbohydrate)	Limited to 2 servings (substituted for carbohydrate)	Not recommended

The Dietary Management of Hyperlipoproteinemia. A Handbook for Physicians and Dietitians. National Heart and Lung Institute, Bethesda, Md., revised 1974.

3. The cholesterol intake is severely restricted in types II and III, moderately restricted for types IV and V, and not restricted for type I.

4. The intake of saturated fat is reduced. Preference is given to fats that are high in polyunsaturated fatty acids. This is especially important for diets for Type IIa.

MEAL PLANNING AND FOOD LISTS

The food allowances for diets for the five types of hyperlipidemias are summarized in Table 25–2. The *Exchange Lists for Meal Planning* (Table A–2) may be used for making food choices. Only low-fat milk and low-fat meat exchanges are used. Fats are selected from those that are high in polyunsaturated fats.

Low-fat desserts. For Types I and II, low-fat desserts may be used as desired within the caloric allowance. For diets IV and V up to two servings of low-fat desserts may be substituted for two bread exchanges. One bread exchange is equivalent to: ¼ cup sherbet or water ice; ½ cup pudding made with skim milk; 1½-inch cube angel food cake; or ⅓ cup gelatin dessert.

Sugars and sweets. These are allowed as desired for Types 1 and 2, and as a substitute for one serving low-fat dessert for Types 4 and 5. One serving low-fat dessert is equivalent to: 1 tablespoon sugar, honey, jelly, or jam; ½ oz jelly beans, hard candy, or mints (not chocolate); or 6 oz sweetened carbonated beverage; or 3 oz fruit flavored drink.

Alcohol. In excessive amounts alcohol increases blood triglyceride levels. None is allowed on diets 1 and 5. On the other three diets it may be used with discretion as a substitute for up to two bread exchanges. One bread exchange is equivalent to: 1 ounce gin, rum, vodka, or whiskey; 1½ oz sweet or dessert wine; 2½ oz dry wine; or 5 oz beer.

Sample menus for the 1800 kcal diet for Types 1 and 2a are shown in Table 25–3.

DIETARY COUNSELING

In most instances the blood lipids are significantly lowered when the patient adheres to his diet. This, in itself, can be important in motivating the patient. But if the effect is to remain, the diet must be used throughout life. Menus for these diets are palatable and easily incorporated into family menus.

Booklets for patients for each of the types of diets are available from the National Heart and Lung Institute and the American Heart Association. They provide detailed information on the purposes of the diet, the lists of foods that may be used, and those to be avoided, typical meal patterns, how to shop for allowed food, how to prepare food, and what to do when eating meals away from home. The *Exchange Lists for Meal Planning* available from The American Dietetic Association may be used in place of these booklets.

TABLE 25–2 TYPICAL ALLOWANCES FOR DIETS FOR TYPES I TO V HYPERLIPOPROTEINEMIAS *
APPROXIMATELY 1800 KCAL †

Exchange List	Food Grouping	Type I	Type IIa	Type IIb and III	Type IV	Type V
1	Milk, nonfat, cups	4	2	2	2	4
2	Vegetables dark green or yellow daily	2	2	ad lib	ad lib	ad lib
3	Fruits citrus or other vitamin-C source daily	3	3	3	6	3
4	Bread, cereal or starchy vegetable	7+	8+	8	8	10
5	Low fat meat, poultry, or fish, ounces	5	6–9 §	6	ad lib	6
	Egg yolk as substitute for 1 oz meat	3/week	none	none	3/week	3/week
6	Fat, teaspoons	none ‡	6–9 §	12	ad lib	6
	Low-fat dessert, servings	ad lib	ad lib	none	2/day or less subst. for dessert	2/day or less subst. for dessert
	Sugars, sweets, servings	ad lib	ad lib	none	subst.	none
	Alcohol	none	with discretion	subst.	subst.	none

* Adapted from *Dietary Management of Hyperlipoproteinemia. A Handbook for Physicians and Dietitians.* National Heart and Lung Institute, Bethesda, Md., revised 1974. Food choices may be made from Exchange Lists for Meal Planning (Table A-2). See also p. 248 for choices for low-fat desserts, sugars, alcohol.

‡ Medium chain triglycerides sometimes prescribed by physician.

§ Use only three 3-oz portions of beef, lamb, pork, ham each week. Use poultry, fish, shellfish (except shrimp), veal for remainder of week. Use 1 teaspoon safflower or corn oil for each ounce of meat.

TABLE 25-3   SAMPLE MENUS FOR TWO TYPES OF MODIFIED-FAT DIETS

Very Low-Fat Diet *(Type 1)*	*Low-Cholesterol Modified-Fat Diet* *(Type 2a)*
Breakfast	*Breakfast*
Stewed apricots	Honeydew melon—1 slice
Cooked or dry cereal	Dry or cooked cereal—¾ cup
Sugar	Sugar—1 teaspoon
Toast—2 slices	Whole-wheat toast—2 slices
Jelly	Safflower oil margarine—2 teaspoons
Skim milk	Jelly—2 teaspoons
Coffee, if desired	Skim milk—1 cup
Luncheon	*Luncheon*
Salad:	Sandwich:
Cottage cheese, uncreamed— ½ cup	Rye bread—2 slices
Peach halves, canned	Sliced turkey—2 oz
Escarole	Mayonnaise—2 teaspoons
Rolls, soft—2	Cabbage-green pepper salad—½ cup
Jelly	Mayonnaise—1 tablespoon
Raspberry sherbet	Banana—1 small
Angel food cake	Skim milk—1 cup
Cocoa made with skim milk, sugar, cocoa	
Dinner	*Dinner*
Grapefruit sections	Broiled flounder—4 oz
Roast leg of veal—3 oz	Safflower or corn oil—1 teaspoon
Baked noodles and tomatoes	Parslied potato—1 small *with*
Asparagus tips	Safflower or corn oil—1 teaspoon
Dinner roll	Mixed diced carrots and celery—½ cup
Jelly	Dinner roll—1
Apple tapioca pudding	Safflower oil margarine—1 teaspoon
Coffee or tea, if desired	Tomato aspic on water cress *with* French dressing—1 tablespoon
	Angel cake—1 small piece
Snack	
Skim milk—1 cup	
Gelatin dessert	

Preparation of meats.   Only low-fat meats are used. All visible fat must be removed. If meats are roasted or broiled, they should be placed on a rack so that the drippings are removed. If the meat is stewed, it may be cooked a day ahead, cooled in the refrigerator, and the fat skimmed off the top of the liquid. Meats, fish, and poultry may be basted with tomato juice, lemon juice, wine, or bouillon, and baked in aluminum foil.

Seasoning vegetables. Lemon juice, vinegar, and herbs lend variety to vegetable flavors. See suggestions for flavoring vegetables on p. 261. When fats are allowed, white sauce may be prepared using nonfat milk.

Using oils and margarine. Safflower, sunflower, and corn oils are used for the type 2 diet; soybean and cottonseed oils are also used with diets for types 3 and 4. Oils may be used in the following ways:

1. As a marinade for meat. Combine the allowed oil with herbs and lemon juice; tomato juice, vinegar, or wine. Brush the meat with oil-herb-juice mixture and allow to stand for several hours or overnight in the refrigerator. Turn the meat often and brush again with the mixture. Drain off liquid from the meat, wipe dry, and broil or roast. Use the liquid for basting.

2. Pan-fry meat, chicken, fish, eggs, pancakes.

3. Substitute oil for solid fat in muffin, biscuit, pancake, and waffle recipes. Use skim milk instead of whole milk.

4. Mix with a tiny pinch of herbs to flavor vegetables; or add to vegetables with a tablespoon or two of water before cooking, cover tightly and cook until tender but still crisp.

5. Add to mashed potatoes with skim milk.

6. Use in mayonnaise, French dressing, and cooked salad dressings.

7. Use in place of solid fats for making white sauces with skim milk.

8. Use for pie crust and chiffon cakes.

Medium-chain triglycerides are sometimes prescribed by the physician for patients on Type I diets to increase their caloric intake. The MCT oil may be used to make salad dressings, in white sauces made with skim milk, or for marinating meat.

REVIEW QUESTIONS AND PROBLEMS

1. From the risks listed on page 244, identify those that apply to yourself or someone you know.

2. A patient has a slightly elevated blood cholesterol, and high blood triglyceride. He is 30 pounds overweight, and has an abnormal glucose tolerance. What changes in the diet would be indicated?

3. Write a day's menu for the patient described in question 2. After he has reached desirable weight, what would be a suitable maintenance diet for him?

4. Name five foods that are high in saturated fat.

5. Why are eggs restricted or omitted on these diets?

6. Why are concentrated sweets and alcohol omitted on some diets?

7. Why would a supplement of vitamin A be prescribed for a patient receiving a very low-fat diet?

8. In any cookbook look up the recipes for biscuits, buttered vegetables, creamed chicken, pie crust. How could you change the recipes so that they would be low in saturated fat and high in polyunsaturated fat?

9. Write a menu for one day for a 1200 kcal diet that is low in cholesterol and very low in fat.

REFERENCES

Buller, A. C.: "Improving Dietary Education for Patients with Hyperlipidemia," *J. Am. Dietet. A.,* **72:**277–81, 1978.

Committee on Nutrition: *Diet and Coronary Heart Disease.* New York: American Heart Association, 1978.

Dietary Management of Hyperlipoproteinemia, booklets for patients, Type I, IIa, IIb, III, IV, and V. Bethesda, Md.: National Heart and Lung Institute, revised 1974.

Eschleman, R., and Winston, M.: *The American Heart Association Cookbook.* New York: David McKay Company, Inc., 1973.

Gotto, A. M., *et al.:* "Prudent Eating after 40," *Geriatrics,* **29:**109–118, May 1974.

Mayer, J.: "The Mysterious Fat Family," *Family Health,* **10:**44–46, August 1978.

Norum, K. R.: "Some Present Concepts Concerning Diet and Prevention of Coronary Heart Disease," *Nutr. Rev.,* **36:**194–98, 1978.

"Updating the Cholesterol Controversy: Verdict—Diet Does Count," *Am. J. Nurs.,* **78:**1681, 1978.

Villet, B.: "Heart Attack: Not for Men Only," *Today's Health,* **53:**24, 1975.

Witschi, J. C., *et al.:* "Family Cooperation and Effectiveness in a Cholesterol-Lowering Diet," *J. Am. Dietet. A.,* **72:**384–89, 1978.

26

CARDIOVASCULAR DISORDERS | NUTRITIONAL PLANNING •
Sodium-Restricted Diets | NOMENCLATURE | SOURCES OF SODIUM | FOOD
SELECTION | DIETARY PLANS | PREPARATION OF FOOD

DISEASES OF THE HEART

Sodium-Restricted Diets

CARDIOVASCULAR DISORDERS

Hypertension (high blood pressure) is a symptom, not a disease. About 23 million Americans are hypertensive; probably half of these are not even aware of the condition. Essential hypertension (cause unknown) accounts for about 90 per cent of all hypertensives. Obesity, cigarette smoking, stress, a sedentary way of life, and high salt intake are believed to increase the risk of hypertension occurring. Hypertension is a leading contributor to heart attack and stroke; it is associated with diseases of the kidney and toxemias of pregnancy.

Hypertension is treated primarily by drugs. Although severe sodium restriction (250 mg sodium daily) is effective in lowering blood pressure, very few individuals are able to adhere to such a rigid diet for any length of time. With medications physicians usually prescribe mild sodium restriction (2000 to 3000 mg sodium). When obesity is present a low-calorie diet should be used until desirable weight is achieved. (See Chapter 22.)

Angina pectoris is the sensation of tightness, pressure, and pain usually in the chest; the pain often spreads to the left shoulder, arm, or hand. It is a sign that the blood supply to the heart muscle is not adequate *(ischemia)*. Any muscle aches when it does not get a sufficient supply of blood. Angina is brought about as a result of the gradual thickening of the blood vessel walls *(arteriosclerosis)*, and the narrowing of the lumen through which the blood flows. The attacks of angina take place after physical exertion, by exposure to a cold wind, through excitement, or during the digestion of a heavy meal. Loss of weight, if obese, and meals that are small and easily digested are helpful measures to these patients.

253

Myocardial infarction is also known as coronary occlusion, coronary thrombosis, coronary, or heart attack. It refers to the damage to heart tissue resulting from the blockage of an artery supplying the heart. The tissue served by that artery is not supplied by the oxygen and nutrients that it needs, and consequently it dies. When a small artery is blocked the area of tissue damage is small, and recovery is good, especially if there is collateral circulation. If a major artery is affected, sudden death follows.

Congestive heart failure occurs when the heart is unable to maintain adequate circulation to the tissues. *Decompensation* is said to have taken place. The reduced level of circulation lowers the excretion of sodium by the kidney. Thus sodium accumulates in the extracellular fluid and holds water with it. The edema is evident in puffiness around the eyes, tightness of rings on the fingers, swelling of the ankles, and then fluid accumulation in the chest cavity, and abdomen. The fluid accumulation further interferes with heart action.

NUTRITIONAL PLANNING

The nutritional care of the patient who has sustained a myocardial infarction must be tailored to the individual's needs. It must include planning for the acute illness, the period of convalescence, and following recovery. Several factors must be considered in planning for the patient's diet, namely shortness of breath, fatigue, abdominal distention, the presence or absence of edema, loss of appetite, and fear of eating.

An essential characteristic of therapy in acute myocardial infarction is rest. (See Fig. 26–1.) A regimen of nutritional care has been described by Christakis and Winston, and is summarized as follows.*

Acute illness. For the first 24 to 48 hours the physician may direct that no food be given by mouth. Then a low-fat liquid diet supplying 500 to 800 kcal (1000 to 1500 ml fluid) is used for two or three days—longer if arrhythmia persists. This diet can include clear soups, weak tea, decaffeinated coffee, ginger ale, fruit juices, and skim milk. Very hot and very cold liquids should be avoided. Only small amounts of liquid are given at one time. The possibility that milk may produce distention because of lactose intolerance should be kept in mind.

Generally it has been considered advisable to feed the acutely ill patient. A recent study, however, has shown that it made little difference whether the patient was fed, or fed himself. Men, especially, preferred to feed themselves.†

Within a few days the patient usually progresses to a soft diet with these characteristics:

1. 1000 to 1200 kcal so that there is minimum circulation required for the digestive-absorptive processes, and to initiate weight loss if obese.

* G. Christakis and M. Winston, "Nutritional Therapy in Acute Myocardial Infarction," *J. Am. Diet. Assoc.*, **63**:233–38, 1973.

† R. Merkel and C. M. Brown, "Evaluating Feeding Activities in a CCU," *Am. J. Nurs.*, **70**:2348–50, 1970.

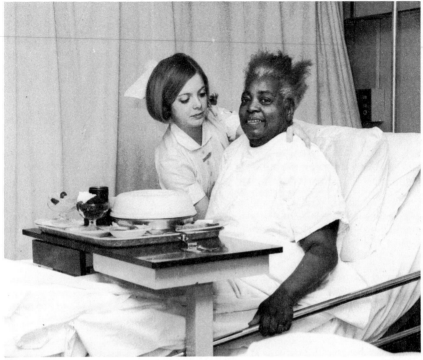

FIGURE 26–1 By adjusting the patient's position, the nurse helps reduce the energy the patient must exert in eating her meal. *(School of Nursing, Thomas Jefferson University, Philadelphia.)*

2. Five to six small, easily digested meals, especially if the patient is dyspneic or has angina.

3. Cholesterol restricted to 300 mg.

4. Low in saturated fat with an increased proportion of polyunsaturated fatty acids. See Chapter 25.

5. Restricted in sodium if there is congestive heart failure.

6. Avoidance of distending foods.

When diuretics are given to the patient with congestive heart failure, the potassium loss may be increased. The physician may request the inclusion of more potassium-rich foods such as plums, prunes, orange juice, potatoes, and other vegetables. The use of a potassium salt as medication is a more reliable way to assure compensation for the losses.

Maintenance diet. As the patient adjusts once again to a normal pattern of living, his diet is based upon his weight status and the blood lipid levels. Gradual weight loss is indicated if the patient is obese; however, some patients do not respond well, physically or psychologically, to weight-losing regimens. A maintenance diet that is restricted to 300 mg cholesterol and that is reduced in its saturated fatty acid content may be useful in reducing the likelihood of a recurrence of the coronary. The selection of the diet to be used on a long-term basis is best determined by the levels of the blood cholesterol and triglycerides about 6 months to a year following the heart attack. See Chapter 25 for diets for hyperlipidemias.

Sodium-Restricted Diets

NOMENCLATURE

Normally the daily sodium intake is 3 to 7 gm (3000 to 7000 mg). A sodium-restricted diet is limited to a specified amount of sodium, and ranges from a mild to severe restriction. Terms such as "salt free," "salt poor," and "low salt" are so indefinite that the patient might well receive a diet with much more sodium than he should have or, perhaps, one with less than he could have.

The levels of sodium restriction described in booklets published by the American Heart Association are

250 mg sodium (11 mEq),* Very Low-Sodium Diet. Used primarily for hospital patients.
500 mg sodium (22 mEq), Strict Low-Sodium Diet. Used primarily for hospital patients.
1000 mg sodium (43 mEq), Moderate Sodium-Restricted Diet. Sometimes used as a maintenance diet for patients at home.
Mild Sodium Restriction. Sodium content of this diet varies from about 2400 to 4500 mg. This is essentially a normal diet but omits salty foods and the use of salt at the table. This is frequently prescribed as a maintenance diet for patients at home.

SOURCES OF SODIUM

Naturally occurring sodium. All living things, plants as well as animals, require some sodium. Hence one would expect to find some sodium in foods as they naturally occur before they are processed by the manufacturer or cooked in the home. Animal foods are relatively high in sodium, and plant foods, with few exceptions are low. You will note in Table 26–1 that 2 cups of milk alone provide almost half the sodium in the calculation for the 500-mg sodium 1800 kcal diet. Meat, fish, and poultry are naturally high in sodium, so their amounts must be controlled on all levels except the mild restriction. Eggs are especially high in sodium, but most of this is in the white and not in the yolk.

Most vegetables are low in sodium, but several, such as beets, spinach, chard, and kale, are "salt-loving" in their growth. They contain too much sodium to be permitted on diets restricted to less than 1000 mg.

* 1 mEq sodium = 23 mg; thus, 250 ÷ 23 = 11 mEq.

Fruits, unsalted cereals, unsalted bread, and unsalted butter as well as oils and sugar contain small amounts of sodium or none at all, and may be used without restriction as far as sodium is concerned.

If all foods in the basic diet (see p. 37) were processed and prepared, and eaten without adding salt or any sodium compound, the sodium content would be about 500 mg.

Salt. The principal source of sodium in the diet is salt used (1) in numerous ways in food processing; for example, bacon, sauerkraut, dried fish, canned vegetables and meats, and many others; (2) in baking and cooking of foods; and (3) at the table. Salt is about 40 per cent sodium. Thus a teaspoon of salt that weighs 6 gm would provide 2400 mg sodium. If a recipe requires one teaspoon of salt and serves six people, you can see that one serving of that food alone would give 400 mg of sodium from the addition of the salt.

Sodium-containing compounds. Numerous compounds containing sodium are used by the manufacturer or in home preparation to improve the flavor or texture of foods. Among the more common ones are:

Baking powder

Baking soda

Monosodium glutamate (MSG)

Sodium acetate

Sodium alginate

Sodium benzoate

Sodium citrate

Sodium propionate

Sodium sulfite

It is not important that you know why each of these compounds is added to foods. But it is essential that you form the habit of looking for the words *sodium, salt,* and *soda* on any label (see Fig. 26–2). However, the label provides no information for such foods as mayonnaise and catsup, which are standardized according to the regulations of the Food and Drug Administration.

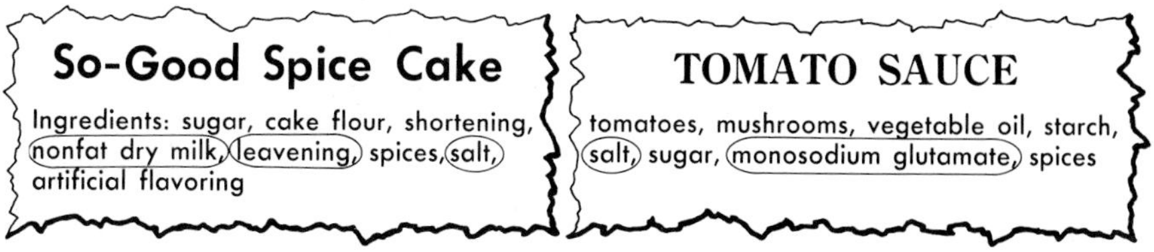

So-Good Spice Cake
Ingredients: sugar, cake flour, shortening, nonfat dry milk, leavening, spices, salt, artificial flavoring

TOMATO SAUCE
tomatoes, mushrooms, vegetable oil, starch, salt, sugar, monosodium glutamate, spices

FIGURE 26–2 Watch for the words "salt" and "sodium" when selecting foods for sodium-restricted diets. Leavenings and nonfat dry milk also contribute much sodium.

Some drinking waters are high in sodium, especially if water softeners are used. Many drugs, such as sedatives, laxatives, and alkalizers, contain sodium. The patient needs to be warned against self-medication with baking soda or various antacids.

FOOD SELECTION

The Exchange Lists for Meal Planning (Table A–2, p. 345) may be modified for sodium-restricted diets. All foods for these diets must be processed and prepared without salt or other sodium compounds. Canned foods, for example, must be eliminated if they contain salt, but dietetic low-sodium canned foods may be used. When using the Exchange Lists the following foods within each list must be avoided:

List 1, Milk and related products: AVOID buttermilk, soda fountain beverages, ice cream, ice milk, sherbet

List 2, Vegetables: AVOID beet greens, beets, carrots, celery, chard, collards, dandelion greens, kale, mustard greens, sauerkraut, spinach, white turnips; any canned vegetables unless canned without salt

List 3, Fruits: AVOID dried fruit if treated with sodium sulfite; maraschino cherries; glazed fruit

List 4, Breads and cereals: AVOID any products containing salt, baking powder, or baking soda; regular yeast breads, muffins, rolls; all dry breakfast cereals except puffed wheat, puffed rice, and shredded wheat; quick breads, muffins, pancakes, waffles; quick bread, biscuit, muffin, pancake, waffle mixes; saltines, graham crackers; self-rising flour; pretzels; popcorn; potato chips; canned baked beans, corn, or Lima beans; frozen Lima beans or peas

List 5, Meat: AVOID fresh or canned shellfish, including clams, crabs, lobsters, oysters, scallops, shrimp; all kinds of cheese; canned, dried, or smoked meat, such as bologna, chipped or corned beef, frankfurters, ham, kosher meat, luncheon meat, sausage, smoked tongue; frozen fish fillets; canned, salted, or smoked fish, including anchovies, caviar, salted and dried cod, herring, sardines; canned salmon, tuna; and peanut butter, except low-sodium

List 6, Fats: AVOID salted butter or margarine; bacon and bacon fat; salt pork; olives; commercial French dressing, mayonnaise, or salad dressing; salted nuts

Miscellaneous foods: AVOID bouillon cubes, commercial candies, catsup, celery salt, chili sauce, garlic salt, sweetened gelatin mixes, meat and steak sauces, prepared horseradish, prepared mustard, monosodium glutamate, onion salt, pickles, pudding mixes, relishes, soy sauce, Worcestershire sauce, barbecue sauce

DIETARY PLANS

The selection of foods for three calorie levels of a 500-mg-sodium diet is shown in Table 26–1. The calculations for sodium in the 1800-calorie diet are based on average values assigned to each food list.

Two sample menus for the 500 mg sodium diet are listed in Table 26–2. The 1000 kcal soft diet illustrates the food choices that might be permitted after the third to fifth day following a myocardial infarction, while the 1800 kcal regular diet might be appropriate for maintenance. When the patient returns to his home, the sodium level might be increased to 2000 mg or so.

TABLE 26–1   500-MG-SODIUM DIET AT THREE CALORIE LEVELS *

Food List	1000 kcal Exchanges	1200 kcal Exchanges	1800 kcal	
			Exchanges	Sodium (mg)
1. Milk, skim	2	2	2	240
2. Vegetables	2–3	2–3	2–3	27
3. Fruit	3	3	3	6
4. Bread	4	4	6	30
5. Meat (3–4 eggs/week)	6	6	7	175
6. Fat	0	4	6	—
Sugars and sweets	0	0	7 teaspoons	——
				478

* *250 mg sodium:* substitute low-sodium milk for regular milk.

1000 mg sodium: measure ¼ teaspoon salt into shaker and use on food during the day; *or* use 2 slices regular bread and 2 teaspoons regular butter in place of 2 slices unsalted bread and 2 teaspoons unsalted butter.

Mild sodium restriction: food may be lightly salted in cooking. Use regular bread and butter. Omit salt at the table. Omit salty foods, such as potato chips, pretzels, pickles, relishes, meat sauces, salty meats, fish and so on.

Unrestricted calories: provide additional calories from fruits, unsalted breads and cereals, unsalted fats, sugars and sweets.

PREPARATION OF FOOD

The booklets prepared by the American Heart Association contain menu suggestions and helpful hints for the preparation of food as well as guides for eating away from home.

Patients who have always used much salt at the table are likely to complain bitterly about the flat taste of the food. Others, who prefer foods only lightly salted, find the diet to be more tolerable. In time most patients find that they can adjust to the restriction of sodium by learning to substitute other flavorings. Salt substitutes are useful to some. Because these compounds may be harmful to patients with damaged kidneys, they should be used only with a physician's prescription.

Many flavoring extracts, spices, and herbs may be used to lend interest to the diet. Usually a dash of spices or a small pinch of herbs is sufficient for most family-size recipes. The flavor should be delicate and subtle rather than strong and overpowering. Meats may be marinated in wine, vinegar, low-sodium French dressing, or sprinkled with lemon juice before cooking. A few suggestions for flavor combinations are provided below.*

* C. H. Robinson, *Proudfit-Robinson's Normal and Therapeutic Nutrition*, 13th ed. (New York: Macmillan Publishing Co., Inc., 1967), pp. 759, 760.

TABLE 26–2 TWO SAMPLE MENUS FOR THE 500-MG SODIUM DIET

1000-kcal Soft Diet * (No salt used in cooking)	1800-kcal Regular Diet (No salt used in cooking)
Breakfast	*Breakfast*
Orange sections	Orange sections
Puffed rice	Shredded wheat
Skim milk—½ cup	Milk, skim—1 cup
No sugar	Sugar—2 teaspoons
Toast, unsalted—1 slice	Soft-cooked egg—1
No butter	Toast, unsalted—1 slice
	Special margarine †, unsalted—2 teaspoons
Luncheon	*Luncheon*
Sliced tender chicken (ground, if necessary)—2 oz	Salad bowl:
Asparagus tips with lemon wedge	Lettuce, endive, escarole, raw cauliflower, green pepper, tomato wedges
Roll, unsalted, soft—1	Sliced chicken strips—2 oz
No butter	French dressing, unsalted—1 tablespoon
Peaches, unsweetened, canned—2 halves	Roll, unsalted—1
Milk, skim—1 cup	Special margarine, unsalted—2 teaspoons
	Marmalade—2 teaspoons
	Milk, skim—1 cup
	Peaches, fresh, sliced
Dinner	*Dinner*
Tender roast beef (ground, if necessary)—3 oz	Roast beef—4 oz
Baked potato without skin—1 small	with currant jelly—1 tablespoon
Peas, canned, unsalted	Potato, baked—1 medium
Milk, skim—½ cup	with chive margarine—2 teaspoons
Banana—½	Fresh peas with mushrooms
	Roll, unsalted—1
	Special margarine, unsalted—2 teaspoons
	Tokay grapes

* Give fruit and milk between meals during early stages of recovery.
† Use margarines or oils high in polyunsaturated fat.

MEAT, POULTRY, FISH, EGGS

Beef: bay leaf, lemon juice, marjoram, dry mustard, mushrooms, nutmeg, onion, green pepper, pepper, sage, thyme; currant or grape jelly

Chicken or turkey: basil, bay leaf, lemon juice, marjoram, onion, pepper, rosemary, sage, sesame seeds, thyme; cranberry sauce

Lamb: curry, garlic, mint, onion, oregano, parsley, rosemary, thyme; mint jelly, broiled pineapple

Pork: garlic, lemon juice, marjoram, sage; applesauce, spiced apples, cranberries

Veal: bay leaf, curry, dill seed, ginger, marjoram, oregano, summer savory; currant jelly; broiled apricots or peaches
Fish: bay leaf, curry, dill, garlic, lemon juice, mushrooms, mustard, onion, paprika, pepper
Eggs: basil, chives, curry, mustard, parsley, green pepper, rosemary, diced tomato

VEGETABLES

Add a dash of sugar while cooking vegetables to bring out flavor.

Asparagus: lemon juice, caraway; unsalted chopped nuts
Green beans: dill, lemon, marjoram, nutmeg, onion, rosemary; slivered almonds
Broccoli: lemon juice, oregano, tarragon
Corn: chives, parsley, green pepper, pimento, tomato
Peas: mint, mushroom, onion, parsley, green pepper
Potatoes: chives, mace, onion, parsley, green pepper
Squash: basil, ginger, mace, onion, oregano
Sweet potatoes: cinnamon, nutmeg; brown sugar
Tomatoes: basil, marjoram, oregano, parsley, sage

Homemade quick breads, biscuits, and muffins may be made by using low-sodium baking powder instead of regular baking powder. For each teaspoon of regular baking powder, it is necessary to use 1½ teaspoons low-sodium baking powder. The salt specified in the recipe should be omitted.

Homemade bread, waffles, and rolls may be made by using yeast and omitting the salt from the recipe. The yeast dough may be rolled out, spread with unsalted butter, and sprinkled with sugar and cinnamon for delicious cinnamon rolls.

REVIEW QUESTIONS AND PROBLEMS

1. What are the circumstances that lead to the formation of edema in patients who have had a heart attack?

2. What is the chief source of sodium in the diet?

3. How do sodium-restricted diets compare with the normal diet in the amounts of sodium contained in them?

4. Classify the following foods as (1) low in sodium; (2) naturally high in sodium; or (3) containing much added salt: oranges, shredded wheat, cornflakes, peaches, catsup, American cheese, skim milk, sardines, peanut butter, potato chips, sugar, fresh peas, canned apricots, canned tuna fish, roast beef, pickles.

5. For a patient with cardiac failure and edema, what factors would be important in dietary care in addition to sodium restriction?

6. How would you change a 500-mg-sodium diet to 250-mg-sodium? To 1000-mg-sodium?

7. List the foods that often cause discomfort and distention for cardiac patients.

8. How could you make each of the following foods more palatable for a sodium-restricted diet: sweet potatoes, frozen green beans, roast pork, unsalted bread?

9. A patient asks if he may use a salt substitute. What should you tell him?

10. A patient with hypertension has been given anti-hypertensive medication and advised to adhere to a mild restriction of sodium. Prepare a list of 15 foods that he should avoid.

11. List the foods that contribute important amounts of sodium in the diets of each of these cultural groups: Chinese; Italian; Greek; blacks.

REFERENCES

American Heart Association: *Your Sodium-Restricted Diet: 500 mg, 1000 mg, Mild Restriction.*

Gordon, E. S.: "Dietary Problems in Hypertension," *Geriatrics,* **29**:139–41, May 1974.

Hemzacek, K. I.: "Dietary Protocol for the Patient Who Has Suffered a Myocardial Infarction," *J. Am. Dietet. A.,* **72**:182–85, 1978.

Long, M., *et al.:* "Hypertension: What Patients Need to Know," *Am. J. Nurs.,* **76**:765–70, 1976.

Peterson, C. R.: "Dietary Counseling for Patients Admitted for Coronary Artery Bypass Graft," *J. Am. Dietet. A.,* **68**:158–59, 1976.

Ramsey, M. A.: "The Failing Heart," *Nursing 72,* **2**:18–23, October 1972.

Reisin, E., *et al.:* "Effect of Weight Loss without Salt Restriction on the Reduction of Blood Pressure in Overweight Hypertensive Patients," *N. Engl. J. Med.,* **298**:1–6, 1978.

Snively, W. D., *et al.:* "Sodium-Restricted Diet: Review and Current Status," *Nurs. Forum,* **13**:59–86, 1974.

DISEASES OF THE KIDNEY

*High-Protein Diet; Diets Controlled for Protein, Potassium, and
Sodium*

STRUCTURAL UNITS OF THE KIDNEY

There are about one million working units called *nephrons* in each kidney.
Each nephron consists of a tuft of capillaries known as the *glomerulus* attached
to a long winding *tubule* that empties into collecting tubules.

The glomerulus filters the blood that circulates through it. Water together
with glucose, amino acids, urea, sodium chloride, and other small molecules
filter into the tubules. Large molecules such as the blood proteins are held
back in the circulation. Each glomerulus filters only a tiny drop of fluid in a
day, but the volume of plasma filtered by the two million glomeruli amounts
to about 125 ml per minute or 180 liters in 24 hours. The amounts of glucose,
sodium chloride, and other substances filtered are equally large; for example,
the sodium chloride filtered is over 1 kilogram which is roughly 100 times
the daily intake of salt!

The winding tubules bring about *selective reabsorption* so that the normal
concentration of substances in the blood is maintained at all times. Normally,
the urine volume ranges from 1000 to 2000 ml, which means that over 99
per cent of the filtered water has been returned to the circulation. Likewise,
all of the glucose and vitamin C, and almost all of the amino acids, sodium,
and other substances have been returned to the blood. For example, if you
eat foods containing more salt than your body needs, the renal excretion of
water and sodium will be increased. On the other hand, if you greatly reduce
your salt intake or if the body sodium is depleted, the excretion in the urine
will be very small.

263

FUNCTIONS OF THE KIDNEY

The overall function of the kidneys is to maintain the normal composition and volume of the blood. This is accomplished by four interrelated activities. (1) Wastes of metabolism are excreted. These include urea, uric acid, creatinine, ammonia, sulfates and other products of metabolism, and toxic substances. (2) The amounts of fluid and electrolytes that are reabsorbed or excreted are exactly regulated so that fluid-electrolyte balance is maintained. The *antidiuretic hormone* (ADH) secreted by the pituitary gland influences the amount of water that will be reabsorbed from the tubules. *Aldosterone* secreted by the adrenal gland controls the relative amounts of sodium that will be reabsorbed or excreted. (3) The final adjustment in acid-base balance is made by the kidney. If there is an increased production of metabolic acids, a more acid urine is secreted. Also, the kidney synthesizes ammonia which neutralizes acid so that there is less loss of base. (4) The kidney synthesizes certain enzymes and hormones. *Renin* is an enzyme that influences the production of aldosterone. Renin also has a powerful effect on blood pressure. *Erythropoietin*, a hormone produced by the kidney, stimulates the bone marrow to produce red blood cells. The kidney converts vitamin D to *vitamin-D hormone*. This hormone is necessary for the absorption of calcium from the intestinal tract, and for the regulation of calcium levels in the blood.

NEPHRITIS

Acute glomerulonephritis (inflammation of the glomeruli) frequently follows a streptococcic infection of the respiratory tract or scarlet fever. It is seen most often in children or young adults. During the acute stage of the illness, there is nausea, vomiting, fever, hypertension, hematuria, and oliguria. The appetite is usually very poor and little is gained by forcing food when the gastrointestinal symptoms are present. The fluid intake is usually restricted. The fluid allowance may be taken in the form of fruit juices, fruit ices, ginger ale, sweetened weak tea, or high-carbohydrate low-electrolyte supplements.* Even these small amounts of carbohydrate help to reduce tissue breakdown.

As soon as the patient is able to eat, a diet providing about 0.5 gm protein per kg for adults (up to 0.75 gm per kg for children) and sufficient calories to maintain weight is given. Most of the protein should be obtained from milk and eggs. Protein foods of low biologic value such as peas, Lima beans, dried peas and beans, nuts, peanut butter, and gelatin are omitted. Sodium restriction is not necessary except when edema is present. Potassium restriction is usually not required. See food allowances for 40 to 60 gm protein diets in Table 27–2 (p. 272).

Chronic glomerulonephritis may be present in a latent stage for years before symptoms are detected. When the kidney function is below 20 to 10 per cent

---

* Controlyte,® Doyle Pharmaceutical Company, Minneapolis, Minnesota. Cal Power,® General Mills, Minneapolis, Minnesota. Polycose,® Ross Laboratories, Columbus, Ohio.

of normal, the patient begins to complain of headache, fatigue, nocturia, and sometimes blurring of the vision. Hypertension, proteinuria, and hematuria may also be present.

Sufficient nutrients to meet body requirements are of utmost importance so that the sense of well-being can be maintained as long as possible. Anemia is relatively common and persistent. Iron salts are usually prescribed, but they do not always correct the anemia.

If the blood urea is only moderately high, about 60 to 70 gm protein are included daily with particular emphasis upon sources of high biologic value. If there is proteinuria, the daily protein intake should be increased by the amount lost in the urine.

Sodium restriction is not necessary except when there is edema, but some physicians routinely prescribe mild restriction. (See Chapter 26.) Because the kidneys are unable to concentrate urine, the fluid and sodium losses can be high. Such losses must be corrected by adequate intakes of fluid and sodium. In these patients a sodium-restricted diet could lead to body loss of sodium, weakness, nausea, and shock.

NEPHROSIS

The nephrotic syndrome includes *lipoid nephrosis,* a rare disease in young children, and the nephrotic phase in some patients with glomerulonephritis. The symptoms characteristic of this syndrome include severe edema, heavy albuminuria, very low serum proteins—especially albumin, high serum lipids—especially cholesterol, anemia, and oliguria.

The diet should furnish sufficient calories for maintenance of weight in adults and normal growth in children. The protein intake needs to be liberal in order to compensate for the large losses in the urine and to correct the level of blood albumin. Many physicians recommend up to 120 gm protein per day for adults and 3 to 4 gm protein per kg for young children.

Medical opinions differ on sodium restriction; some recommend 1000 to 2000 mg sodium if there is severe edema. It is questionable whether severe sodium restriction is of any value if it means that the patient will not eat. Cholesterol restriction is set at 300 mg daily by some physicians, while others do not restrict the cholesterol intake.

High-protein diet. As in all therapeutic diets, the planning for high protein intake begins with the normal diet. The basic diet outlined on p. 37 furnishes about 70 gm protein. To achieve a level of 120 gm protein means that concentrated sources of protein would be useful so that there is not excessive bulk to be consumed. If the patient likes meat, fish, or poultry the modest amounts in the basic diet may be increased by 2 or 3 ounces.

Additonal milk is usually included. One way to increase the protein in the diet at low cost and with little increase in volume of the diet is to use nonfat dry milk. Depending upon the brand used, 4 to 5 tablespoons added to 8 oz milk will double the amount of protein. Nonfat dry milk may also be added to mashed potatoes, cream sauces, cream soups, baked custard, and other foods.

Many patients who require a high-protein diet have poor appetites. It is better to start with the patient's present food intake and to gradually increase the protein and calorie intake. The portions served should be of such size that the patient is able to eat all the foods offered. A bedtime snack is a good way to increase protein and calorie intakes. Two examples of such snacks are:

Sandwich
  2 slices bread
  2 teaspoons butter, mayonnaise
  1½ oz. roast beef
  1 oz cheese
Milk, 1 cup

Protein, 29 gm; calories, 585

High-protein milk shake (tall glass)
  1 cup milk
  4–5 tablespoons nonfat dry milk
  2 tablespoons chocolate syrup

Protein, 16 gm; calories, 345

Food allowances to provide approximately 120 gm protein and 2500 kcal:

  4 cups milk
  1 egg
7–9 oz meat, poultry, fish, cheese
3–4 servings vegetables
    1 green leafy or deep yellow
    1 raw
    1 potato or substitute
  3 servings fruit, including 1 citrus fruit
6–7 servings cereals, breads
Butter, margarine, salad dressings
Sugar, jelly, jam
Desserts such as puddings, custard, ice cream

The following menu illustrates the kinds and amounts of foods used for a diet providing 120 gm protein and 2500 kcal:

Breakfast
Stewed prunes
Wheat flakes *with*
Milk, 1 cup
Sugar
Toast, enriched, 1 slice
Butter or margarine
Jelly
Coffee with cream, sugar

Luncheon
Cold sliced ham, bologna, cheese, 3 oz
Potato salad
Lettuce, sliced tomato
Mayonnaise
Roll
Butter or margarine
Fresh peach ice cream
Cookie
Milk, 1 cup
Tea, if desired

Dinner	*Bedtime*

Dinner

Swiss steak, 4 oz
Parsley buttered noodles
French green beans with slivered almonds
Grapefruit avocado salad on water cress
French dressing
Dinner roll with butter or margarine
Floating Island
Milk, 1 cup
Tea or coffee, if desired

Bedtime

Egg salad sandwich
Milk, 1 cup

RENAL FAILURE

Clinical findings. Renal failure indicates that the kidneys are no longer able to fulfill their functions adequately. *Uremia* refers to the retention of urea and other constituents in the blood together with the pattern of symptoms that accompany such retention. *Azotemia* refers specifically to the accumulation of nitrogenous constituents in the blood. When the glomerular filtration rate (GFR) is less than 10 ml per minute (normal is 125 ml per minute) and the blood urea nitrogen (BUN) is 80 mg per 100 ml or more, symptoms of uremia appear. With appropriate dietary management these symptoms can be controlled. When the GFR is 3 ml per minute, dietary modification alone is not adequate and dialysis is needed.

Acute renal failure sometimes occurs from the trauma associated with burns, accidents, or surgery, or from the ingestion of poisons. These patients are oliguric or even anuric. It is an emergency situation that often requires dialysis.

Chronic renal failure is the final outcome of chronic glomerulonephritis or may be associated with poor circulation because of extensive atherosclerosis or cardiac failure.

In renal failure the patient has an elevated blood urea nitrogen, acidosis, anemia, and usually excretes little or no urine. These changes produce gastrointestinal upsets such as anorexia, nausea, vomiting, bad breath, and ulcerations of the mouth. These symptoms make it difficult for the patient to eat.

Other symptoms include headache, muscle twitchings, sometimes blurred vision, and serious interference with heart function. The inability to excrete sodium and water can lead to congestive heart failure. Elevation of the serum potassium can block heart action leading to death.

Because the kidney is unable to produce active vitamin D the absorption of calcium is reduced. The serum calcium is below normal, and abnormal amounts of calcium are released from bone leading to *renal osteodystrophy*. On the other hand the serum phosphorus level is elevated. This causes further release of calcium and phosphorus from bone, resulting in a vicious cycle.

Planning nutrient levels. The diet in renal failure is planned individually for each patient. It takes into account the symptoms, the blood levels of urea and electrolytes, and the nutritional status. Laboratory studies from time to time determine whether the diet needs to be adjusted for one or more nutrients. The diet may be controlled for some or all of these factors: protein, potassium, sodium, phosphorus, and fluids. For patients who are awaiting renal dialysis or who are unable to receive dialysis, the diet is more severely restricted than for patients who are dialyzed at periodic intervals.

Energy. Any breakdown of body tissues releases both nitrogen and potassium to the circulation. In severe renal insufficiency this can lead to dangerous increases in the blood levels. Therefore, it is essential to prevent this by giving 35 to 45 kcal per kg (about 2000 to 3000 kcal daily). Carbohydrates and fats are the principal sources of energy.

Protein. Most frequently protein is restricted to less than 0.5 gm per kg body weight for patients who are not on dialysis. An intake of 40 gm protein is common, but it may be as low as 20 gm. For patients on dialysis a protein intake of 60 to 70 gm is usual. On diets severely restricted in protein the essential amino acids are supplied from milk and eggs. The body can synthesize nonessential amino acids from the excess nitrogenous constituents in the blood.

Potassium. In severe renal failure the serum concentration of potassium is sometimes at dangerously high levels. This can be minimized by giving a diet restricted in potassium; 40 mEq (1560 mg) is often prescribed.

When the urine volume is still adequate, potassium is excreted without too much difficulty and restriction is not necessary. If potassium-losing diuretics are used, additional potassium may be needed to maintain normal serum levels.

Sodium. Restriction of sodium ranging from 500 mg to 2000 mg is ordered if there is edema and hypertension. Some patients are "salt losers." If they are placed on a sodium-restricted diet they will lose more sodium than they are ingesting, and they will become dehydrated.

Phosphorus. When blood levels of phosphorus are elevated, aluminum hydroxide gel is often prescribed to bind the phosphate in the intestinal tract. A phosphorus-restricted diet (1000 to 1500 mg) may also be ordered.

Minerals and vitamins. The protein-restricted diets do not provide recommended daily allowances of calcium, iron, vitamin B complex, and vitamin D. Supplements of these nutrients should be prescribed.

Fluid. When there is oliguria the fluid intake is restricted to the daily volume in the urine plus about 500 to 700 ml which represents the approximate loss from the skin, lungs, and bowel. For example, a urinary excretion of 250 ml daily would permit a fluid intake of 750 ml. This includes all the water present in foods as well as that in beverages. A 100-gm portion of fruits and vegetables supplies 80 to 90 ml water, and 100 ml of milk is equal to 87 ml water. See Table A–1 for per cent of water in foods.

Food lists and meal plans. A *protein-free electrolyte-free diet* may be used for a few days if the patient is anuric. This supplies sufficient calories to prevent tissue breakdown. Calories are furnished by hard candies and butter balls consisting of a mixture of butter and sugar flavored to improve palatability. A number

TABLE 27–1 PROTEIN, SODIUM, AND POTASSIUM VALUES FOR FOOD LISTS

Food List	Household Measure	Weight gm	Protein gm	Sodium * mg	Potassium mg
Milk, whole or nonfat	1 cup	240	8	120	335
Milk, low sodium	1 cup	240	8	7	600
Meat, poultry, fish, cooked	1 ounce	30	7	25	100
Egg	1	50	7	60	65
Cheese, American, salted	1 ounce	30	7	210	25
Cheese, cottage, salted	1 ounce	30	7	85	25
Fruits, list 1	½ cup	100	less than 0.5	2	85–145
Fruits, list 2	½ cup	100	1	2	135–200
Vegetables, list 1	½ cup	100	1	9	110–190
list 2	½ cup	100	2	9	160–245
list 3	½ cup	100	3	9	210
Bread, low sodium	1 slice	30	2	5	30
Bread, regular	1 slice	30	2	160	30
Bread, low-protein, low-electrolyte	1 slice	30	0.1	9	3
Butter, unsalted	1 teaspoon	5	tr	tr	tr
Butter, salted	1 teaspoon	5	tr	50	tr

* Except for cheese, regular bread, and salted butter, the values listed for sodium are those that apply when no salt is used in processing or preparation of the food. Also, certain high-sodium items in the meat and vegetable lists would be omitted if the diet is restricted in sodium.

of high-carbohydrate supplements that contain no protein or electrolytes are commercially available. (See p. 264.)

Sources of protein. Almost all of the protein in the restricted diets must come from milk, eggs, and meat. Cereals, bread, rice, macaroni, spaghetti, and noodles are usually depended upon as good sources of calories. However, 6 to 8 servings of these foods a day would account for 15 to 25 gm protein, which is not of high biologic value. Obviously not much of these foods could be used on diets restricted to 40 gm protein or less.

Special flours and breads have been developed by food processors that are protein-free and low in potassium and sodium.† Recipes for using these products have been developed by the manufacturers. The absence of protein in the flour means that breads will not have the texture qualities provided by gluten, and they are generally less acceptable to the patient. Jellies, unsalted butter and margarine, and honey improve the palatability as well as enhancing the caloric intake. The nurse must emphasize to the patient that it is important

† Dietetic Paygel-P, General Mills, Minneapolis, Minnesota.
Cellu Wheat Starch and Cellu Low Protein Baking Mix, Chicago Dietetic Supply House, LaGrange, Illinois.

FOOD LISTS FOR CONTROLLED PROTEIN, SODIUM, AND POTASSIUM DIETS *

Milk List

Buttermilk, unsalted
Evaporated milk, reconstituted
Low sodium milk
Nonfat dry milk, reconstituted
Skim milk
Whole milk

Meat or Substitute List

Beef, chicken, duck, lamb, liver, pork, tongue (unsalted), turkey, veal
Cod, flatfish (flounder or sole), kingfish (whiting), haddock, perch, canned salmon and tuna (omit on sodium-restricted diet)
Clams, crab, lobster, scallops, shrimp (all omitted on sodium-restricted diet)
Egg
Cheese—Cheddar, cottage, American, Swiss (omit on sodium-restricted diet)

Fruit, List 1

Apple, raw   1 small
Grapes, European   12
½ cup servings of: applesauce, pears, pineapple, diced watermelon
½ cup of juices: apple, grape, peach nectar, pear nectar, orange-apricot, pineapple-grapefruit, pineapple-orange

With liberal potassium allowance
(145 mg potassium per serving)
½ cup of: apricot nectar, pineapple juice, canned fruit cocktail, purple plums

Fruit, List 2

Pear, raw   1 small
Tangerine   1 small

Fruit, List 2 (Continued)

½ cup servings of fresh or frozen blackberries, blueberries, boysenberries, canned cherries, figs; canned or fresh grapefruit; frozen red raspberries

With liberal potassium allowance
(200 mg potassium per serving)
Orange   1 small
Peach, raw   1 small
Plums, fresh   2 medium
Strawberries, fresh ⅔ cup
½ cup servings of cantaloupe, honeydew, frozen melon balls, fresh or frozen rhubarb
½ cup of these juices: grapefruit, grapefruit-orange, orange, tomato

Vegetables, List 1

1 gm protein, 110 mg potassium per serving
½ cup of raw cabbage, cucumber, lettuce, onion, tomato

1 gm protein, 125 mg potassium per serving
½ cup servings of canned green or wax beans, carrots (+),† spinach (+); fresh cooked cabbage, eggplant, mustard greens, onions, summer squash

Liberal potassium allowance: 1 gm protein, 190 mg potassium per serving
½ cup servings of canned beets (+), rutabagas, tomatoes; fresh cooked carrots (+), turnips (+), frozen summer squash, winter squash

Vegetables, List 2

2 gm protein, 160 mg potassium per serving
½ cup servings of canned asparagus; fresh or frozen green or wax beans, okra

---

* Adapted from Robinson, C. H., and Lawler, M. R.: *Normal and Therapeutic Nutrition*, 15th ed., Macmillan Publishing Co., Inc., 1977, pp. 560–63.
† Vegetables marked with (+) are omitted when the diet is restricted in sodium.

Vegetables, List 2 (Continued)

Liberal potassium allowance: 2 gm protein, 245 mg potassium per serving

½ cup servings of fresh or frozen cauliflower; cooked dandelion greens (+); potato, boiled (pared before cooking), or mashed

Vegetables, List 3

3 gm protein, 210 mg potassium per serving
½ cup servings of kale (+); frozen asparagus, broccoli, collards (+), mixed vegetables (+), whole kernel corn

Bread and substitutes

Bread	1 slice
Cereals, dry	1 cup
Cornflakes, Puffed	
Rice, Puffed Wheat,	
shredded wheat	
Cereals, cooked	½ cup
cornmeal, farina,	
oatmeal, rice,	
rolled wheat	
Crackers, soda	3 squares
Flour	2 tablespoons
Grits	1 cup

Bread and substitutes (Continued)

Macaroni, noodles, or spaghetti	¼ cup
Rice	½ cup

Fats

Butter
Cream (1 ounce contains 35 mg potassium)
Fat or cooking oil
Margarine
Salad dressings: French or mayonnaise

Miscellaneous

Cornstarch
Flavoring extracts
Ginger ale
Hard candies
Herbs (see suggestions p. 260)
Honey
Jam or jelly
Jellybeans
Rice starch
Spices (see suggestions p. 260)
Sugar, white, confectioners'
Syrup
Tapioca
Vinegar
Wheat starch

to consume all the food allowed on the diet; it is not sufficient to restrict protein alone.

Sources of potassium. The normal intake of potassium varies from 3000 to 8000 mg, being at the higher levels when protein and calorie intakes are high. Protein-rich foods are also good sources of potassium. Therefore, diets restricted in protein will also contain less potassium.

Potassium salts are quite soluble in water. Stewed meats will have less potassium than broiled or roasted meats, providing that the stewing liquid is not consumed.

Vegetables and fruits are also good sources of potassium, but there is a wide variability from one food to another. Canned fruits and vegetables contain less potassium than fresh if the liquid is drained from the product. Boiled potatoes will have less potassium than baked or fried potatoes. The potassium content of a potato can be reduced by (1) cutting the potato into small pieces, (2) immersing the potato in water for ½ hour before cooking, and (3) boiling in fresh water to cover.

Sources of phosphorus. Milk, eggs, meat, poultry, fish, nuts, whole-grain breads and cereals, dried beans and peas, dried fruits, chocolate, and cocoa are rich sources of phosphorus. When the diet is restricted in phosphorus, controlled amounts of milk, eggs, meat, fish, and poultry are allowed. Enriched bread or low-protein bread may be used.

Diet lists. The plan of diets described here is but one of many that have been developed in hospitals throughout the country. Although the principles described above apply to all diet plans, the food lists differ somewhat. Table 27–1, p. 269, summarizes the values to be used in calculating diets.

TABLE 27–2 SUGGESTED DAILY MEAL PATTERN FOR CONTROLLED
PROTEIN, SODIUM, AND POTASSIUM DIET

		Protein		
	Measure	*20 gm*	*40 gm*	*60 gm*
Breakfast				
Fruit, list 1	1 exchange	1	1	1
Egg	1	—	1	1
Cereal	1 exchange	1	1	1
Low-protein bread	1 slice	2	—	—
Bread, enriched	1 slice	—	1	1
Milk	cup	¼	¼	¼
Lunch				
Egg	1	1	—	—
Meat or equivalent	1 ounce	—	1	2
Bread or substitute	1 exchange	—	1	2
Low-protein bread	1 slice	2	—	—
Vegetable, list 1	1 exchange	—	1	1
Milk	cup	—	½	½
Low-protein dessert	1 serving	1	1	1
Fruit, list 1	1 exchange	1	1	1
Dinner				
Meat or equivalent	1 ounce	—	1	2
Bread or substitute	1 exchange	1	1	2
Low-protein bread	1 slice	2	—	—
Vegetable, list 1	1 exchange	1	—	—
Vegetable, list 2	1 exchange	—	1	1
Fruit, list 2	1 exchange	—	1	2
Milk	cup	½	—	—
Low-protein dessert	1 serving	1	—	—

Manual of Diets, Department of Dietetics, Hospital of St. Raphael, Veterans Administration Hospital, Yale–New Haven Hospital, New Haven, Conn.

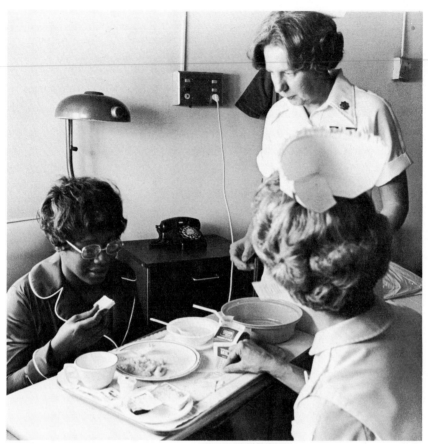

FIGURE 27–1 Patients with chronic renal failure often have poor appetites. They may need assistance as well as encouragement to consume sufficient food to meet caloric requirements. The nurse and dietitian must also explain the nature of the diet to the patient. *(Department of Nursing, Delaware County Community College, Media, Pennsylvania.)*

Fruits have been grouped into two lists, one providing less thant 0.5 gm protein per serving, and one containing 1.0 gm per serving. There are three lists of vegetables, furnishing 1.0, 2.0, and 3.0 gm protein respectively. Within the fruit and vegetable lists are foods that may be used when potassium restriction is less severe.

The daily allowance for protein is divided approximately evenly in the three meals so that there is maximum utilization. These patients cannot afford to cheat on their diets. To do so means that the body is overloaded with nitrogen, potassium, sodium, and fluid. On the other hand there is decided improvement of the appetite and sense of well-being when the patient consumes all the foods planned for his controlled diet. (See Table 27–2 and Fig. 27–1.)

URINARY CALCULI

Most kidney stones contain calcium as calcium carbonate, phosphate, or oxalate. There are also uric acid stones and cystine stones. Some stones dissolve in acid and some in alkali. Medications are usually prescribed to increase the acidity or alkalinity of the urine. Diet alone does not sufficiently change the pH of the urine, but modifications are sometimes prescribed so that the diet will not counteract the effectiveness of the medication.

A *calcium- and phosphorus-restricted diet* limits milk to 1½ cups or less, and eliminates cheese and all foods prepared with milk.

If an *acid-ash diet* is ordered the emphasis is upon meat, eggs, fish, poultry, cereals, and breads, macaroni and other pastas, rice, cranberry juice, prunes, and plums. The amounts of milk, vegetables, and fruits are included at levels suggested in the basic diet. (See p. 37.)

For oxalate and uric acid stones an *alkaline-ash diet* is sometimes ordered. This diet restricts the amount of eggs, meat, cereals, and breads, and emphasis is placed upon milk, fruits, and vegetables.

Butter, margarine, shortenings, oils, sugar, hard candies, gumdrops, honey, and pure starches are neutral and may be used on either acid-ash or alkaline-ash diets.

A diet restricted in oxalate is sometimes ordered, but its effectiveness is unknown. Such a diet would eliminate almonds, beets and beet greens, cashew nuts, chard, chocolate, cocoa, coffee, corn, currants, endive, figs, Concord grapes, okra, plums, potatoes, raspberries, rhubarb, spinach, sweet potatoes, tea, and tomatoes.

Uric acid stones are sometimes a complication of gout. (See p. 240.)

REVIEW QUESTIONS AND PROBLEMS

1. What changes take place in the composition of urine of the normal individual in these situations: a diet containing many salty foods is eaten; a diet containing very little salt is eaten; the protein intake is about 100 gm or more each day?

2. What problems might arise for the patient with chronic renal failure in the three situations listed in question 1?

3. Why is it so important to emphasize liberal intakes of carbohydrate and fat by patients with renal failure?

4. An increase in fluid intake is usually recommended when a high-protein diet is ordered. Why?

5. What would be the total fluid intake from the following meal: 1 egg, 2 slices bread, ½ cup green beans, ½ cup applesauce, ½ cup milk? See Table A–1 (p. 322) for information on water contents of food.

6. A patient on a potassium-restricted diet is told not to use the juices from canned vegetables and fruits. Why?

7. A patient on a potassium-restricted diet is advised that he may include a small potato in his diet two or three times a week. What directions should be given for the preparation of the potato?

8. Using the 60 gm-protein diet plan in Table 27–2 and the food exchange lists, plan a menu for one day that is low in potassium and sodium.

9. In the sample menu for the high-protein diet on page 266 arrange the food items under these four headings: acid ash; alkaline ash; neutral; and high in oxalates.

10. Which foods would be emphasized for a patient with renal calculi that are more soluble in acid?

REFERENCES

Anderson, C. F., et al.: "Nutritional Therapy for Adults with Renal Disease," JAMA, 223:68–75, 1973.

Burton, B. T.: "Current Concepts of Nutrition and Diet in Diseases of the Kidney. Part II. Dietary Regimen in Specific Kidney Disorders," J. Am. Dietet. A., 65:627–33, 1974.

Corea, A. L.: "Current Trends in Diet and Drug Therapy for the Dialysis Patient," Nurs. Clin. North Am., 10:469–79, 1975.

Hamburger, R. J.: "Management of Uremia," Am. Fam. Physician, 16:125–32, September 1977.

Sanderson, M.: "Diet and Dialysis," Nurs. Times, 72:1774–75, 1976.

Santopietro, M-C. S.: "Meeting the Emotional Needs of Hemodialysis Patients and Their Spouses," Am. J. Nurs., 75:629–32, 1975.

DISEASES OF THE

GASTROINTESTINAL TRACT

Bland Fiber-Restricted Diet; High-Fiber Diet;
Very Low-Residue Diet

The dietary modifications for diseases of the gastrointestinal tract are discussed in three chapters: peptic ulcer, hiatus hernia, constipation, and diverticulitis in this chapter; diseases of malabsorption in Chapter 29; and diseases of the liver, gallbladder, and pancreas in Chapter 30. Since any diseases of the gastrointestinal tract are closely associated with function, the student should first review the normal digestive processes (see Chapter 3).

General Dietary Considerations

The planning of the diets for diseases of the gastrointestinal tract must consider: (1) the nutritional status of the individual; (2) the adequacy of the proposed diet; (3) the secretion of enzymes, gastric juice, and bile; (4) the motility of the tract; (5) the integrity of the absorbing surfaces of the intestines; (6) stress factors such as anxiety, fear, pressure of work, grief, and others; and (7) individual beliefs and tolerances regarding food.

For some diseases there is a physiologic basis for the dietary modification; for example, lactose intolerance, gluten-induced enteropathy, cirrhosis of the liver, and pancreatic insufficiency. For other pathologic conditions there is no sound rationale for diet therapy. The diets used for such conditions are often based on tradition and are generally regarded as conservative and restricted. Recent clinical research has indicated that for many conditions such as peptic ulcer essentially normal diets are just as effective as those more limited in food choice. The trend in many conditions is toward liberalization of diet.

276

DIETARY FIBER

The terms "fiber" and "residue" are often misused. *Dietary fiber* consists of the indigestible parts of plants. It includes cellulose, hemicellulose, lignin, gums, pectins, and mucilages occurring in the cell structure of plants. *Residue* refers to the bulk remaining in the lower part of the gastrointestinal tract. It includes the dietary fibers, cells sloughed off from the intestinal mucosa, and intestinal bacteria and their residues. For example, milk contains no dietary fiber, but the lactose in milk is favorable to the growth of certain types of bacteria in the intestine.

Sources of fiber. The structural parts of plants are important sources of fiber. The fiber content of overripe vegetables such as peas and corn is higher than that of young, tender peas or succulent corn. Bran, whole-grain breads and cereals, legumes, vegetables, and fruits are emphasized in high-fiber diets.

Fiber and motility. A high-fiber diet increases peristalsis, shortens the length of time that food wastes remain in the colon, and increases stool volume. A low-fiber intake reduces peristalsis, increases the pressure within the lumen of the colon, increases transit time through the intestinal tract, and results in small, dry stools.

Modifying fiber content of diets. The fiber content may range from high, to low, to fiber-free. The diet is progressively reduced in fiber content in the following ways:

1. Selecting only young tender vegetables.

2. Omitting those foods that have seeds, tough skins, or much structural fiber; for example, berries, celery, corn, cabbage, stalks of asparagus, mature beans, and peas.

3. Peeling fruits and vegetables, such as apples, pears, potatoes, stalks of broccoli.

4. Cooking foods to soften the fiber.

5. Pressing foods through a sieve (puréeing or straining).

6. Using refined cereals and white breads in place of whole-grain cereals and breads.

7. Omitting fruits and vegetables entirely; using only strained juices.

Strained fruits and vegetables and ground meats are extremely unpopular. They have lost appeal in appearance, texture, and in flavor, and are generally regarded as baby foods. These restrictions are now seldom used for patients with peptic ulcer, colitis, or diverticulitis except in early stages of treatment. On the other hand, strained foods are useful for patients with bleeding esophageal varices, for blenderized tube feedings, and for preparation for gastrointestinal surgery.

FOOD AND GASTRIC ACIDITY

The sight, smell, and taste of food stimulates the secretion of gastric juice. Foods have a pH of 5 to 7 which is much less acid than gastric juice. Thus, no foods, including citrus and other acid-tasting fruits, are sufficiently acid to change the acidity of the stomach contents.

Protein-rich foods neutralize gastric acid. Hence, the use of milk for many years has been emphasized. The neutralizing effect lasts for only ½ to 2 hours, and diet alone cannot be depended upon to fully neutralize the acids that are formed.

Fats reduce acid production and also decrease motility. The long-used regimen of milk and cream feedings for peptic ulcer were therefore intended to neutralize and to reduce acid production. Because saturated fats may increase the risk of atherosclerosis, cream is now seldom used.

Gastric acid production is increased by coffee, tea, alcohol, and tobacco; meat extractives as in meat soups, gravies, sauces; and spices such as chili powder, black pepper, mustard seed, and nutmeg. Other spices and herbs have no appreciable effect on acid production.

FOOD TOLERANCE

Many people believe that certain foods cause discomfort such as heartburn, abdominal distention, and flatulence. Among foods commonly cited are strongly flavored vegetables that contain sulfur compounds—broccoli, Brussels sprouts, cabbage, cauliflower, cucumber, leeks, onions, radishes, and turnips; melons; and dry beans. Tolerance to these foods is highly individual, and one person may eat onions with relish and no subsequent problems, while another experiences discomfort after eating even a small quantity. Therefore, these foods should not be arbitrarily excluded for all patients, but should be allowed according to individual tolerance.

Patients with gastrointestinal disturbances are often nervous, anxious, overly concerned about their work, and tense. Their emotions strongly influence the digestion of foods. They also have many preconceived ideas about foods that they have heard from relatives or friends. Perhaps in no disease condition is individualization of diet more important than it is for diseases of the gastrointestinal tract. On the other hand, some firmness is often necessary to emphasize the need for nutritional adequacy.

Rapid eating, incomplete mastication, and failure to rest are frequently noted in these patients. They need to learn to take time for meals, to eat slowly, to relax before and after meals, and to look for diversions that can relieve the pressures and anxieties.

Peptic Ulcer

CLINICAL FINDINGS

A peptic ulcer is an erosion of the gastrointestinal mucosa. It may be found in the esophagus, stomach, and most often in the duodenum. Pain is caused by contact of the hydrochloric acid with the eroded surface. The pain is described as dull, gnawing, burning, or even piercing. The patient with a peptic ulcer is often anxious, tense, emotional, and one who strives for perfection in whatever he does. Usually there is increased secretion of gastric juice and increased motility. Many patients who have restricted their intake to relatively few foods have low blood proteins, anemia, and weight loss.

TREATMENT

The objective of treatment is to heal the ulcer. Physical and mental rest are crucial not only during the acute illness but subsequent to full healing. Most patients require some guidance in modifying their life style so that there is less stress both at home and at work.

The physician prescribes one or more of these drugs: *antacids* to neutralize acid; *anticholinergic* agents to reduce acid secretion; and *antispasmodics* to reduce motility. Antacids interfere with iron absorption, and iron supplements may be prescribed to correct or prevent anemia.

The objectives of dietary management are to maintain good nutrition; to supply the nutrients needed to heal the ulcer, protein and ascorbic acid being especially important; and to provide foods that give the patient satisfaction and comfort.

LIBERAL DIET

Many physicians now prescribe a so-called liberal diet, which is essentially a normal diet, at the very beginning of therapy. However, if the ulcer is located in the esophagus or if the ulcer is bleeding a more conservative approach is recommended.

The liberal diet may follow the description of the normal diet (see p. 205) but with emphasis on these points:

1. Based upon a diet history, individualize the diet according to the patient's food habits and preferences. Explain fully the reasons for any modifications that should be made in this pattern. (See Fig. 28–1.)

2. Regulate energy intake according to weight status; those who have lost weight should have a daily caloric intake about 500 kcal above their normal requirement.

3. Include recommended amounts of foods from the four food groups to ensure nutritive adequacy.

4. Use moderation in food selection; avoid excessive use of any one food group; for example, milk, high-fiber foods, and so on.

5. Allow all foods which the patient tolerates, except for items listed in number 6. Some can tolerate all strongly flavored vegetables while others experience discomfort with the inclusion of one or more of this class.

6. Omit alcohol, tobacco; meat soups, meat extractives; pepper, chili powder,

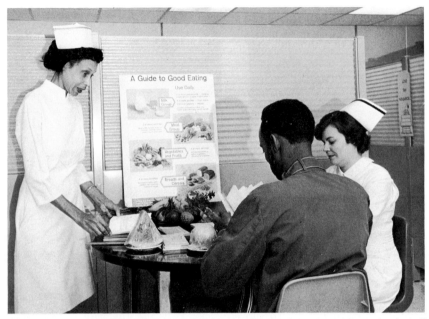

FIGURE 28–1 A patient convalescing from peptic ulcer learns, to his surprise, that he will be able to enjoy most foods from a normal diet. Selecting a nutritionally adequate diet is important. The nurse will be able to reinforce the instruction from time to time. *(Dietetic Service, Veterans Administration Hospital, Coatesville, Pennsylvania. Photo by J. Josephs.)*

mustard, and nutmeg. Small amounts of coffee or tea with milk are usually permitted.

7. Eat small meals and include midmorning, midafternoon, and evening snacks. Small meals reduce the distention of the stomach and thus reduce acid flow. Protein in each of the six feedings temporarily neutralizes acid.

8. Rest before and after meals. Eat slowly in a pleasant environment. Avoid conversations that are emotionally upsetting.

BLAND FIBER-RESTRICTED DIET

Some patients progress more rapidly when they are placed on a conservative regimen. In part this may be explained by their need to have someone who gives them close guidance, even with an authoritarian approach. Also, it may stem from ideas they have long held that ulcers should be treated with a very strict diet. Acute illness is not the best time to change these ideas. The restricted diet is more appropriate for bleeding ulcers and ulcers of the esophagus.

The conventional approach to diet allows a limited selection of food at first and progressing through three or four stages to a normal diet. A moderately liberal progression is described below.

Stage 1. Milk at two-hourly intervals: 180 ml (6 oz). In addition at mealtimes

1 serving (3 to 4 oz) of any one of these foods: strained cream soup, eggs, cottage cheese, white potato, white toast or crackers, refined cereals.

Stage 2. Milk is given on awakening, midmorning, midafternoon, and before bedtime: 240 ml (8 oz). At mealtime the total volume of food is about 350–450 gm (12–16 oz). All foods of stage 1 are used. In addition allow tender meat, poultry, fish, prepared any way except fried; fruit juices, banana, orange or grapefruit sections, canned fruits except berries; cooked or canned tender asparagus, wax or green beans, beets, spinach, sweet potato, winter squash. The following menu is typical of allowances for stage 2:

On Awakening
Milk—8 oz

Breakfast
Oatmeal
Milk, sugar
Egg—1
Enriched toast
Butter or margarine
Orange juice—½ cup

Midmorning
Milk—8 oz
Crackers—2

Luncheon
Cream of pea soup—½ cup
Crackers—2
Chicken-noodle casserole
White bread
Butter or margarine
Canned peaches
Milk

Midafternoon
Vanilla pudding
Milk

Dinner
Roast beef—3 oz
Mashed potato
Asparagus tips
Bread or roll
Butter or margarine
Vanilla ice cream
Milk

Bedtime
Milk shake
Plain sugar cookies

Stage 3. Six feedings a day are continued. The foods allowed on the soft diet, p. 207, are used with two exceptions: broth, meat soups, and gravies are omitted; and coffee is limited to 1 cup per day and is diluted with milk.

Stage 4. Normal (liberal) diet; see p. 205.

Other Diseases of the Gastrointestinal Tract

HIATUS HERNIA

Hiatus hernia is an abnormal gap in the diaphragm so that parts of the stomach and other organs slip into the chest cavity. It is found in about 10 per cent of all people, although most of them have no symptoms. Patients complain of heartburn because of the reflux of gastric juice into the esophagus. Those who are obese should lose weight, since excessive weight causes increased pressure, just as do tight garments. A normal diet is usually tolerated, although some patients omit certain foods to which they are intolerant. Small meals with midmorning and midafternoon snacks are better than three large meals. No food should be taken for several hours prior to bedtime. If the symptoms are severe the bland fiber-restricted diet, stages 2 and 3, described on p. 281 should be tried.

CONSTIPATION

Atonic constipation occurs more frequently in elderly persons and those who are physically handicapped. They have little exercise and often confine their food selection to low-fiber foods. In addition they may drink little liquid, resort to the use of laxatives, and have irregular habits of elimination. Obviously these practices must be changed to correct the constipation. Unless the physician indicates otherwise, the patient should be encouraged to drink at least 1200 to 1500 ml fluid daily; to exercise as the condition warrants; and to develop regular habits of elimination.

High-fiber diet. This is essentially a normal diet with emphasis on foods rich in fiber. The fiber content of the diet should be increased gradually by initiating first one and then another of the following:

1. Add 1 to 2 tablespoons bran to breakfast cereal, or mix with milk or juice. Bran may also be included in muffins and breads.

2. Substitute at least four servings whole-grain bread and cereals for refined cereals and white bread.

3. Include at least four servings of vegetables and fruit daily. Raw carrots, lettuce, potatoes with skins, apples with peel, oranges, and stewed dried fruits should be encouraged.

4. When planning menus, include raw vegetable salads, and fruits for dessert.

DIVERTICULITIS

Diverticulosis is the presence of tiny sacs or pouches in the intestinal wall, most often in the colon. The diverticuli become filled with food wastes and bacteria, but produce no symptoms until they become infected and inflamed *(diverticulitis)*. Once inflamed, severe pain and even perforation may occur.

Long continued use of low-fiber diets is believed to contribute to the development of diverticuli. The swallowing of air together with the gases resulting from the overproduction of bacteria in the intestines leads to increased gas pressure. Diets that are low in fiber cause the colon to contract more tightly; this further increases the gas pressure. The walls of the colon then bulge out to form the diverticulum.

Treatment. During the acute stage bed rest, antibiotics, and a clear-liquid diet followed by a very low-residue diet are prescribed. Surgery is sometimes indicated.

The second stage in dietary management is a gradual increase in fiber content until a high-fiber intake is achieved (see p. 282). Patients are likely to be fearful of increasing their fiber intake because they may have been told that a low-fiber diet is essential to treatment. They need to understand that a high-fiber intake results in lowering the pressure that builds up in the colon, that fiber increases the bulk of the stool, that there is a shorter time for food wastes and bacterial growth to accumulate, and that elimination is improved. Some persons experience flatulence at first, but this is not cause for discontinuing the diet. The adjustment is more readily made if fiber intake is increased over a period of weeks. For example, the patient might modify his diet only by adding a táblespoon of bran to his breakfast cereal; a few days to a week later he might add a second tablespoon or so on.

Very low-residue diet.   This diet is designed to furnish a minimum of fiber and also lead to a minimum of residue in the intestinal tract. The diet allows tender meats, poultry, fish, eggs, white bread, macaroni, noodles, simple desserts, clear soups, tea, and coffee. It omits all fruits, fruit juices, vegetables, and usually milk. Such a diet is obviously lacking in calcium, iron, and vitamins, and should be used for only a few days. A typical menu follows:

Breakfast	*Luncheon*	*Dinner*
Cream of wheat	Tomato bouillon	Small club steak
Milk for cereal	Crackers	Baked potato without skin;
Sugar	Roast chicken	butter
Soft-cooked egg	Buttered rice	Roll with butter
White toast	White bread or roll	Whipped raspberry gelatin
Butter	Butter or margarine	Plain sugar cookies
Coffee	White cake with icing	Tea with lemon and sugar
	Tea with lemon and sugar	

REVIEW QUESTIONS AND PROBLEMS

1. What are the sources of fiber in the diet? What is meant by residue?

2. What are some factors that explain the intolerances that people have to foods?

3. Take a survey of five people you know to find out what foods they do not tolerate. What reasons do they give for any intolerance they have?

4. What is the relationship of fiber and strongly flavored vegetables to the discomfort that patients with gastrointestinal diseases often describe?

5. What are the advantages of a liberal diet in the treatment of patients with peptic ulcer? When would a progressive regimen be better?

6. Write a menu for one day for a patient who carries his lunch to work and who is following a bland fiber-restricted diet, stage 3.

7. A high-fiber diet is recommended for reducing the incidence of diverticulitis. Explain why such a diet would be useful.

REFERENCES

American Dietetic Association: "Position Paper on Bland Diet in the Treatment of Chronic Duodenal Ulcer Disease," *J. Am. Dietet. A.,* **59:**244–45, 1971.

Bass, L.: "More Fiber—Less Constipation," *Am. J. Nurs.,* **77:**254–55, 1977.

Burkitt, D. P., *et al.:* "Dietary Fiber and Disease," *J.A.M.A.,* **229:**1068–74, 1974.

Douglas, A. P.: "Diarrhoea," *Nurs. Times,* **71:**2022–23, 1975.

Eastwood, M.: "Diverticular Disease," *Nurs. Times,* **71:**68, 1975.

Friedmam, G. D., *et al.:* "Cigarettes, Alcohol, Coffee and Peptic Ulcer," *N. Engl. J. Med.,* **290:**469–73, 1974.

Given, B., and Simmons, S.: "Care of the Patient with Gastric Ulcer," *Am. J. Nurs.,* **70:**1472–75, 1970.

Plumley, P. F., and Francis, B.: "Dietary Mangement of Diverticular Disease," *J. Am. Dietet. A.,* **63:**527–30, 1973.

Spiro, H. M.: The Rough and the Smooth, Some Reflections on Diet Therapy," *N. Engl. J. Med.,* **293:**83–85, 1975.

MALABSORPTION DISORDERS

Lactose-Restricted Diet; Gluten-Restricted Diet

Malabsorption is a general term that describes incomplete absorption of one or more nutrients. Among the causes are increased motility of the gastrointestinal tract; inadequate supply or absence of pancreatic or intestinal enzymes or bile; defect in the structure of the villi so that the area of absorbing surface is reduced; and allergy. Symptoms that are usually present include anorexia, abdominal distention, diarrhea, muscle wasting and weight loss because of inability to absorb nutrients, and vitamin and mineral deficiencies.

DIARRHEA

Diarrhea is the frequent passage of liquid or semisolid stools. In acute diarrhea fluids and electrolytes may be given intravenously to allow the gastrointestinal tract to rest. After the first 24 hours progression is made according to the patient's tolerance to a very low-residue diet (p. 283), soft diet (p. 207), and regular diet.

Prolonged diarrhea leads to serious losses of fluids, electrolytes, proteins, fats, carbohydrates, and vitamins. These losses must be corrected by adequate fluid intake, mineral and vitamin supplements, and a high-calorie high-protein diet. In addition gluten restriction is required for gluten-induced enteropathy and lactose restriction or omission for lactase deficiency.

ULCERATIVE COLITIS

This is an inflammation of the colon, occurring more frequently in young adults. The causes are unknown. Many of the patients are nervous, worried,

285

and emotionally unstable. Any upsets aggravate the condition. In severe colitis there is much loss of water, electrolytes, and protein in the numerous stools. Abdominal discomfort, weight loss, dehydration, anemia, and general weakness are outstanding.

Dietary management. Because tissue-wasting is great a diet that supplies 2500–3500 kcal and 100–150 gm protein is required. Supplements of iron and vitamins are usually indicated. Many of these patients have moderate to severe lactose intolerance (see below) and require calcium supplements as well. Initially a very low-residue diet is prescribed with progression to a soft fiber-restricted diet.

The nurse and the dietitian must convince the patient of their interest in his welfare by frequent visits, especially at mealtime. They must be prepared to listen to many complaints, to reassure the patient of the importance of diet in his recovery, and to assist in the selection of the diet from a list of appropriate foods. (See Fig. 29–1.)

LACTOSE INTOLERANCE

Congenital lactase deficiency. A small percentage of infants are born with a lack of lactase and therefore are unable to digest the lactose in milk. These

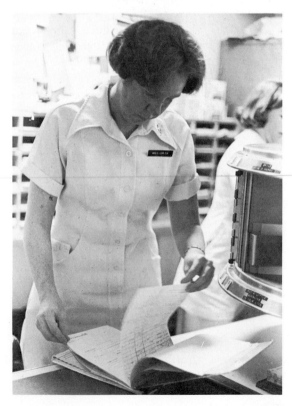

FIGURE 29–1 A nurse reviews the patient's chart and makes notations regarding the acceptance of his diet. *(Department of Nursing, Delaware County Community College, Media, Pennsylvania.)*

infants become severely ill within a few days of birth. They must be given a formula that is free of all sources of lactose, such as meat-base, soybean, or amino acid hydrolysate.*

Acquired lactase deficiency. Many individuals have adequate levels of lactase during infancy and preschool years but lose some of the ability to digest lactose in later years. The deficiency occurs frequently in Oriental and African populations and in the Middle East. It occurs in only a small per cent of Caucasians.

Lactose intolerance is sometimes seen in patients who consume large amounts of milk; for example, with excessive use of milk in diets for peptic ulcer and in tube feedings. Deficiency also occurs in some patients with ulcerative colitis, gluten-induced enteropathy, cystic fibrosis, kwashiorkor, following gastrectomy, and with therapy including neomycin or colchicine.

Lactose-restricted diet. Most children and adults with lactase deficiency can tolerate small amounts of lactose, and the diet should be adjusted to the individual's tolerance. For example, a child may tolerate ½ cup of milk at a time but have symptoms of bloating, flatulence, cramps, and diarrhea when he drinks greater amounts of milk at each meal. Some people also tolerate the small amounts of lactose in cheeses and in butter and margarine that contains milk. Others tolerate fermented milks such as buttermilk and yogurt. A commercial preparation of lactase is available for addition to milk to convert the lactose to the sugars that can be absorbed.†

When there is total absence of lactase, a rare occurrence, the diet must be planned to eliminate all sources of lactose. Calcium supplements must be prescribed for such dietary restriction. The foods to avoid include:

Milk in all forms: fresh; evaporated; dry; fermented; malted
Beverages containing milk or milk powder: Cocomalt; cocoa, chocolate, Ovaltine
Breads and rolls made with milk; sweet rolls; bread mixes; griddle cakes; waffles; zwieback
Cereals: any containing nonfat milk powder. READ LABELS
Desserts: any made with milk, including cakes, cookies, custard, ice cream, pies made
    with milk, puddings, sherbets
Fats: butter and margarines that contain milk, cream, cream substitutes
Meat: frankfurters and luncheon meats with milk powder. READ LABELS
Sauces and soups: cream; dried soup mixes
Sweets: caramel or chocolate candy
Vegetables; seasoned with butter or margarine; with cream sauces

GLUTEN-INDUCED ENTEROPATHY

Gluten-induced enteropathy is also known as *celiac disease* in children and *nontropical sprue* in adults. Gluten occurs in wheat, oats, rye, and barley. When

* Mul-Soy® and CHO-Free Formula®, Syntex Laboratories, Palo Alto, California; MBF (Meat-Base Formula), Gerber Products, Fremont, Michigan; Isomil®, Ross Laboratories, Columbus, Ohio; Nutramigen® and ProSobee®, Mead Johnson & Company, Evansville, Indiana.
† Lact-Aid®. SugarLo Company, Atlantic City, New Jersey.

gluten is ingested changes occur in the epithelial cells of the jejunum, and absorption of sugars, fats, and amino acids is greatly reduced. The stools are bulky, foamy, and foul; they have a high percentage of fat (steatorrhea) and there are serious losses of all nutrients. Many signs of malnutrition are present in the untreated patient: weight loss, muscle wasting, protruding abdomen, sore mouth, bone pain, increased fractures, peripheral neuritis, and prolonged bleeding time.

Dietary management. The elimination of all sources of gluten in the diet brings about remarkable improvement. This means that all products containing wheat, rye, oats, or barley must be omitted from the diet. The diet must be continued indefinitely. Even small amounts of wheat as that used for thickening gravy produces harmful symptoms. The patient requires much counseling regarding the foods that he may have, how to prepare them, how to interpret labels, and so on. The characteristics of a gluten-restricted diet follow.

Gluten-Restricted Diet

The diet excludes all sources of wheat, rye, oats, and barley. Read labels carefully.

Aqueous multivitamins are usually prescribed in addition to the diet.

The diet may be progressed gradually; that is, small amounts of unsaturated fats may be used at first, adding harder fats later. Fiber may be reduced initially by using only cooked fruits and vegetables. Strongly flavored vegetables may be poorly tolerated at first.

INCLUDE THESE FOODS, OR THEIR NUTRITIVE EQUIVALENTS, DAILY:

2–4 cups milk
6–8 ounces (cooked weight) lean meat, fish, or poultry; eggs; cheese
    4 vegetables including:
        1 dark green or deep yellow
        1 potato
        2 other vegetables
        Other to be served raw, if tolerated
    3 fruits including:
        1–2 servings citrus fruit or other good source ascorbic acid
        1–2 other fruits
    4 servings bread and cereals; corn, rice, soybean, gluten-free wheat starch
        NO WHEAT, RYE, OATS, BARLEY
2 tablespoons fat
Additional calories are provided by using more of the foods listed, desserts, soups, sweets

FOODS ALLOWED	FOODS TO AVOID
Beverages—carbonated, cocoa, coffee, fruit juices, milk, tea	*Beverages*—ale, beer, instant coffee containing cereal, malted milk, Postum, products containing cereal

FOODS ALLOWED	FOODS TO AVOID
Breads—cornbread, muffins, and pone with no wheat flour; breads made with cornmeal, cornstarch, potato, rice, soybean, wheat starch flour	*Breads*—all containing any wheat, rye, oats, or barley; bread crumbs, muffins, pancakes, rolls, rusks, waffles, zwieback; all commercial yeast and quick bread mixes; all crackers, pretzels, Ry-Krisp
Cereals—cooked cornmeal, Cream of Rice, hominy or grits, rice; ready to eat: corn or rice cereals such as cornflakes, rice flakes, Puffed Rice	*Cereals*—cooked or ready-to-eat breakfast cereals containing wheat, oats, barley, macaroni, noodles, pasta, spaghetti, wheat germ
Cheese—cottage; later, other cheeses	
Desserts—custard, fruit ice, fruit whips, plain or fruit ice cream (homemade), plain or fruit gelatin, meringues; homemade puddings—cornstarch, rice, tapioca; rennet desserts; sherbet; cakes and cookies made with allowed flours	*Desserts*—cake, cookies, doughnuts, pastries, pie; bisques, commercial ice cream, ice cream cones; prepared mixes containing wheat, rye, oats, or barley; puddings thickened with wheat flour
Eggs—as desired	
Fats—oil: corn, cottonseed, olive, sesame, soybean; French dressing, pure mayonnaise, salad dressing with cornstarch thickening	*Fats*—salad dressing with flour thickening
Later addition: butter, cream, margarine, peanut oil, vegetable shortening	
Flour—cornmeal, potato, rice, soybean, gluten-free wheat starch	*Flour*—barley, oat, rye, wheat—bread, cake, entire wheat, graham, self-rising, whole wheat, wheat germ
Fruits—all cooked, canned, and juices; fresh and frozen as tolerated, avoiding skin and seeds initially	*Fruits*—prunes, plums, and their juices; those with skins and seeds at first
Meat—all lean meats, poultry, fish: baked, broiled, roasted, stewed	*Meat*—breaded, creamed, croquettes, luncheon meats unless pure meat, meat loaf, stuffings with bread, scrapple, thickened stew
Introduce fatty meats, fish, and poultry gradually	
Milk—all kinds	
Soups—broth, bouillon, cream if thickened with cornstarch, vegetable	*Soups*—thickened with flour; containing barley, noodles, etc.
Sweets—candy, honey, jam, jelly, marmalade, marshmallows, molasses, syrup, sugar	*Sweets*—candies containing wheat products
Vegetables—cooked or canned: buttered; fresh as tolerated	*Vegetables*—creamed if thickened with wheat, oat, rye, or barley products. Strongly flavored if they produce discomfort.
Miscellaneous—gravy and sauces thickened with cornstarch; olives, peanut butter, pickles, popcorn, potato chips	*Miscellaneous*—gravies and sauces thickened with flours not permitted

TYPICAL MENU FOR GLUTEN-RESTRICTED DIET

Breakfast

Tomato juice
Puffed rice with milk, sugar
Poached egg
Corn sticks (cornmeal; no wheat flour)
Butter, jelly
Coffee with cream, sugar

Luncheon

Baked breast of chicken (egg-cornflake crust)
Savory rice
Buttered spinach

Celery and carrot sticks
Vanilla tapioca pudding with sliced orange sections
Milk

Dinner

Pot roast of beef *with*
Gravy (thickened with cornstarch)
Parsley potato
Mashed winter squash
Tossed green salad
French dressing
Fruit gelatin
Coffee or tea

REVIEW QUESTIONS AND PROBLEMS

1. What symptoms would lead you to suspect that an individual may have an intolerance to lactose? What causes this intolerance?

2. What substitutes are used in formulas for infants who have lactase deficiency?

3. Modify the following dinner menu so that it is suitable for (a) a young adult who needs a lactose-free diet; (b) a young woman with ulcerative colitis who needs a high-protein very low-residue diet; (c) a man with sprue for whom a gluten-restricted diet has been ordered.

Cream of tomato soup with crackers
Roast chicken with stuffing, gravy
Mashed potatoes
Creamed spinach
Dinner roll
Butter
Mixed vegetable salad with blue cheese dressing
Angel food cake with sliced peaches
Coffee; cream; sugar

REFERENCES

Bayless, T. M.: "Disaccharidase Deficiency," *J. Am. Dietet. A.,* 60:478–82, 1972.

Commentary: "Lactose, Milk Intolerance, and Feeding Programs," *J. Am. Dietet. A.,* 61:242–42, 1972.

Darlow, G. M.: "Coeliac Disease," *Nurs. Times,* 71:806–808, 1975.

Jackson, B.: "Ulcerative Colitis from an Etiological Perspective," *Am. J. Nurs.,* 73:258–61, 1973.

McCreery, M.: "Diet: First-Line Defense Against Celiac Disease," *R.N.,* 39:50–52, February 1976.

Reif, L.: "Managing a Life with Chronic Disease," *Am. J. Nurs.*, **73**:258–61, 1973.

Rosenberg, F. H.: "Lactose Intolerance," *Am. J. Nurs.*, **77**:823–24, 1977.

Stephenson, L. S., *et al.:* "Milk Consumption by Black and by White Pupils in Two Primary Schools," *J. Am. Dietet. A.*, **71**:258–62, 1977.

30

DISEASES OF THE LIVER,

GALLBLADDER, AND PANCREAS

FUNCTIONS OF THE LIVER

The liver is probably the most complex organ in the body with numerous functions that are listed only briefly here. It synthesizes plasma proteins, hemoglobin, prothrombin, heparin, glycogen, lipoproteins, phospholipids, cholesterol, and numerous other substances. It stores glycogen, iron, copper, and vitamins A and D. It participates in the metabolism of nutrients by the removal of the amino group from amino acids, the synthesis of urea, the release of glycogen to maintain normal blood sugar levels, the formation of bile for the normal digestion of fats, the oxidation of fatty acids, and the conversion of carotene to vitamin A. It detoxifies poisons that would otherwise be harmful to the body. With such a variety of functions it is evident that any disease can seriously interfere with nutritional status and health.

HEPATITIS

Hepatitis is an inflammation of the liver. Among the causes are viral infection transmitted by contaminated food or water; infection following transfusion of blood products that contain the virus; alcoholism; drug addiction; and poisonings by such agents as carbon tetrachloride.

Among the symptoms that interfere with food intake are anorexia, nausea, vomiting, fever, abdominal discomfort, and diarrhea. Weight loss is often great. Bed rest and diet therapy are the principal treatment.

Dietary management. A nutritionally adequate diet is an important aspect of therapy, since poor nutritional status can result in permanent damage to

292

the liver. Because of nausea and vomiting in the early stages it may be necessary to resort to parenteral fluids or to tube feedings.

The appetite usually remains poor, so that the nurse and dietitian must be sure that the diet is attractive and appealing to the taste, and must use a good deal of persuasion to get the patient to eat. Each meal should include only the amounts of food that the patient can be expected to eat. Six small meals are better than three overly large meals. The diet is based upon the following considerations.

1. As soon as the patient is able to eat a full-fluid diet (see p. 206) six or more feedings may be given initially followed by a soft diet (see p. 207) and then a regular diet.

2. If weight loss is great and if there are other signs of malnutrition, the caloric intake should be increased to 3000 kcal or more, and the protein to 100 gm or more. See Chapter 22 for high-calorie diet.

3. Most patients tolerate a normal fat intake, although fried foods are sometimes omitted. When there is obstruction of the biliary tract a low-fat intake is necessary.

4. A liberal carbohydrate intake enhances the caloric intake and also assures a continuous synthesis of glycogen.

CIRRHOSIS

This is a chronic disease with considerable loss of liver cells, fatty infiltration, and fibrosis. It is sometimes the outcome of inadequately treated hepatitis, and more often is associated with chronic alcoholism. Among the changes frequently seen are anemia, prolonged bleeding time, lowered serum albumin, and jaundice. In severe damage ascites, esophageal varices, and hepatic coma are dangerous complications.

Dietary management. A normal diet is satisfactory for patients in whom there are no complications. When a patient is poorly nourished, a high-calorie diet is indicated. The protein allowance should be about 1 gm per kg (60 to 80 gm for the adult). Mineral and vitamin supplements are sometimes prescribed. As in hepatitis, many patients with cirrhosis have poor appetites, and the nurse and dietitian must be prepared to improve food intake by counseling the patient concerning the importance of the diet, by adjusting menus to the patient's likes and dislikes, and sometimes by resorting to supplementary foods rich in nutrients. (See Fig. 30–1.)

Ascites is the accumulation of massive amounts of fluid in the abdomen. When it is present the normal diet must be restricted in sodium to about 250 mg daily (see p. 256). This level of restriction requires the use of low-sodium milk, the preparation of all food without salt or other sodium-containing compounds, and selection of foods that are naturally low in sodium. Because of the distention of the abdomen, patients are unable to eat large amounts of food at one time. Thus, six meals daily are indicated.

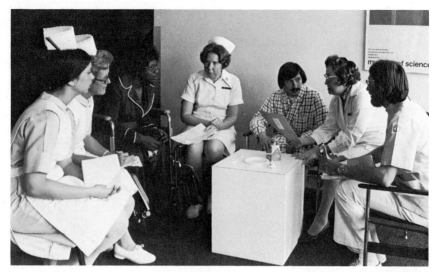

FIGURE 30–1   In a clinical conference the patient's nutritional needs are discussed. The patient should have an opportunity to present his problems and to participate in the planning of his diet. *(Department of Nursing, Delaware County Community College, Media, Pennsylvania.)*

Esophageal varices is the engorgement of the veins of the lower esophagus that results from shunting of the portal blood. If the veins rupture severe hemorrhage results. The veins may be irritated by coarse, fibrous foods, by swallowing a large bolus of food, or by coffee, tea, tobacco, pepper, and chili seasoning. Small, frequent feedings of a soft fiber-restricted diet (see p. 207) are used. If further restriction seems indicated a full-fluid or very low-residue diet (see pp. 206, 283) is used.

HEPATIC COMA

This is a complication of severe liver disease caused by a high blood level of ammonia. The ammonia is produced in the intestinal tract by bacterial action. It is especially likely to occur following gastrointestinal hemorrhage, surgery, or the use of a high-protein diet in severe liver disease. The ammonia that enters the general circulation from the intestinal tract is toxic to the central nervous system so that the typical symptoms are drowsiness, irritability, restlessness, poor coordination of the arms and legs, fecal odor to the breath, and eventually loss of consciousness.

Dietary management.   The administration of antibiotics to reduce bacterial growth and hence the production of ammonia in the intestines is often sufficient to correct the condition. If this is not adequate, the diet is modified as follows:

1. Sufficient calories from carbohydrate and fat to prevent tissue breakdown; about 1500 to 2000 kcal.

2. Protein-free to low-protein diet—about 20 to 30 gm protein—for a few days. See low-protein diet, p. 272.

With improvement the diet is cautiously increased by 10 gm protein every few days until a normal diet is again achieved. Many patients use a 40 to 50 gm-protein diet for long periods of time.

DISEASES OF THE GALLBLADDER

Function. The gallbladder concentrates the bile and stores it. Upon entering the duodenum, fat stimulates the secretion of a hormone, *cholecystokinin*. This hormone is carried by the blood stream to the gallbladder and forces contraction, so that the bile is released into the common duct and then into the duodenum. Bile emulsifies fats so that they can be hydrolyzed by the fat-splitting enzymes, the lipases. If there is any interference with the flow of bile, fat digestion is impaired.

Inflammation of the gallbladder is known as *cholecystitis*, and formation of gallstones is *cholelithiasis*. Stones are often present without symptoms. If the gallbladder is inflamed or if there are stones blocking the flow of bile, there is pain when the gallbladder contracts.

Dietary modification. The aim of diet therapy is to reduce the discomfort by minimizing the contraction of the gallbladder. In acute cholecystitis no food is given for the first 12 to 24 hours. A clear-fluid diet (p. 205) is followed by a soft very low-fat diet, allowing only 20 to 30 gm fat per day. This allows skim milk, 5 to 6 ounces of very lean meat, fish, or poultry, not over 3 eggs per week, and customary amounts of breads, cereals, fruits, and vegetables. This food allowance is low in cholesterol, but it is not known whether cholesterol restriction reduces the formation of stones or not. (See very low-fat diet, p. 250.)

Once the acute attack subsides, the patient is progressed gradually to a diet that includes 50 to 60 gm fat daily. Such an allowance permits the use of whole milk (2 cups) and 2 to 3 teaspoons butter or margarine in addition to foods allowed on the very low-fat diet. Obesity is frequent in patients with gallbladder disease, and a low-calorie low-fat diet should be used.

Many patients with gallbladder disease complain of abdominal discomfort when they eat certain foods such as eggs, legumes, melons, berries, and strongly flavored vegetables. Although these foods need not be omitted for all patients, the individual tolerances should be respected.

PANCREATITIS

Disease of the pancreas interferes with the normal production of pancreatic enzymes, and therefore the digestion of fats, protein, and starches is reduced. Undigested fat, starch, and protein are present in the stools in increased amounts.

Fat-soluble vitamins are poorly absorbed. Such losses if not corrected lead to general malnutrition.

Acute pancreatitis is often accompanied by severe pain, distention, nausea, vomiting, and constipation. Nothing is given by mouth initially, but fluids and electrolytes are replaced parenterally. Then the diet is progressed from clear fluids to a soft diet as tolerated.

Chronic pancreatitis is often caused by alcoholism. A disorder of lipid metabolism is also associated with pancreatitis and abdominal pain. (See Type 1 and 5 hyperlipoproteinemias, Chapter 25.) The pain is often severe with the ingestion of fat or alcohol. Pancreatic extract may be used to aid digestion. The maintenance diet is very low in fat—20 to 30 gm per day, and high in protein and carbohydrate to supply calories. (See pp. 246–51 for fat-restricted diet, types 1 and 5.)

CYSTIC FIBROSIS

This is an inherited disease that affects the exocrine glands (glands that excrete to the outside of the body). There is excessive secretion of thick mucus which often blocks the ducts of the liver, pancreas, and lungs. Large amounts of sodium chloride are excreted in the perspiration.

If the pancreatic ducts are blocked, the pancreatic enzymes cannot reach the duodenum, and malabsorption is often severe. The child appears haggard, shows signs of tissue wasting, has a large protruding abdomen, and excretes large, foul stools with much fat, starch, and protein.

Dietary management. In pancreatic dysfunction pancreatic extract is given before each meal to aid digestion. A high-calorie high-protein diet is essential. If fats cannot be tolerated medium-chain triglycerides (MCT) are useful to increase the calorie intake. MCT is an oil available in a pharmacy that can be used for food preparation.* Because the oil is made up of short-chain fatty acids, it is more readily absorbed. Supplements of the B-complex vitamins, ascorbic acid, and water-soluble preparations of vitamins A and D are usually required. Additional salt intake is required when skin losses of salt are great. Patients find it difficult to eat if their breathing is affected. They must eat slowly and should be given small meals at frequent intervals.

REVIEW QUESTIONS AND PROBLEMS

1. Prepare a table that summarizes the dietary changes made for each of these conditions: hepatitis; hepatic coma; esophageal varices; ascites; cholecystitis; cystic fibrosis. Use these headings in your table: calories; protein; fat; carbohydrate; sodium; texture.

2. Plan a menu for a young man who has hepatitis. Include at least 100 gm protein and 3000 kcal.

* Mead Johnson & Company, Evansville, Indiana.

3. Modify the menu you have planned in question 2 so that it will provide no more than 250 mg sodium. What reasons can you give for restricting sodium?

4. What symptoms would suggest to you that a patient may have impending hepatic coma? Plan a 20 gm protein 1500 kcal diet for such a patient.

REFERENCES

Burnette, B. A.: "Family Adjustment to Cystic Fibrosis," *Am. J. Nurs.*, 75:1986–89, 1975.
Davidson, C. S.: "Dietary Treatment of Hepatic Diseases," *J. Am. Dietet. A.*, 62:515–19, 1973.
Hunt, M. M.: "Dietary Care of Patients with Cystic Fibrosis," *Dietetic Currents*, 3: May/June 1976, (Ross Laboratories).
Illingworth, C.: "Gallstones," *Nurs. Times*, 66:167–68, 1970.
Luke, B.: "The Nutritional Implications of Alcohol Abuse," *R.N.*, 39:32–34, April 1976.
Simmons, S., and Given, B.: "Acute Pancreatitis," *Am. J. Nurs.*, 71:934–39, 1971.

31

NUTRITION AND DIET IN CANCER

Cancer is defined by the American Cancer Society as a "disorderly growth of the body's tissue cells." *Malignant tumor* and *neoplasm* are other terms for cancer. Tumor cells can break away from the original site, enter the circulation, and become attached to another tissue and grow; this is known as *metastasis*.

INCIDENCE

Cancer is a major health problem in the United States. About 1000 people die daily from cancer, and one of every four persons will develop cancer some time during his lifetime. With early detection the American Cancer Society estimates that more than 100,000 lives could be saved each year.

Lung cancer ranks first as a cause of death from cancer in American males, and breast cancer first in females. Cancer of the colon and rectum is the second leading cause of death from cancer in both males and females. For some reason not yet clearly understood the incidence of stomach cancer in the United States has been declining.

CANCER SIGNALS

It behooves all persons to be familiar with the seven signals listed by the American Cancer Society that could indicate the presence of cancer.

1. Unusual bleeding or discharge
2. Lump or thickening in the breast or elsewhere

3. A sore that does not heal
4. Change in bowel or bladder habits
5. Hoarseness or cough
6. Indigestion or difficulty in swallowing
7. Change in size or color of a wart or mole.

The Society urges that a physician be consulted if any of these signs persist for more than two weeks, and immediately if there is unusual bleeding.

EFFECTS OF CANCER ON NUTRITIONAL STATUS

Weight loss, weakness, and loss of appetite are important findings as the cancer progresses. The tumor uses nutrients from the diet for its growth so that the normal cells do not receive their full quota. If the diet itself is inadequate, the normal cells will be further depleted to nourish the tumor cells.

Vomiting and diarrhea are frequently present in patients with cancer. The loss of appetite, nausea, and vomiting reduce the food intake. Malnutrition is further aggravated by diarrhea which leads to reduced absorption of nutrients, and increased fluid and electrolyte loss.

The location of the tumor has specific effects on nutrition and metabolism. For example, pancreatic tumor interferes with fat digestion and absorption; thyroid tumor affects the calcium levels in the blood; tumors of the esophagus or small intestine may lead to obstruction; and tumors of the liver or kidney to failure of these organs.

TREATMENT

Radiation, chemotherapy, and surgery are used singly or in combination. Immunotherapy has recently been used in combination with one or more of these. The purpose of radiation or chemotherapy is to destroy abnormal cells. Unfortunately, these therapies also have toxic effects on normal cells, leading to a variety of undesirable side effects. By surgery all or part of the tumor is removed. Specific nutritional considerations prior to and following surgery are discussed in Chapter 32.

Treatment team. The treatment team includes the patient, physician, nurse, dietitian, and some members of the family. Depending upon the problems that arise, other members of the team include the dentist, surgeon, psychologist, physical and occupational therapists, pharmacist, chaplain, and social worker.

The patient is the key member of the team. Without the patient's participation success is not possible. The focus is on the patient as a person—not just on the treatment of the cancer. The team members must keep the patient informed about the therapy that is planned and being given, what to expect because of the treatment, and what is expected of him. At all times it is essential that the team members keep in touch with each other so that they can coordinate their efforts for the best possible care.

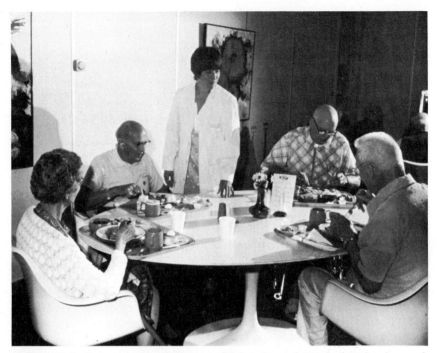

FIGURE 31-1 Patients in a nursing home are likely to have a better food intake when meals are eaten in a group setting. Here a dietitian checks on meal acceptance. *(Dietetic Service, Veterans Administration Medical Center, Bay Pines, Florida.)*

Nutritional support. Patients often express certain concerns relating diet to their illness. They may fear that something they ate caused the cancer. Or someone may have told them that megadoses of vitamins or some bizarre diet would cure the cancer. Or the patient may say: "If only I could eat, I would get better."

The nurse, dietetic technician, and dietitian share responsibility for meeting the nutritional needs of the patient. (See Fig. 31–1.) Specific responsibilities are these:

1. Counseling the patient regarding the essentials of good nutrition.

2. Instituting good nutritional practices before or at the initiation of therapy so that a pattern of diet has been established before adverse effects of therapy are felt.

3. Respecting the patient's likes and dislikes, and recognizing the changes in taste and appetite that occur.

4. Individualizing the diet with respect to the kinds of foods, size of feedings, and interval feedings.

5. Giving continuous encouragement at meal times and even gently coaxing the patient so that he consumes as much of his food as possible.

6. Recording food intake.

7. Monitoring the patient's weight.

8. Alerting the physician regarding poor food intake and weight loss so that nutritional measures can be taken before malnutrition becomes an added problem.

The nurse and the dietitian are likely to be the first to know that the patient has pain on chewing or swallowing, or that nausea prevents food intake. With this knowledge the physician may prescribe a local anesthetic to be used in the mouth before meals, or an antiemetic to reduce the nausea, or a zinc supplement to improve appetite.

DIETARY ADJUSTMENTS

The cancer itself interferes with appetite and food intake. Radiation and chemotherapy contribute to lack of appetite, changes in the sense of taste, sore mouth, nausea, and vomiting so that food intake is reduced. Vomiting and diarrhea interfere with the absorption of nutrients and lead to fluid and electrolyte imbalance. Chemotherapeutic agents can also cause hemorrhagic colitis or cystitis.

Even though the therapy prescribed may reduce or stop tumor growth, severe malnutrition can interfere with recovery. Foods from the regular diet should be used whenever they are tolerated because this helps to maintain morale as well as enhancing nutrition. When foods become tasteless, or unpleasant to the taste, the attractive appearance and aroma of food are more important than ever. Milk, eggnogs, and milk shakes or commercial food supplements should be given between meals as additional sources of calories and protein. It is a good idea to start these feedings before therapy begins so that the patient has accepted them as a pattern throughout his treatment.

With chemotherapy or radiation of head and neck areas the mouth becomes very sore so that chewing or swallowing can be extremely painful. The consistency of the diet must be modified according to individual need: soft-fiber restricted diet (see p. 207), soft diet with all foods ground or puréed; or full-fluid diet (see p. 206) sipped through a straw. Foods that are spicy, or sour such as citrus fruits or with vinegar, coarse in texture, or very hot or very cold should be avoided. When oral food intake is inadequate, nasogastric or gastrostomy tube feedings (see p. 308) may be used. Hyperalimentation (see p. 308) is sometimes used to maintain nutritional status.

Radiation of head and neck areas. Radiation brings about an altered sense of taste, extremely dry mouth, and lack of appetite. Exposure of the salivary glands to radiation leads to a reduced flow of thick, viscous saliva so that swallowing becomes difficult. Selecting moist foods, or mixing dry foods with sauces and gravies will aid in swallowing. Tilting the head back while eating also makes swallowing easier. The reduction in the saliva leads to great increase in tooth decay. Therefore foods high in sugar content must be avoided—candy, cake, cookies, jellies, soft drinks containing sugar, and coffee or tea with sugar.

Radiation of abdomen, pelvis. The adverse effects of radiation include small bowel enteritis, diarrhea, and malabsorption. Usually a soft fiber-restricted diet or very low-residue diet is prescribed. Lactase deficiency is sometimes present, in which case milk should be omitted.

An *elemental diet* may be prescribed if diarrhea persists. This is a diet developed commercially that leaves a minimum of residue and that requires a minimum of digestion.* Elemental diets are unpalatable, but are taken better if they are mixed with some rum or fruit juices. They should be served very cold. These diets are also *hyperosmolar* which means that they will draw additional fluid into the intestines so that cramping occurs. To avoid this effect the diet should be given at half strength for the first two days, three fourths strength for the next two days, and full strength by the fifth day. They should always be sipped slowly to avoid the gas pains.

Dietary counseling. Individual or group counseling are used. One advantage of group counseling is that patients can encourage and help each other to improve their food intakes. Patients need to know how the food groups contribute to the various nutrients; tips on increasing the caloric and protein content of the diet; the importance of chewing food well and relaxing to avoid gastrointestinal discomfort; the advantages of frequent small meals; and how to prepare food at home.

IS DIET A RISK FACTOR IN CANCER?

Many substances in the air, soil, water, and foods gain entrance to the body through the skin, lungs, and alimentary canal. A few of these substances are known to be carcinogenic; for example cigarette smoke and asbestos. Much publicity has been given to the possibility that the level of fat, fiber, or other nutrients or the use of food additives could increase the risk of cancer. The publicity often implies that there is proof, beyond any doubt, of the harmful effects of these substances. This is not true, and people are unnecessarily fearful. Let us look at some of the factors that might increase risk.

Molds. *Mycotoxins* are certain types of molds that are believed to produce cancer. *Aflatoxin*, one of these molds, grows on peanuts and grains that lie on moist ground or are stored at high humidity. The aflatoxin is prevalent in Africa and is believed to be responsible for some of the liver cancer seen there. These molds do not pose any threat in the United States because of controls in harvesting and storage of crops, and because of continuous inspection by the U.S. Food and Drug Administration.

Additives. By federal law no additive may be used in food if it produces cancer in animals at any level of feeding. Usually the amount needed to produce the cancer in the test animals is so high that it would be impossible for a person to consume a corresponding amount based upon his body size. Some food colorings and cyclamates were banned a few years ago, and nitrates and

---

* Vivonex® Standard; Vivonex® High Nitrogen, Eaton Laboratories, Norwich, New York. Precision High Nitrogen Diet®; Precision Isotonic Diet, The Doyle Pharmaceutical Company, Minneapolis, Minnesota.

nitrites used in preservation of frankfurters, bacon, and luncheon meats will be gradually eliminated. Although these substances, fed at very high levels, produced cancer in animals, there is no proof that any person has contracted cancer as a result of eating foods with these additives.

Theory regarding fat.   Colon cancer and breast cancer have been correlated with a high fat intake, but correlation does not mean cause! Japanese living in Japan who eat a low-fat diet have a low incidence of colon and breast cancer. Japanese immigrants to Hawaii where they consume more fat have an increased incidence of cancer; those of the second generation have a still higher incidence. In California, the Seventh Day Adventists who do not eat meat (also do not smoke or use alcohol) have less colon cancer than do other Californians.

The theory concerning fat is as follows; fat in the diet increases bile and sterol production. Bile acids and sterols are believed to break down to substances that could be carcinogenic. Continuous exposure of the intestinal wall to these substances could be harmful.

The low-fiber theory.   According to some British physicians, there is a relationship between a low-fiber diet and a high incidence of colon cancer. African tribes who consume a high-fiber diet have little colon cancer; people of western Europe and the United States whose diets are low in fiber have colon cancer more frequently.

These physicians have developed this theory: low-fiber diets remain in the intestinal tract a long time. There is much bacterial action and a much longer exposure of the intestinal lining to any harmful substances. High-fiber diets, on the other hand produce a softer, bulkier stool with a more rapid elimination time; hence, there is less bacterial action and less exposure to the intestinal wall.

Based on these theories, is there anything that the healthy person can do to reduce the risk of cancer from diet? A sensible approach is to maintain good nutrition by choosing a wide variety of foods; to reduce the intake of fat; and to increase moderately the intake of fiber. These are reasonable steps to good nutrition, but they are no guarantee that they reduce the risk of cancer.

REVIEW QUESTIONS AND PROBLEMS

1. State three reasons why maintaining good nutrition is especially important for the cancer patient.

2. List some ways that you could help a patient who has a poor appetite to improve his food intake.

3. A patient who has had mouth radiation complains that he cannot swallow some of the food on his dinner tray. What changes can be made to ease the swallowing problem?

4. What is meant by an elemental diet? When is it used? Examine the label on a can that contains such a formula. What are the ingredients? How should the diet be given?

5. Why is a low-sugar diet ordered for a patient who has had radiation of the mouth? What are some foods that should be omitted?

REFERENCES

Bruya, M., and Madeira, N.: "Stomatitis after Chemotherapy," *Am. J. Nurs.*, 75:1349–52, 1975.

Carson, J. A. S.: "Nutrition in a Team Approach to Rehabilitation of the Patient with Cancer," *J. Am. Dietet. A.*, 72:407–409, 1978.

Elliott, C. S.: "Radiation Therapy: How You Can Help," *Nurs. '76*, 6:34–41, September 1976.

Hegedus, S., and Pelham, M.: "Dietetics in a Cancer Hospital," *J. Am. Dietet. A.*, 67:235–40, 1975.

Pelham, M. C., and Wollard, J. J.: "Nutritional Support of Cancer Patients," *Dietetic Currents* (Ross Laboratories, Columbus, O), 5 (No. 3), May–June, 1978.

Trowbridge, J., and Carl, W.: "Oral Care of the Patient Having Head and Neck Irradiation," *Am. J. Nurs.*, 75:2146, 1975.

32

METABOLISM FOLLOWING SURGERY | NUTRIENT REQUIREMENTS |
PREOPERATIVE DIET | POSTOPERATIVE DIET | PARENTERAL NUTRITION |
TUBE FEEDINGS · Diet for Special Surgical Procedures |
POSTGASTRECTOMY REGIMEN | INTESTINAL SURGERY | BURNS

NUTRITION IN SURGICAL CONDITIONS

Tube Feedings; High-Protein, High-Fat Diet
(for Dumping Syndrome)

Good nutrition prior to surgery leads to effective wound healing, increases resistance to infection, shortens the period of convalescence, and lowers the mortality rate. On the other hand, poor nutrition prior to surgery results in excessive weight loss, poor wound healing, edema or dehydration, reduced motility of the gastrointestinal tract, and decubitus ulcers. The level of serum proteins, hemoglobin, and electrolytes are often reduced. Poorly nourished patients are at greater risk during and following surgery.

METABOLISM FOLLOWING SURGERY

Catabolism and then anabolism are the normal reactions to surgery, trauma from an accident, hemorrhage, or burns. The *catabolic phase* usually lasts for a few days. Increased amounts of pituitary and adrenal hormones are secreted. As a result, sodium and water are often retained. There is a loss of body cells, and consequently an increase in the excretion of nitrogen and potassium. The acid-base balance may be disturbed. Peristalsis is reduced or even absent.

Wound healing represents the *anabolic phase.* Tissue cells are replaced, leading to positive nitrogen and potassium balance. Sodium and water losses return to normal and the body returns to its normal state of hydration. Peristalsis gradually returns to normal. This phase occurs despite the initial poor intake of food, and only emphasizes the importance of good nutrition prior to surgery or injury.

305

NUTRIENT REQUIREMENTS

Energy, protein, and ascorbic acid are major needs for rapid wound healing and convalescence from surgery. (See Fig. 32–1.)

Energy. If the caloric intake is inadequate, protein will be used to supply energy rather than for wound repair and tissue building. Even very small amounts of glucose as in a parenteral feeding can have some protein-sparing effect. The caloric requirements are very high when there is fever or in patients with severe burns.

Protein. Protein is essential for normal wound healing, to protect the liver against possible injury, and to increase the resistance to infection. For well-nourished individuals a normal protein intake is adequate. When there has been malabsorption, or following severe injury, the protein need may be well over 100 gm daily.

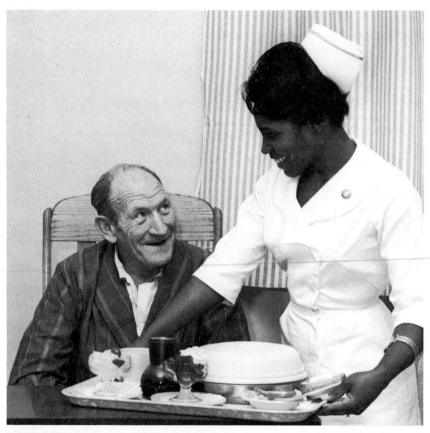

FIGURE 32–1   Nurse gives encouragement to patient to consume the high-calorie high-protein diet needed during stress of injury or surgery. *(School of Nursing, Thomas Jefferson University, Philadelphia.)*

Fluid-electrolyte balance. Each day a significant amount of fluid is lost from the body (see p. 92). Ordinarily this is replaced not only by beverages but also by the food intake. In surgical procedures the losses are further increased through exudates, hemorrhage, and vomiting. The intake is usually decreased because of inability to eat.

Fluid and electrolyte imbalances must be corrected prior to surgery because of the great risks that accompany dehydration and acidosis. Fluids are given orally and parenterally as indicated. Subsequent to surgery parenteral fluids are given until the patient can take satisfactory amounts of fluids and food by mouth. The nurse should note the total intake and excretion of fluid.

Vitamins. Ascorbic acid is especially important for wound healing. The surgeon sometimes prescribes a supplement in addition to the vitamin C provided by the diet. Vitamin K is also of special concern. Failure to synthesize vitamin K in the intestine may occur when antibiotics are given; or the liver may be unable to convert vitamin K to prothrombin. Either deficiency increases the likelihood of abnormal bleeding. When the caloric requirements are greatly increased, as in burns, there is a corresponding increase in the need for B-complex vitamins.

PREOPERATIVE DIET

Sometimes it is possible to improve the state of nutrition prior to surgery. Obesity presents a hazard to surgery. Whenever possible, the obese patient should lose some weight before surgery is attempted. Other patients are malnourished prior to surgery because of lack of appetite, pain, digestive discomfort, or fear of eating. If surgery can be delayed for a time, a high-calorie, high-protein diet is of value even for a week or two. Patients with metabolic diseases such as diabetes mellitus must be in metabolic balance before surgery is attempted.

Usually no food is allowed after the evening meal on the day before surgery. However, if surgery is planned for late afternoon or if a local anesthetic is to be used, a light breakfast is sometimes ordered. Fluids are generally permitted until midnight preceding the day of operation.

Prior to surgery on the gastrointestinal tract a very low-residue diet is often ordered for several days in order to reduce the intestinal residue to a minimum (see p. 302). *Synthetic low-residue diets** (also known as *elemental diets* or *chemically-defined diets*) are replacing the low-residue diet in many hospitals. These diets contain simple carbohydrates, amino acids, essential fatty acids, minerals, and vitamins. They are easily absorbed and leave no residue in the intestinal tract. They are available in several flavors. They are more acceptable if served cold and should be sipped slowly. The nurse must be certain that the patient fully ingests each feeding.

* *Precision*, The Doyle Pharmaceutical Company, Minneapolis, Minnesota. *Vivonex*, Eaton Laboratories, Norwich, New York. *Vital*, Ross Laboratories, Columbus, Ohio.

POSTOPERATIVE DIET

The dietary progression depends upon the nature of the surgery. Food and fluids cannot be given orally until peristalsis has returned. Parenteral fluids maintain fluid and electrolyte balances.

When gastric secretions have begun and peristalsis resumes, clear fluids are given with the initial amounts being 30 to 60 ml. Warm fluids such as tea and broth are better than cold fluids. Patients respond better to solid foods than to liquid foods, and a very low-residue diet given in small amounts is usually the first order. Foods that are high in protein and fat are less distending than those high in carbohydrate. The patient should eat slowly and in small amounts to reduce the amount of air that is swallowed. The diet progresses to a soft fiber-restricted diet and then a regular diet, usually within a few days of surgery.

PARENTERAL NUTRITION

Parenteral fluids may consist of physiologic saline or with additions of 5 per cent glucose, amino acids, electrolytes, vitamins, and medications. They are not nutritionally adequate, but they maintain fluid and electrolyte balance during the immediate postoperative period. One liter of 5 per cent glucose contains 50 gm glucose or 200 kcal. Even 400 kcal in a day can be beneficial in reducing tissue breakdown.

Total parenteral nutrition (hyperalimentation). A number of situations arise in which oral or tube feedings cannot be used for several weeks; for example, prolonged coma, severe uncontrolled malabsorption, extensive burns, and gastrointestinal fistulas. By techniques developed within the last decade a nutritionally adequate hypertonic solution consisting of glucose, protein hydrolysates, minerals, and vitamins can be given by means of an indwelling catheter into the superior vena cava. The high rate of blood flow brings about rapid dilution of the solution, and full nutritional requirements can be met indefinitely.

TUBE FEEDINGS

A tube feeding is a nutritionally adequate allowance of liquefied foods that can be administered through a tube in the stomach or duodenum. A tube feeding is used in paralysis or obstruction of the esophagus, in anorexia nervosa, following mouth or gastric surgery, in severe burns, for unconscious patients, or in any situation where the patient is unable to chew or swallow.

Most hospitals now use commercial tube feedings, including blenderized feedings, milk-base formulas, lactose-free formulas, and synthetic residue-free formulas. (See Table A-7.)

A milk-base formula may be prepared in the hospital or home. It is a calculated recipe that consists of whole or skim milk, eggs, some form of carbohydrate such as strained cooked cereal, sugar, or molasses, and vitamin supplements.

The protein content is sometimes increased by adding nonfat dry milk, and the calories can be increased by substituting cream for part of the milk.

A blenderized formula consists of strained baby meats, fruits, and vegetables in addition to the foods used in a milk-based formula. These formulas are generally better tolerated than milk-based formulas. They may also be varied from day to day to change the flavor, which many patients say they can taste. When there is intolerance to milk, an adequate formula can be developed that is milk-free.

Tube feedings are generally planned to supply one kilocalorie per milliliter. Thus a daily intake of 2 liters will furnish 2000 kcal.

The nurse should observe the patient carefully for the first few days after initiating a tube feeding, and be aware of complaints such as a feeling of fullness, gas, regurgitation, cramping, and diarrhea. Most if not all of these can be avoided by taking certain precautions. Initially tube feedings should be given at half to two-thirds strength, and in small volumes such as 30 to 60 ml every hour. When it is evident that the patient tolerates the feeding, the concentration and the volume can be gradually increased until the desired calorie level is reached.

Some tube feedings are not well tolerated because they contain excess sugars, amino acids, and electrolytes that draw fluid from the blood circulation into the intestine. The patient complains of weakness and distention. When the protein intake needs to be high it is important that adequate fluids be supplied so that the nitrogenous wastes can be efficiently excreted by the kidney. Some patients do not tolerate lactose and require feedings that do not contain milk.

Tube feedings are an excellent medium for bacterial growth. Feedings should be kept under constant refrigeration once they have been prepared or when a proprietary product has been opened. Any formula remaining at the end of a 24-hour period should be discarded. The tubes must be thoroughly flushed out.

Diet for Special Surgical Procedures

POSTGASTRECTOMY REGIMEN

Following gastrectomy a number of problems arise. In the absence of the gastric juices the entire digestion of protein must occur in the small intestine. Fat is less well utilized because of inadequate mixing of food with digestive juices. In the absence of gastric juice, iron is less well absorbed and iron-deficiency anemia occurs more often. Since the intrinsic factor is no longer produced from the stomach, the absorption of vitamin B_{12} does not occur. Several years later the patient will have pernicious anemia unless vitamin B_{12} is given by injection.

Immediately following gastrectomy, 30 to 60 ml of clear fluids are given hourly. By the third day a full-fluid or very low-residue diet is usually allowed. The foods are introduced gradually, however, keeping meals very small and at frequent intervals. Eggs, custards, cereals, milk, cream soups, and fruit purées are introduced first; then cottage cheese, tender chicken, and puréed vegetables are added. The emphasis is upon foods high in protein and fat and low in carbohydrate. Fluids are better tolerated if they are taken between meals.

Dumping syndrome. Certain patients who have had a gastrectomy complain of nausea, weakness, sweating, and dizziness shortly after meals. Vomiting, diarrhea, and weight loss are common.

The condition is caused by rapid entry of the food material directly into the intestinal tract. The large amount of carbohydrate draws water from the blood circulation into the small intestine and thus reduces the circulating blood volume. The sugars are rapidly absorbed into the blood. This causes too much insulin to be produced, and in a short time the blood sugar drops to very low levels. Thus the patient has the symptoms of insulin shock and also the symptoms that accompany reduction of the circulating blood volume.

The diet used for this condition is summarized as follows:

1. Give small meals every two hours consisting of meat, fish, poultry, eggs, or cheese with butter, margarine, or bacon.

2. As improvement occurs, add one to two small servings of one of these: bread, crackers, cereals, vegetables, and finally unsweetened fruits. Gradually increase the amounts and variety of these foods until the diet approaches a normal pattern.

3. Omit fluids at mealtime; they may be taken after at least 45 minutes have elapsed.

4. Omit very cold foods.

TYPICAL MENU FOR INITIAL STAGE

Breakfast, Noon, or Evening	*Midmorning, Midafternoon, Bedtime*
2 beef patties, or roast meat, chicken, fish, steaks, chops, or 2 to 3 eggs	3 oz meat, fish, poultry
2 to 3 pats butter or margarine	2 to 3 pats butter or margarine

TYPICAL MENU FOR FIRST PROGRESSION

Breakfast	*Midmorning, Midafternoon, Bedtime*
2 scrambled eggs	2 oz meat, fish, poultry
2 strips bacon	2 pats butter
½ piece toast with butter	2 thin slices bread for sandwich

Luncheon or Dinner

4 oz meat, poultry, or fish
1 small serving green or yellow vegetable
½ slice bread with butter or margarine

5. Avoid sugar, jelly, jam, syrup, candy, soft drinks, sweetened fruit, gravies, sauces, cakes, cookies, pastries, ice cream, and other sweetened foods.

6. Relax and rest before and after meals.

INTESTINAL SURGERY

Patients who have had an ileostomy or colostomy require a great deal of emotional support and continued assurance that the foods given to them can be safely eaten. The nurse also observes carefully the tolerance the patient has to the foods that are offered.

Ileostomy.   Following removal of a section of the ileum (ileectomy) a permanent opening in the abdominal wall (ileostomy) is provided through which digestive wastes are eliminated. The waste material is fluid and continuous and the losses of fluid, sodium, potassium, and nutrients are considerable. Fat absorption is poor and vitamin B_{12} absorption is reduced or absent.

Clear fluids are given following surgery and then a very low-residue diet is introduced. Gradually foods containing a little fiber are added one by one to the low-residue diet, testing each food thoroughly for tolerance before adding a second. Weight loss is common and a high-protein high-calorie diet modified in fiber content is needed. Periodic injections of vitamin B_{12} will be required to prevent pernicious anemia later in life.

Colostomy.   A colostomy consists in attaching the proximal end of the resected colon to the opening in the abdominal wall. There is some ability to absorb water so that feces are more formed than in the ileostomy, and some bowel regularity can be established. Initially these patients are given a clear fluid and then a very low-residue diet. Most of them are eventually able to eat an essentially normal diet.

Short bowel syndrome.   Massive resection of the intestine seriously reduces the amount of nutrient that can be absorbed. In this syndrome the section of bowel remaining is generally less than 2.5 m (8 ft). Food materials move so rapidly through the remaining bowel that there is insufficient time for digestion and absorption of nutrients. If the jejunum has been removed some absorption can take place from the ileum. The jejunum, on the other hand, has only a small capacity to absorb water and electrolytes and cannot make up for a missing ileum.

Among the life-threatening problems following massive resection are severe changes in fluid and electrolyte balance, diarrhea, steatorrhea, extensive weight loss, and severe malnutrition. Following surgery total parenteral nutrition is used for two to three months (see p. 308). After this period a synthetic low-residue diet may be used (see p. 302). Gradually small feedings of low-fiber carbohydrate foods (50 to 100 gm daily) are introduced, after which small amounts of protein-rich low-fat foods are given. Fats are usually poorly tolerated, and the day's intake is often restricted to 40 gm or less.

Weight loss is usually extreme. Great increases are required for intake of energy, protein, minerals, and vitamins. Up to 175 gm protein and 5000 kcal may be needed to prevent further weight loss. Medium-chain triglycerides are sometimes used to increase the caloric intake. They must be introduced gradually. (See p. 251.)

BURNS

Fluid, electrolyte, and protein losses are tremendous from the burned surfaces. Edema at the burn site, failure to obtain satisfactory skin growth, atony of the gastrointestinal tract, vomiting, and diarrhea are frequently encountered. The excretion of large amounts of nitrogen, potassium, and other wastes places a tremendous load upon the kidneys. Large intakes of fluid are required to hold these wastes in solution and to replace body fluids.

Intravenous feedings including total parenteral nutrition are used until the patient is able to take oral feedings. When peristalsis is adequate tube feedings may be used instead of, or in addition to, oral feedings. A diet supplying 3000 to 5000 kcal and 150 gm or more of protein is usually needed (see pp. 224 and 265). Up to 1.0 gm ascorbic acid is often prescribed, as are also supplements of the B-complex vitamins.

Burned patients are in severe pain and sometimes lose the will to live. The fear of scarring and loss of attractive appearance can be overwhelming. The hospital stay is long and costly, and there may be great concern about how bills can be paid. These patients require great emotional support. When they are able to eat, the nurse and dietitian must encourage the patient to do so, as well as to drink sufficient fluids to permit adequate excretion of wastes. The patient's likes and dislikes, as well as tolerances for specific foods, must be taken into account when planning menus. Some patients will take oral supplements from commercial products better than those that are prepared in the hospital because they view these products as a specific prescription.

REVIEW QUESTIONS AND PROBLEMS

1. What is meant by blenderized tube feeding; elemental diet; milk-base formula?

2. What nutrients are especially important to promote wound healing?

3. Why is vitamin K of special importance in surgery?

4. Patients following surgery often complain of gastric fullness and cramping. What are some reasons for these symptoms? What dietary procedures may reduce them?

5. List several precautions that should be observed in using a tube feeding.

6. Why are injections of vitamin B_{12} essential for patients who have had a gastrectomy? for those who have had massive intestinal resection?

7. When does the dumping syndrome occur? What are the symptoms? What are the important characteristics of the diet?

8. What is meant by the short bowel syndrome? What plans must be made for nutritional care?

9. Study the charts of four patients who have had surgery. Prepare a summary that shows the nature of the surgery, the postoperative orders for parenteral fluids, vitamin and mineral supplements, and diet. Indicate the postoperative days when each order was initiated.

REFERENCES

Amos, A.: "Parenteral Nutrition. 2. The Nurse's Role," *Nurs. Times,* 72:1153–55, 1976.

Gormican, A.: "Tube Feeding," *Dietetic Currents,* 2: May/June 1975 (Ross Laboratories).

Goy, J. A. E.: "Parenteral Nutrition. 1. Theoretical Aspects," *Nurs. Times,* 72:1150–52, 1976.

Kark, R. M.: "Liquid Formula and Chemically Defined Diets," *J. Am. Dietet. A.,* 64:476–79, 1974.

Kubo, W. M., *et al.:* "Fluid and Electrolyte Problems of Tube-Fed Patients," *Am. J. Nurs.,* 76:912–16, 1976.

Lamanske, J.: "Helping the Ileostomy Patient to Help Himself," *Nursing 77,* 7:34–39, January 1977.

Law, D. H.: "Current Concepts in Nutrition. Total Parenteral Nutrition," *N. Engl. J. Med.,* 297:1104–1107, 1977.

MacFadyen, B. V., and Dudrick, S. J.: "Total Parenteral Nutrition of the Critically Ill Patient," *Dietetic Currents,* 5: January/February 1978 (Ross Laboratories).

Pennisi, V. M.: "Monitoring the Nutritional Care of Burned Patients," *J. Am. Dietet. A.,* 69:531–33, 1976.

Walike, B. C.: "Nasogastric Tube Feeding: The Nursing Perspective," *Dietetic Currents,* 2: November/December 1975 (Ross Laboratories).

Weber, B.: "Eating with a Trach," *Am. J. Nurs.,* 74:1439, 1974.

FOOD ALLERGIES AND SKIN DISORDERS

NATURE OF ALLERGIES

A homemaker ate a piece of chocolate cake and a few hours later developed a migraine-type headache. A 10-year old boy began to wheeze while eating in a restaurant; his fork had a tiny trace of egg on it. A girl ordered a seafood casserole in a restaurant and almost immediately after tasting it began to tremble, perspire, and later had severe vomiting and diarrhea. A newborn baby developed severe eczema within a few days after starting his milk formula. All of these individuals were allergic to some food. About one in every 6 persons, or roughly 32 million Americans has an allergy to some substance. Less than one third of these are caused by foods.

Allergy is an abnormal reaction of the body's antibody-antigen defense mechanism. There appears to be an excessive production of immunoglobulin E (IgE) which in turn over-reacts with the allergen (antigen) to produce the symptoms. An *allergen* is the substance that sets off the reaction. In most instances the allergen is protein in nature, but nonprotein substances such as aspirin can also cause reactions.

The tendency to allergy is inherited. If one parent is allergic, there is a 50 per cent chance that the child will be allergic. If both parents are allergic, the change of allergy in the child increases to 75 per cent. The child does not inherit allergy to the same substances, nor does he have the same symptoms as his parents.

Allergies are initiated in four ways: (1) by contact with foods, drugs, aerosol sprays, pesticides, poison ivy, hair, molds; (2) by ingestion of foods, drugs; (3)

314

by inhalation of pollens, dust, cosmetics, sprays, molds, perfumes; (4) by injection of vaccines, serums, hormones, antibiotics, insect bites.

Food allergens. The most frequent food allergens are milk, wheat, eggs, fish, shellfish, citrus fruits, strawberries, tomatoes, and chocolate. Milk is the most frequent allergen in infants. Other foods to which people are sometimes sensitive are pork, nuts, peanut butter, peas, corn, onion, garlic, cabbage, and potatoes. Foods that belong to the same botanic class are likely to produce reactions; for example, oranges, grapefruit, and lemons, or cabbage, cauliflower, and broccoli.

SYMPTOMS

The symptoms are as varied as the causes. Any kind of physical or emotional stress—anger, fear, fatigue, illness, family or school problems—often provokes the allergic reaction or makes it more severe.

There may be only one symptom such as a skin rash or headache, or a combination of symptoms such as itching, diarrhea, and asthma. The response is almost immediate in those who are severely allergic, but is delayed for hours or even days in persons who are mildly allergic.

The skin, the eyes, the respiratory, gastrointestinal, urinary, or nervous systems may be affected. Changes observed in the skin include hives, eczema, fever blisters, itching, and edema. The eyes could be red, swollen, itchy, or burning. If the mucous membranes of the gastrointestinal tract are affected, symptoms such as bad breath, nausea, vomiting, stomatitis, abdominal distention, cramps, diarrhea, or constipation might be present. Nervous system changes include migraine, anxiety, fatigue, and muscle and joint aching.

DIAGNOSIS

Diet history. Severe, immediate reactions can usually be identified readily, but the more mild, delayed reactions are often not diagnosed for relatively long periods of time, and only after detailed study of the diet. Whenever food allergy is suspected, a comprehensive diet history is essential. The patient, or the patient's parent, should keep a complete food diary for a period of time as well as a record of the occurrence of symptoms. Sometimes the correlation of the dietary record and the symptoms establishes the cause of the allergy. More often these records help to determine which elimination diets might be most useful.

Skin tests. Suspected substances may be exposed to the skin to determine whether they cause redness or swelling at the point of contact. By themselves, skin tests are not too reliable for they may give false-positive or false-negative reactions. They can be useful for indicating the elimination diets to be tried first.

Elimination diets. Based upon the dietary history, food diary, and/or skin tests, a diet that eliminates the foods likely to produce allergy is tried. One of the widely used systems of elimination diets is that developed by Dr. Albert Rowe. The *cereal-free elimination diet* excludes all cereal grains, milk, eggs, beef, pork (except bacon), fish, and some fruits and vegetables. If the patient is symptom free on this diet, foods are added, one at a time, every three to five days in this sequence: fruits and vegetables, rice, oats, corn, rye, wheat, beef. If any food produces a symptom, it is removed from the list of permitted foods. The *fruit-free, cereal-free* diet eliminates all cereal grains, fruits, spices, and condiments.

TREATMENT

Infants are frequently allergic to cow's milk. Some of them can tolerate goat's milk, while others need milk-free formulas in which the protein is furnished by soybeans, meat, or casein hydrolysate.* The tolerance to milk often improves as the child grows older.

Building on the elimination diet. When the offending foods have been identified, the simplest treatment is to avoid those foods. This is not difficult when such foods as strawberries or chocolate are the allergens. Because of the wide occurrence of milk, eggs, and wheat in many foods, it is much more difficult to plan a diet that will avoid recurrences.

Let us suppose that a patient remained symptom-free on a given elimination diet. Then, all foods on that diet become the starting point for building the diet. Cautiously, *one food at a time* is added to the diet, and the patient's reactions are observed for a few days. If the added food provokes no reaction, it is added to the list of the foods allowed, and another food is tested in the same way.

Hyposensitization. When an important food such as milk or wheat is producing symptoms, hyposensitization (also known as desensitization) is practical. It consists in giving the patient minute amounts of the offending substance. For example, a drop of milk might be diluted in a pint of water, and a few drops of this dilution fed once a day. If there is no reaction after a few days, the patient is given a slightly greater amount of the dilution. If reactions do occur, it is necessary to move back to an amount that does not produce symptoms. Because additions must be made so gradually, the hyposensitization requires weeks, months, or even longer.

PATIENT COUNSELING

Many foods contain minute amounts of substances to which some people react. The patient must have detailed lists of foods to use, and foods to avoid.

* Soybean isolates: *Isomil*, Ross Laboratories, Columbus, Ohio; *ProSobee*, Mead Johnson & Company, Evanston, Indiana; *Mul-Soy*, Syntex Laboratories, Palo Alto, California. *MBF (Meat-Base Formula)*, Gerber Products Company, Fremont, Michigan. Casein hydrolysate: *Nutramigen*, Mead Johnson & Company, Evanston, Indiana.

The meal pattern should fit in with the family's pattern, and must be one that assures nutritional adequacy. An allergy to milk means that another source of calcium, usually a calcium supplement, must be provided. Soybean substitutes for milk are sometimes fortified with calcium. Allergy to citrus fruits means that other foods that are good sources of ascorbid acid must be emphasized. When there is allergy to wheat it is sometimes necessary to emphasize adequate caloric intake.

A number of recipe booklets are available for patients who are allergic to milk, eggs, or wheat. Rye, corn, rice, soy, or potato flours may be used instead of wheat flour; however, they do not contain the gluten in wheat and the textures of products made with these flours are quite different from those to which people are accustomed.

Reading labels on food packages and cans, and interpreting the information is absolutely essential. The foods that contain milk have been listed for the lactose-free diet (p. 287). Foods to avoid for egg-free and wheat-free diets follow.

DIET WITHOUT EGGS—FOODS TO AVOID

Eggs in any form
Beverages—Cocomalt, eggnog, malted beverages, Ovaltine, root beer
Breads and rolls containing eggs—crust glazed with egg, French toast, sweet rolls, griddle cakes, muffins, waffles, pretzels, zwieback
Desserts—cake, cookies, custard, doughnuts, ice cream, sherbet, meringue, cream-filled pies—coconut, cream, custard, lemon, pumpkin, puddings
Meats—meat loaf or meat balls; breaded meats dipped in egg
Noodles
Salad dressings—cooked dressing, mayonnaise
Sauces—Hollandaise
Soups—broth, bouillon, consommé (if cleared with egg)
Sweets—many cake icings, candies: cream, chocolate, fondant, marshmallow, nougat

DIET WITHOUT WHEAT—FOODS TO AVOID

Beverages—Cocomalt, malted milk, instant coffee with added cereal grain, coffee substitutes; beer, gin, whiskey
Breads, crackers, rolls—all breads including wheat, hot breads and muffins; baking powder biscuits; gluten bread; matzoth, pretzels, zwieback; white and graham crackers; griddle cakes, waffles
Note: bread, crackers, or wafers made of 100 per cent rye, corn, rice, soy, or potato flours may be used.
Cereals—bran, bran flakes, Cheerios, Cream of Wheat, farina, Grape-Nuts, Kix, Maltex, Muffets, New oats, Pablum, Pep, Pettijohn's, Puffed Wheat, Ralston cereals, Shredded Wheat, Special K, Total, Wheatena, wheat flakes, wheat germ, Wheaties, Wheat Chex, and others (Read ingredient list on labels.)
Desserts—cake or cookies, homemade, from mixes, or bakery; doughnuts, ice cream, ice-cream cones, pies, puddings
Flour—white, whole wheat, graham

Gravies and sauces thickened with flour. May use cornstarch thickening.

Meats—prepared with flour, bread, or cracker crumbs such as croquettes and meat loaf; stews thickened with flour or made with dumplings; frankfurters, luncheon meats, or sausage in which wheat had been used as a filler; canned meat dishes such as stew, chili

Pastas—macaroni, noodles, spaghetti, vermicelli, and so on

Salad dressings—thickened with flour

Soups—commercially canned (Read ingredient label.)

Asthma. Patients who have severe asthma are often unable to consume sufficient food at meals to meet their nutritional needs. Midmorning and midafternoon snacks help to assure adequate food intake, but a late evening feeding is not advisable. The patient is advised to eat his meals slowly. Any kind of stress at meal time should be avoided.

SKIN DISEASES

Nutritional deficiencies. Among the skin disorders resulting from nutritional deficiencies are *keratinization* in severe vitamin A deficiency, *cheilosis* in riboflavin deficiency, and *dermatitis* in niacin deficiency. (See Chapters 11 and 12.) Eczema is a frequent disorder in infants. Usually it is a symptom of allergy, but deficiencies of linoleic acid or vitamin B_6 also result in eczema.

Acne vulgaris. This is a chronic inflammation of the sebaceous glands accompanied by pimples and blackheads. It is especially trying during the adolescent period.

The treatment has been described as "confusing, contradictory, and controversial." Chocolate, candies, sweets, fried foods, rich desserts are often blamed for the condition, but research has shown that they apparently have little effect. Although there is no harm in the restriction of these foods, it is probably futile to expect improvement in the skin condition if they are omitted. The most positive approach that can be taken is to emphasize the need for a nutritionally adequate diet and to stress principles of hygiene such as skin cleanliness, exercise, elimination, and regular hours of rest.

REVIEW QUESTIONS AND PROBLEMS

1. Define: allergy, allergen, elimination diet, hyposensitization.
2. What is the role of heredity in allergy?
3. List six foods that frequently produce allergy.
4. Plan a menu for a day for a young man who is allergic to wheat; for a 10-year-old boy who is allergic to eggs.
5. Prepare a list of good sources of ascorbic acid for a patient who is allergic to citrus fruits.
6. What nutritional problems should you anticipate for a person who is allergic to milk? How would you avoid these problems?

REFERENCES

Allergy Recipes. Chicago, IL: The American Dietetic Association, 1969.

Baking for People with Food Allergies. Home and Garden Bulletin No. 147. Washington, D.C.: U.S. Department of Agriculture, 1976.

Cole, D.: "Feeding Allergic Patients," *Hospitals,* **45**:95–100, February 16, 1971.

Mayer, J.: "Food Allergies," *Postgrad. Med.,* **47**:230–33, June 1970.

Speer, F.: "Food Allergy: The 10 Common Offenders," *Am. Fam. Physician,* **13**:106–12, February 1976.

Wood, M. N.: "Eating Well on a Wheat-Free Diet," *Today's Health,* **48**:60–63, February 1970.

APPENDIXES

Table A–1. Nutritive Values of the Edible Part of Foods*

[Dashes in the columns for nutrients show that no suitable value could be found although there is reason to believe that a measurable amount of the nutrient may be present]

No.	Food, Approximate Measure, and Weight (in grams)	Measure	gm	Water per cent	Food Energy calories	Protein gm	Fat gm	Fatty Acids: Saturated (total) gm	Fatty Acids: Unsaturated: Oleic gm	Fatty Acids: Unsaturated: Linoleic gm	Carbohydrate gm	Calcium mg	Iron mg	Vitamin A Value I.U.	Thiamin mg	Riboflavin mg	Niacin mg	Ascorbic Acid mg
	Milk, Cheese, Cream, Imitation Cream; Related Products																	
	Milk:																	
	Fluid:																	
1	Whole, 3.5% fat	1 cup	244	87	160	9	9	5	3	Trace	12	288	0.1	350	0.07	0.41	0.2	2
2	Nonfat (skim)	1 cup	245	90	90	9	Trace	—	—	—	12	296	0.1	10	0.09	0.44	0.2	2
3	Partly skimmed, 2% nonfat milk solids added	1 cup	246	87	145	10	5	3	2	Trace	15	352	0.1	200	0.10	0.52	0.2	2
	Canned, concentrated, undiluted:																	
4	Evaporated, unsweetened	1 cup	252	74	345	18	20	11	7	1	24	635	0.3	810	0.10	0.86	0.5	3
5	Condensed, sweetened	1 cup	306	27	980	25	27	15	9	1	166	802	0.3	1,100	0.24	1.16	0.6	3
	Dry, nonfat instant:																	
6	Low-density (1 1/3 cups needed for reconstitution to 1 qt)	1 cup	68	4	245	24	Trace	—	—	—	35	879	0.4	120	0.24	1.21	0.6	5
7	High-density (7/8 cup needed for reconstitution to 1 qt)	1 cup	104	4	375	37	1	—	—	—	54	1,345	0.6	130	0.36	1.85	0.9	7
	Buttermilk:																	
8	Fluid, cultured, made from skim milk	1 cup	245	90	90	9	Trace	—	—	—	12	296	0.1	10	0.10	0.44	0.2	2
9	Dried, packaged	1 cup	120	3	465	41	6	3	2	Trace	60	1,498	0.7	260	0.31	2.06	1.1	—
	Cheese:																	
	Natural:																	
	Blue or Roquefort type:																	
10	Ounce	1 oz.	28	40	105	6	9	5	3	Trace	1	89	0.1	350	0.01	0.17	0.3	0
11	Cubic inch	1 cu. in.	17	40	65	4	5	3	2	Trace	Trace	54	0.1	210	0.01	0.11	0.2	0
12	Camembert, packaged in 4-oz pkg. with 3 wedges per pkg.	1 wedge	38	52	115	7	9	5	3	Trace	1	40	0.2	380	0.02	0.29	0.3	0
	Cheddar:																	
13	Ounce	1 oz	28	37	115	7	9	5	3	Trace	1	213	0.3	370	0.01	0.13	Trace	0
14	Cubic inch	1 cu in	17	37	70	4	6	3	2	Trace	Trace	129	0.2	230	0.01	0.08	Trace	0
	Cottage, large or small curd:																	
	Creamed:																	
15	Package of 12 oz, net wt.	1 pkg	340	78	360	46	14	8	5	Trace	10	320	1.0	580	0.10	0.85	0.3	0
16	Cup, curd pressed down	1 cup	245	78	260	33	10	6	3	Trace	7	230	0.7	420	0.07	0.61	0.2	0
	Uncreamed:																	
17	Package of 12 oz net wt.	1 pkg	340	79	290	58	1	1	Trace	Trace	9	306	1.4	30	0.10	0.95	0.3	0
18	Cup, curd pressed down	1 cup	200	79	170	34	1	Trace	Trace	Trace	5	180	0.8	20	0.06	0.56	0.2	0

Cream:

No.	Food	Measure	Grams	Water (%)	Food energy (cal)	Protein (g)	Fat (g)	Saturated (total) (g)	Oleic (g)	Linoleic (g)	Carbohydrate (g)	Calcium (mg)	Iron (mg)	Vitamin A (I.U.)	Thiamin (mg)	Riboflavin (mg)	Niacin (mg)	Ascorbic acid (mg)
	Cream:																	
19	Package of 8 oz. net wt.	1 pkg	227	51	850	18	86	48	28	3	5	141	0.5	3,500	0.05	0.54	0.2	0
20	Package of 3 oz. net wt.	1 pkg	85	51	320	7	32	18	11	1	2	53	0.2	1,310	0.02	0.20	0.1	0
21	Cubic inch	1 cu in	16	51	60	1	6	3	2	Trace	Trace	10	Trace	250	Trace	0.04	Trace	0
	Parmesan, grated:																	
22	Cup, pressed down	1 cup	140	17	655	60	43	24	14	1	5	1,893	0.7	1,760	0.03	1.22	0.3	0
23	Tablespoon	1 tbsp	5	17	25	2	2	1	Trace	Trace	Trace	68	Trace	60	Trace	0.04	Trace	0
24	Ounce	1 oz	28	17	130	12	9	5	3	Trace	1	383	0.1	360	0.01	0.25	0.1	0
	Swiss:																	
25	Ounce	1 oz	28	39	105	8	8	4	3	Trace	1	262	0.3	320	Trace	0.11	Trace	0
26	Cubic inch	1 cu in	15	39	55	4	4	2	1	Trace	Trace	139	0.1	170	Trace	0.06	Trace	0
	Pasteurized processed cheese: American:																	
27	Ounce	1 oz	28	40	105	7	9	5	3	Trace	1	198	0.3	350	0.01	0.12	Trace	0
28	Cubic inch	1 cu in	18	40	65	4	5	3	2	Trace	Trace	122	0.2	210	Trace	0.07	Trace	0
	Swiss:																	
29	Ounce	1 oz	28	40	100	8	8	4	3	Trace	1	251	0.3	310	Trace	0.11	Trace	0
30	Cubic inch	1 cu in	18	40	65	5	5	3	2	Trace	Trace	159	0.2	200	Trace	0.07	Trace	0
	Pasteurized process cheese food, American:																	
31	Tablespoon	1 tbsp	14	43	45	3	3	2	1	Trace	1	80	0.1	140	Trace	0.08	Trace	0
32	Cubic inch	1 cu in	18	43	60	4	4	2	1	Trace	1	100	0.1	170	Trace	0.10	Trace	0
33	Pasteurized process cheese spread, American	1 oz	28	49	80	5	6	3	2	Trace	2	160	0.2	250	Trace	0.15	Trace	0
	Cream:																	
34	Half-and-half (cream and milk)	1 cup	242	80	325	8	28	15	9	1	11	261	0.1	1,160	0.07	0.39	0.1	2
35	Half-and-half	1 tbsp	15	80	20	1	2	1	1	Trace	1	16	Trace	70	Trace	0.02	Trace	Trace
36	Light, coffee or table	1 cup	240	72	505	7	49	27	16	1	10	245	0.1	2,020	0.07	0.36	0.1	2
37	Light, coffee or table	1 tbsp	15	72	30	1	3	2	1	Trace	1	15	Trace	130	Trace	0.02	Trace	Trace
38	Sour	1 cup	230	72	485	7	47	26	16	1	10	235	0.1	1,930	0.07	0.35	0.1	2
39	Sour	1 tbsp	12	72	25	1	2	1	1	Trace	1	12	Trace	100	Trace	0.02	Trace	Trace
40	Whipped topping (pressurized)	1 cup	60	62	155	2	14	8	5	Trace	6	67	—	570	—	0.04	—	—
41	Whipped topping (pressurized)	1 tbsp	3	62	10	Trace	1	Trace	Trace	Trace	Trace	3	—	30	—	Trace	—	—
	Whipping, unwhipped (volume about double when whipped):																	
42	Light	1 cup	239	62	715	6	75	41	25	2	9	203	0.1	3,060	0.05	0.29	0.1	2
43	Light	1 tbsp	15	62	45	Trace	5	3	2	Trace	1	13	Trace	190	Trace	0.02	Trace	Trace
44	Heavy	1 cup	238	57	840	5	90	50	30	3	7	179	0.1	3,670	0.05	0.26	0.1	2
45	Heavy	1 tbsp	15	57	55	Trace	6	3	2	Trace	1	11	Trace	230	Trace	0.02	Trace	Trace
	Imitation cream products (made with vegetable fat): Creamers:																	
46	Powdered	1 cup	94	2	505	4	33	31	1	0	52	21	0.6	200[2]	—	—	Trace	—
47	Powdered	1 tsp	2	2	10	Trace	1	Trace	Trace	0	1	1	Trace	Trace[2]	—	—	—	—
48	Liquid (frozen)	1 cup	245	77	345	2	27	25	1	0	25	29	—	100[2]	—	0	—	—
49	Liquid (frozen)	1 tbsp	15	77	20	Trace	2	1	Trace	Trace	2	2	—	10	—	0	—	—
50	Sour dressing (imitation sour cream) made with nonfat dry milk	1 cup	235	72	440	8	38	35	1	Trace	17	277	0.1	Trace	0.07	0.38	0.2	1
51	Sour dressing (imitation sour cream) made with nonfat dry milk	1 tbsp	12	72	20	Trace	2	2	Trace	Trace	1	14	Trace	Trace	Trace	Trace	Trace	Trace
	Whipped topping:																	
52	Pressurized	1 cup	70	61	190	1	17	15	1	0	9	5	—	340[2]	—	0	—	—
53	Pressurized	1 tbsp	4	61	10	Trace	1	1	Trace	Trace	Trace	Trace	—	20[2]	—	0	—	—

*Nutritive Value of Foods, Home and Garden Bulletin No. 72, U.S. Department of Agriculture, Washington, D.C., 1970.

[1] Value applies to unfortified product; value for fortified low-density product would be 1500 I.U. and the fortified high-density product would be 2290 I.U.

[2] Contributed largely from beta-carotene used for coloring.

Table A-1. (Cont.)

Food, Approximate Measure, and Weight (in grams)		gm	Water per cent	Food Energy calories	Pro-tein gm	Fat gm	Fatty Acids Satu-rated (total) gm	Unsaturated Oleic gm	Lin-oleic gm	Carbo-hy-drate gm	Cal-cium mg	Iron mg	Vita-min A Value I.U.	Thia-min mg	Ribo-flavin mg	Niacin mg	Ascor-bic Acid mg
Whipped topping (cont.)																	
54	Frozen 1 cup	75	52	230	1	20	18	Trace	0	15	5	—	2560	—	0	—	—
55	Powdered, made with 1 tbsp	4	52	10	Trace	1	1	Trace	0	1	Trace	—	230	—	0	—	—
56	whole milk 1 cup	75	58	175	3	12	10	1	Trace	15	62	Trace	2330	0.02	0.08	0.1	Trace
57	1 tbsp	4	58	10	Trace	1	1	Trace	Trace	1	3	Trace	220	Trace	Trace	Trace	Trace
	Milk beverages:																
58	Cocoa, homemade 1 cup	250	79	245	10	12	7	4	Trace	27	295	1.0	400	0.10	0.45	0.5	3
59	Chocolate-flavored drink made with skim milk and 2% added butterfat 1 cup	250	83	190	8	6	3	2	Trace	27	270	0.5	210	0.10	0.40	0.3	3
	Malted milk:																
60	Dry powder, approx. 3 heaping teaspoons per ounce 1 oz	28	3	115	4	2	—	—	—	20	82	0.6	290	0.09	0.15	0.1	0
61	Beverage 1 cup	235	78	245	11	10	7	5	1	28	317	0.7	590	0.14	0.49	0.2	2
	Milk desserts:																
62	Custard 1 cup	265	77	305	14	15	7	5	1	29	297	1.1	930	0.11	0.50	0.3	1
	Ice cream:																
63	Regular (approx. 10% fat) 1/2 gal	1,064	63	2,055	48	113	62	37	3	221	1,553	0.5	4,680	0.43	2.23	1.1	11
64	1 cup	133	63	255	6	14	8	5	Trace	28	194	0.1	590	0.05	0.28	0.1	1
65	3-fl-oz cup	50	63	95	2	5	3	2	Trace	10	73	Trace	220	0.02	0.11	0.1	1
66	Rich (approx. 16% fat) 1/2 gal	1,188	63	2,635	31	191	105	63	6	214	927	0.2	7,840	0.24	1.31	1.2	12
67	1 cup	148	63	330	4	24	13	8	1	27	115	Trace	980	0.03	0.16	0.1	1
	Ice milk:																
68	Hardened 1/2 gal	1,048	67	1,595	50	53	29	17	2	235	1,635	1.0	2,200	0.52	2.31	1.0	10
69	1 cup	131	67	200	6	7	4	2	Trace	29	204	0.1	280	0.07	0.29	0.1	1
70	Soft-serve 1 cup	175	67	265	8	9	5	3	Trace	39	273	0.2	370	0.09	0.39	0.2	2
	Yoghurt:																
71	Made from partially skimmed milk 1 cup	245	89	125	8	4	2	1	Trace	13	294	0.1	170	0.10	0.44	0.2	2
72	Made from whole milk 1 cup	245	88	150	7	8	5	3	Trace	12	272	0.1	340	0.07	0.39	0.2	2
	Eggs																
	Eggs, large, 24 ounces per dozen: Raw or cooked in shell or with nothing added:																
73	Whole, without shell 1 egg	50	74	80	6	6	2	3	Trace	Trace	27	1.1	590	0.05	0.15	Trace	0
74	White of egg 1 white	33	88	15	4	Trace	—	—	—	Trace	3	Trace	0	Trace	0.09	Trace	0
75	Yolk of egg 1 yolk	17	51	60	3	5	2	2	Trace	Trace	24	0.9	580	0.04	0.07	Trace	0
76	Scrambled with milk and fat 1 egg	64	72	110	7	8	3	3	Trace	1	51	1.1	690	0.05	0.18	Trace	0
	Meat, Poultry, Fish, Shellfish; Related Products																
77	Bacon (20 slices per lb raw), broiled or fried crisp 2 slices	15	8	90	5	8	3	4	1	1	2	0.5	0	0.08	0.05	0.8	—
	Beef,[3] cooked: Cuts braised, simmered, or pot-roasted:																
78	Lean and fat 3 ounces	85	53	245	23	16	8	7	Trace	0	10	2.9	30	0.04	0.18	3.5	—

No.	Food, approximate measure	Grams	Water (%)	Food energy (cal)	Protein (g)	Fat (g)	Saturated fat (g)	Oleic (g)	Linoleic (g)	Carbohydrate (g)	Calcium (mg)	Iron (mg)	Vitamin A (IU)	Thiamin (mg)	Riboflavin (mg)	Niacin (mg)	Ascorbic acid (mg)
79	Lean only — 2.5 ounces	72	62	140	22	5	2	2	Trace	0	10	2.7	10	0.04	0.16	3.3	—
	Hamburger (ground beef), broiled:																
80	Lean — 3 ounces	85	60	185	23	10	5	4	Trace	0	10	3.0	20	0.08	0.20	5.1	—
81	Regular — 3 ounces	85	54	245	21	17	8	8	Trace	0	9	2.7	30	0.07	0.18	4.6	—
	Roast, oven-cooked, no liquid added:																
	Relatively fat, such as rib:																	
82	Lean and fat — 3 ounces	85	40	375	17	34	16	15	1	0	8	2.2	70	0.05	0.13	3.1	—
83	Lean only — 1.8 ounces	51	57	125	14	7	3	3	Trace	0	6	1.8	10	0.04	0.11	2.6	—
	Relatively lean, such as heel of round:																	
84	Lean and fat — 3 ounces	85	62	165	25	7	3	3	Trace	0	11	3.2	10	0.06	0.19	4.5	—
85	Lean only — 2.7 ounces	78	65	125	24	3	1	1	Trace	0	10	3.0	Trace	0.06	0.18	4.3	—
	Steak, broiled:																	
	Relatively fat, such as sirloin:																	
86	Lean and fat — 3 ounces	85	44	330	20	27	13	12	1	0	9	2.5	50	0.05	0.16	4.0	—
87	Lean only — 2.0 ounces	56	59	115	18	4	2	2	Trace	0	7	2.2	10	0.05	0.14	3.6	—
	Relatively lean, such as round:																	
88	Lean and fat — 3 ounces	85	55	220	24	13	6	6	Trace	0	10	3.0	20	0.07	0.19	4.8	—
89	Lean only — 2.4 ounces	68	61	130	21	4	2	2	Trace	0	9	2.5	10	0.06	0.16	4.1	—
	Beef, canned:																	
90	Corned beef — 3 ounces	85	59	185	22	10	5	4	Trace	0	17	3.7	20	0.01	0.20	2.9	—
91	Corned beef hash — 3 ounces	85	67	155	7	10	5	4	Trace	9	11	1.7	—	0.01	0.08	1.8	—
92	Beef, dried or chipped — 2 ounces	57	48	115	19	4	2	2	Trace	0	11	2.9	—	0.04	0.18	2.2	—
93	Beef and vegetable stew — 1 cup	235	82	210	15	10	5	4	Trace	15	28	2.8	2,310	0.13	0.17	4.4	15
94	Beef potpie, baked 4 1/4-inch diam., weight about 8 ounces before baking — 1 pie	227	55	560	23	33	9	20	2	43	32	4.1	1,860	0.25	0.27	4.5	7
	Chicken, cooked:																	
95	Flesh only, broiled — 3 ounces	85	71	115	20	3	1	1	1	0	8	1.4	80	0.05	0.16	7.4	—
	Breast, fried, 1/2 breast:																	
96	With bone — 3.3 ounces	94	58	155	25	5	1	2	1	1	9	1.3	70	0.04	0.17	11.2	—
97	Flesh and skin only — 2.7 ounces	76	58	155	25	5	1	2	1	1	9	1.3	70	0.04	0.17	11.2	—
	Drumstick, fried:																	
98	With bone — 2.1 ounces	59	55	90	12	4	1	2	1	Trace	6	0.9	50	0.03	0.15	2.7	—
99	Flesh and skin only — 1.3 ounces	38	55	90	12	4	1	2	1	Trace	6	0.9	50	0.03	0.15	2.7	—
100	Chicken, canned, boneless — 3 ounces	85	65	170	18	10	3	4	2	0	18	1.3	200	0.03	0.11	3.7	3
101	Chicken potpie, baked 4 1/4-inch diam., weight before baking about 8 ounces — 1 pie	227	57	535	23	31	10	15	3	42	68	3.0	3,020	0.25	0.26	4.1	5
	Chili con carne, canned:																	
102	With beans — 1 cup	250	72	335	19	15	7	7	Trace	30	80	4.2	150	0.08	0.18	3.2	—
103	Without beans — 1 cup	255	67	510	26	38	18	17	1	15	97	3.6	380	0.05	0.31	5.6	—
104	Heart, beef, lean, braised — 3 ounces	85	61	160	27	5	—	—	1	1	5	5.0	20	0.21	1.04	6.5	1
	Lamb[3] cooked:																	
105	Chop, thick, with bone, broiled — 1 chop 4.8 ounces	137	47	400	25	33	18	12	1	0	10	1.5	—	0.14	0.25	5.6	—
106	Lean and fat — 4.0 ounces	112	47	400	25	33	18	12	1	0	10	1.5	—	0.14	0.25	5.6	—
107	Lean only — 2.6 ounces	74	62	140	21	6	3	2	Trace	0	9	1.5	—	0.11	0.20	4.5	—
	Leg, roasted:																	
108	Lean and fat — 3 ounces	85	54	235	22	16	9	6	Trace	0	9	1.4	—	0.13	0.23	4.7	—
109	Lean only — 2.5 ounces	71	62	130	20	5	3	2	Trace	0	9	1.4	—	0.12	0.21	4.4	—
	Shoulder, roasted:																	
110	Lean and fat — 3 ounces	85	50	285	18	23	13	8	1	0	9	1.0	—	0.11	0.20	4.0	—
111	Lean only — 2.3 ounces	64	61	130	17	6	3	2	Trace	0	8	1.0	—	0.10	0.18	3.7	—
112	Liver, beef, fried — 2 ounces	57	57	130	15	6	—	—	—	3	6	5.0	30,280	0.15	2.37	9.4	15

[2] Contributed largely from beta-carotene used for coloring.
[3] Outer layer of fat on the cut was removed to within approximately 1/2-inch of the lean. Deposits of fat within the cut were not removed.

Table A-1. (Cont.)

	Food, Approximate Measure, and Weight (in grams)			Water per cent	Food Energy calories	Protein gm	Fat gm	Fatty Acids Saturated (total) gm	Fatty Acids Unsaturated Oleic gm	Fatty Acids Unsaturated Linoleic gm	Carbohydrate gm	Calcium mg	Iron mg	Vitamin A Value I.U.	Thiamin mg	Riboflavin mg	Niacin mg	Ascorbic Acid mg
113	Pork, cured, cooked: Ham, light cure, lean and fat, roasted	3 ounces	85	54	245	18	19	7	8	2	0	8	2.2	0	0.40	0.16	3.1	—
	Luncheon meat:																	
114	Boiled ham, sliced	2 ounces	57	59	135	11	10	4	4	1	0	6	1.6	0	0.25	0.09	1.5	—
115	Canned, spiced or unspiced	2 ounces	57	55	165	8	14	5	6	1	1	5	1.2	0	0.18	0.12	1.6	—
	Pork, fresh,³ cooked:																	
116	Chop, thick, with bone	1 chop, 3.5 ounces	98	42	260	16	21	8	9	2	0	8	2.2	0	0.63	0.18	3.8	—
117	Lean and fat	2.3 ounces	66	42	260	16	21	8	9	2	0	8	2.2	0	0.63	0.18	3.8	—
118	Lean only	1.7 ounces	48	53	130	15	7	2	3	1	0	7	1.9	0	0.54	0.16	3.3	—
	Roast, oven-cooked, no liquid added:																	
119	Lean and fat	3 ounces	85	46	310	21	24	9	10	2	0	9	2.7	0	0.78	0.22	4.7	—
120	Lean only	2.4 ounces	68	55	175	20	10	3	4	1	0	9	2.6	0	0.73	0.21	4.4	—
	Cuts, simmered:																	
121	Lean and fat	3 ounces	85	46	320	20	26	9	11	2	0	8	2.5	0	0.46	0.21	4.1	—
122	Lean only	2.2 ounces	63	60	135	18	6	2	3	1	0	8	2.3	0	0.42	0.19	3.7	—
	Sausage:																	
123	Bologna, slice, 3-in diam. by 1/8 inch	2 slices	26	56	80	3	7	—	—	—	Trace	2	0.5	—	0.04	0.06	0.7	—
124	Braunschweiger, slice 2-in diam. by 1/4 inch	2 slices	20	53	65	3	5	—	—	—	Trace	2	1.2	1,310	0.03	0.29	1.6	—
125	Deviled ham, canned	1 tbsp	13	51	45	2	4	2	2	Trace	0	1	0.3	—	0.02	0.01	0.2	—
126	Frankfurter, heated (8 per lb purchased pkg)	1 frank	56	57	170	7	15	—	—	—	1	3	0.8	—	0.08	0.11	1.4	—
127	Pork links, cooked (16 links per lb raw)	2 links	26	35	125	5	11	4	5	1	Trace	2	0.6	0	0.21	0.09	1.0	—
128	Salami, dry type	1 oz	28	30	130	7	11	—	—	—	Trace	4	1.0	—	0.10	0.07	1.5	—
129	Salami, cooked	1 oz	28	51	90	5	7	—	—	—	Trace	3	0.7	—	0.07	0.07	1.2	—
130	Vienna, canned (7 sausages per 5-oz can)	1 sausage	16	63	40	2	3	—	—	—	Trace	1	0.3	—	0.01	0.02	0.4	—
	Veal, medium fat, cooked, bone removed:																	
131	Cutlet	3 oz	85	60	185	23	9	5	4	Trace	0	9	2.7	—	0.06	0.21	4.6	—
132	Roast	3 oz	85	55	230	23	14	7	6	Trace	0	10	2.9	—	0.11	0.26	6.6	—
	Fish and shellfish:																	
133	Bluefish, baked with table fat	3 oz	85	68	135	22	4	—	—	—	0	25	0.6	40	0.09	0.08	1.6	—
	Clams:																	
134	Raw, meat only	3 oz	85	82	65	11	1	—	—	—	2	59	5.2	90	0.08	0.15	1.1	8
135	Canned, solids and liquid	3 oz	85	86	45	7	1	—	—	—	2	47	3.5	—	0.01	0.09	0.9	—
136	Crabmeat, canned	3 oz	85	77	85	15	2	—	—	—	1	38	0.7	—	0.07	0.07	1.6	—
137	Fish sticks, breaded, cooked, frozen; stick 3 3/4 by 1 by 1/2 inch	10 sticks or 8 oz pkg.	227	66	400	38	20	5	4	10	15	25	0.9	—	0.09	0.16	3.6	—
138	Haddock, breaded, fried	3 oz	85	66	140	17	5	1	3	Trace	5	34	1.0	—	0.03	0.06	2.7	2
139	Ocean perch, breaded, fried	3 oz	85	59	195	16	11	—	—	—	6	28	1.1	—	0.08	0.09	1.5	—
140	Oysters, raw, meat only (13–19 med. selects)	1 cup	240	85	160	20	4	—	—	—	8	226	13.2	740	0.33	0.43	6.0	—

326

141	Salmon, pink, canned	3 oz	85	71	120	17	5	1	1	Trace	0	167[4]	0.7	60	0.03	0.16	6.8	—
142	Sardines, Atlantic, canned in oil, drained solids	3 oz	85	62	175	20	9	—	—	—	0	372	2.5	190	0.02	0.17	4.6	—
143	Shad, baked with table fat and bacon	3 oz	85	64	170	20	10	—	—	—	0	20	0.5	20	0.11	0.22	7.3	—
144	Shrimp, canned, meat	3 oz	85	70	100	21	1	—	—	—	1	98	2.6	50	0.01	0.03	1.5	—
145	Swordfish, broiled with butter or margarine	3 oz	85	65	150	24	5	—	—	—	0	23	1.1	1,750	0.03	0.04	9.3	—
146	Tuna, canned in oil, drained solids	3 oz	85	61	170	24	7	2	1	1	0	7	1.6	70	0.04	0.10	10.1	—
	Mature Dry Beans and Peas, Nuts, Peanuts; Related Products																	
147	Almonds, shelled, whole kernels	1 cup	142	5	850	26	77	6	52	15	28	332	6.7	0	0.34	1.31	5.0	Trace
	Beans, dry:																	
	Common varieties as Great Northern, navy and others:																	
	Cooked, drained:																	
148	Great Northern	1 cup	180	69	210	14	1	—	—	—	38	90	4.9	0	0.25	0.13	1.3	0
149	Navy (pea)	1 cup	190	69	225	15	1	—	—	—	40	95	5.1	0	0.27	0.13	1.3	0
	Canned, solids and liquid:																	
	White with—																	
150	Frankfurters (sliced)	1 cup	255	71	365	19	18	—	—	—	32	94	4.8	330	0.18	0.15	3.3	Trace
151	Pork and tomato sauce	1 cup	255	71	310	16	7	2	3	1	49	138	4.6	330	0.20	0.08	1.5	5
152	Pork and sweet sauce	1 cup	255	66	385	16	12	4	5	1	54	161	5.9	—	0.15	0.10	1.3	—
153	Red kidney	1 cup	255	76	230	15	1	—	—	—	42	74	4.6	10	0.13	0.10	1.5	—
154	Lima, cooked, drained	1 cup	190	64	260	16	1	—	—	—	49	55	5.9	—	0.25	0.11	1.3	—
155	Cashew nuts, roasted	1 cup	140	5	785	24	64	11	45	4	41	53	5.3	140	0.60	0.35	2.5	—
	Coconut, fresh, meat only:																	
156	Pieces, approx. 2 by 2 by 1/2 inch	1 piece	45	51	155	2	16	14	1	Trace	4	6	0.8	0	0.02	0.01	0.2	1
157	Shredded or grated, firmly packed	1 cup	130	51	450	5	46	39	3	Trace	12	17	2.2	0	0.07	0.03	0.7	4
158	Cowpeas or blackeye peas, dry, cooked	1 cup	248	80	190	13	1	—	—	—	34	42	3.2	20	0.41	0.11	1.1	Trace
159	Peanuts, roasted, salted, halves	1 cup	144	2	840	37	72	16	31	21	27	107	3.0	—	0.46	0.19	24.7	0
160	Peanut butter	1 tbsp	16	2	95	4	8	2	4	2	3	9	0.3	—	0.02	0.02	2.4	0
161	Peas, split, dry, cooked	1 cup	250	70	290	20	1	—	—	—	52	28	4.2	100	0.37	0.22	2.2	—
162	Pecans, halves	1 cup	108	3	740	10	77	5	48	15	16	79	2.6	140	0.93	0.14	1.0	2
163	Walnuts, black or native, chopped	1 cup	126	3	790	26	75	4	26	36	19	Trace	7.6	380	0.28	0.14	0.9	—
	Vegetables and Vegetable Products																	
	Asparagus, green:																	
	Cooked, drained:																	
164	Spears, 1/2-in. diam. at base	4 spears	60	94	10	1	Trace	—	—	—	2	13	0.4	540	0.10	0.11	0.8	16
165	Pieces, 1 1/2 to 2-in. lengths	1 cup	145	94	30	3	Trace	—	—	—	5	30	0.9	1,310	0.23	0.26	2.0	38
166	Canned, solids and liquid	1 cup	244	94	45	5	1	—	—	—	7	44	4.1	1,240	0.15	0.22	2.0	37

[3]Outer layer of fat on the cut was removed to within approximately 1/2-inch of the lean. Deposits of fat within the cut were not removed.
[4]If bones are discarded, value will be greatly reduced.

Table A–1. (Cont.)

Food, Approximate Measure, and Weight (in grams)		gm	Water per cent	Food Energy calories	Pro-tein gm	Fat gm	Fatty Acids Satu-rated (total) gm	Unsaturated Oleic gm	Lin-oleic gm	Carbo-hy-drate gm	Cal-cium mg	Iron mg	Vita-min A Value I.U.	Thia-min mg	Ribo-flavin mg	Niacin mg	Ascor-bic Acid mg
Beans:																	
167	Lima, immature seeds, cooked, drained	1 cup	170	71	190	13	1	—	—	—	34	80	4.3	480	0.31	0.17	2.2	29
	Snap:																	
	Green:																	
168	Cooked, drained	1 cup	125	92	30	2	Trace	—	—	—	7	63	0.8	680	0.09	0.11	0.6	15
169	Canned, solids and liquid	1 cup	239	94	45	2	Trace	—	—	—	10	81	2.9	690	0.07	0.10	0.7	10
	Yellow or wax:																	
170	Cooked, drained	1 cup	125	93	30	2	Trace	—	—	—	6	63	0.8	290	0.09	0.11	0.6	16
171	Canned, solids and liquid	1 cup	239	94	45	2	1	—	—	—	10	81	2.9	140	0.07	0.10	0.7	12
172	Sprouted mung beans, cooked, drained	1 cup	125	91	35	4	Trace	—	—	—	7	21	1.1	30	0.11	0.13	0.9	8
	Beets:																	
	Cooked, drained, peeled:																	
173	Whole beets, 2-in. diam.	2 beets	100	91	30	1	Trace	—	—	—	7	14	0.5	20	0.03	0.04	0.3	6
174	Diced or sliced	1 cup	170	91	55	2	Trace	—	—	—	12	24	0.9	30	0.05	0.07	0.5	10
175	Canned, solids and liquid	1 cup	246	90	85	2	Trace	—	—	—	19	34	1.5	20	0.02	0.05	0.2	7
176	Beet greens, leaves and stems, cooked, drained	1 cup	145	94	25	3	Trace	—	—	—	5	144	2.8	7,400	0.10	0.22	0.4	22
	Blackeye peas. See Cowpeas																	
	Broccoli, cooked, drained:																	
177	Whole stalks, medium size	1 stalk	180	91	45	6	1	—	—	—	8	158	1.4	4,500	0.16	0.36	1.4	162
178	Stalks cut into 1/2-in pieces	1 cup	155	91	40	5	1	—	—	—	7	136	1.2	3,880	0.14	0.31	1.2	140
179	Chopped, yield from 10-oz frozen pkg	1 3/8 cups	250	92	65	7	1	—	—	—	12	135	1.8	6,500	0.15	0.30	1.3	143
180	Brussels sprouts, 7–8 sprouts (1 1/4 to 1 1/2 in diam.) per cup, cooked	1 cup	155	88	55	7	1	—	—	—	10	50	1.7	810	0.12	0.22	1.2	135
	Cabbage:																	
	Common varieties:																	
	Raw:																	
181	Coarsely shredded or sliced	1 cup	70	92	15	1	Trace	—	—	—	4	34	0.3	90	0.04	0.04	0.2	33
182	Finely shredded or chopped	1 cup	90	92	20	1	Trace	—	—	—	5	44	0.4	120	0.05	0.05	0.3	42
183	Cooked	1 cup	145	94	30	2	Trace	—	—	—	6	64	0.4	190	0.06	0.06	0.4	48
184	Red, raw, coarsely shredded	1 cup	70	90	20	1	Trace	—	—	—	5	29	0.6	30	0.06	0.04	0.3	43
185	Savoy, raw, coarsely shredded	1 cup	70	92	15	2	Trace	—	—	—	3	47	0.6	140	0.04	0.06	0.2	39
186	Cabbage, celery or Chinese raw, cut in 1-in pieces	1 cup	75	95	10	1	Trace	—	—	—	2	32	0.5	110	0.04	0.03	0.5	19
187	Cabbage, spoon (or pakchoy), cooked	1 cup	170	95	25	2	Trace	—	—	—	4	252	1.0	5,270	0.07	0.14	1.2	26
	Carrots:																	
	Raw:																	
188	Whole, 5 1/2 by 1 inch, (25 thin strips)	1 carrot	50	88	20	1	Trace	—	—	—	5	18	0.4	5,500	0.03	0.03	0.3	4

No.	Food, approximate measure	Measure	Grams	Water (%)	Food energy (cal.)	Protein (g)	Fat (g)	Saturated (g)	Oleic (g)	Linoleic (g)	Carbohydrate (g)	Calcium (mg)	Iron (mg)	Vitamin A (I.U.)	Thiamine (mg)	Riboflavin (mg)	Niacin (mg)	Ascorbic acid (mg)
189	Grated	1 cup	110	88	45	1	Trace	—	—	—	11	41	0.8	12,100	0.06	0.06	0.7	9
190	Cooked, diced	1 cup	145	91	45	1	Trace	—	—	—	10	48	0.9	15,220	0.08	0.07	0.7	9
191	Canned, strained or chopped (baby food)	1 ounce	28	92	10	Trace	Trace	—	—	—	2	7	0.1	3,690	0.01	0.01	0.1	1
192	Cauliflower, cooked, flower-buds	1 cup	120	93	25	3	Trace	—	—	—	5	25	0.8	70	0.11	0.10	0.7	66
193	Celery, raw: Stalk, large outer, 8 by about 1 1/2 inches, at root end	1 stalk	40	94	5	Trace	Trace	—	—	—	2	16	0.1	100	0.01	0.01	0.1	4
194	Pieces, diced	1 cup	100	94	15	1	Trace	—	—	—	4	39	0.3	240	0.03	0.03	0.3	9
195	Collards, cooked	1 cup	190	91	55	5	1	—	—	—	9	289	1.1	10,260	0.27	0.37	2.4	87
196	Corn sweet: Cooked, ear 5 by 1 3/4 inches[5]	1 ear	140	74	70	3	1	—	—	—	16	2	0.5	[6]310	0.09	0.08	1.0	7
197	Canned, solids and liquid	1 cup	256	81	170	5	2	—	—	—	40	10	1.0	[6]690	0.07	0.12	2.3	13
198	Cowpeas, cooked immature seeds	1 cup	160	72	175	13	1	—	—	—	29	38	3.4	560	0.49	0.18	2.3	28
	Cucumbers, 10-ounce; 7 1/2 by about 2 inches:																	
199	Raw, pared	1 cucumber	207	96	30	1	Trace	—	—	—	7	35	0.6	Trace	0.07	0.09	0.4	23
200	Raw, pared, center slice 1/8-inch thick	6 slices	50	96	5	Trace	Trace	—	—	—	2	8	0.2	Trace	0.02	0.02	0.1	6
201	Dandelion greens, cooked	1 cup	180	90	60	4	1	—	—	—	12	252	3.2	21,060	0.24	0.29	—	32
202	Endive, curly (including escarole)	2 ounces	57	93	10	1	Trace	—	—	—	2	46	1.0	1,870	0.04	0.08	0.3	6
203	Kale, leaves including stems, cooked	1 cup	110	91	30	4	1	—	—	—	4	147	1.3	8,140	—	—	—	68
	Lettuce, raw:																	
204	Butterhead, as Boston types; head, 4-inch diameter	1 head	220	95	30	3	Trace	—	—	—	6	77	4.4	2,130	0.14	0.13	0.6	18
205	Crisphead, as Iceberg; head, 4 3/4 inch diameter	1 head	454	96	60	4	Trace	—	—	—	13	91	2.3	1,500	0.29	0.27	1.3	29
206	Looseleaf, or bunching varieties, leaves	2 large	50	94	10	1	Trace	—	—	—	2	34	0.7	950	0.03	0.04	0.2	9
207	Mushrooms, canned, solids and liquid	1 cup	244	93	40	5	Trace	—	—	—	6	15	1.2	Trace	0.04	0.60	4.8	4
208	Mustard greens, cooked	1 cup	140	93	35	3	1	—	—	—	6	193	2.5	8,120	0.11	0.19	0.9	68
209	Okra, cooked, pod 3 by 5/8 inch	8 pods	85	91	25	2	Trace	—	—	—	5	78	0.4	420	0.11	0.15	0.8	17
	Onions: Mature:																	
210	Raw, onion 2 1/2-inch diameter	1 onion	110	89	40	2	Trace	—	—	—	10	30	0.6	40	0.04	0.04	0.2	11
211	Cooked	1 cup	210	92	60	3	Trace	—	—	—	14	50	0.8	80	0.06	0.06	0.4	14
212	Young green, small, without tops	6 onions	50	88	20	1	Trace	—	—	—	5	20	0.3	Trace	0.02	0.02	0.2	12
213	Parsley, raw, chopped	1 tablespoon	4	85	Trace	Trace	Trace	—	—	—	Trace	8	0.2	340	Trace	0.01	Trace	7
214	Parsnips, cooked	1 cup	155	82	100	2	1	—	—	—	23	70	0.9	50	0.11	0.12	0.2	16
	Peas, green:																	
215	Cooked	1 cup	160	82	115	9	1	—	—	—	19	37	2.9	860	0.44	0.17	3.7	33
216	Canned, solids and liquid	1 cup	249	83	165	9	1	—	—	—	31	50	4.2	1,120	0.23	0.13	2.2	22
217	Canned, strained (baby food)	1 ounce	28	86	15	1	Trace	—	—	—	3	3	0.4	[6]140	0.02	0.02	0.4	3

[5] Measure and weight apply to entire vegetable or fruit including parts not usually eaten.
[6] Based on yellow varieties; white varieties contain only a trace of cryptoxanthin and carotenes, the pigments in corn that have biologic activity.

Table A-1. (Cont.)

	Food, Approximate Measure, and Weight (in grams)		gm	Water per cent	Food Energy calories	Pro-tein gm	Fat gm	Fatty Acids Satu-rated (total) gm	Unsaturated Oleic gm	Lin-oleic gm	Carbo-hy-drate gm	Cal-cium mg	Iron mg	Vita-min A Value I.U.	Thia-min mg	Ribo-flavin mg	Niacin mg	Ascor-bic Acid mg
218	Peppers, hot, red, without seeds, dried (ground chili powder, added seasonings)	1 tablespoon	15	8	50	2	2	—	—	—	8	40	2.3	9,750	0.03	0.17	1.3	2
	Peppers, sweet:																	
	Raw, about 5 per pound:																	
219	Green pod without stem and seeds	1 pod	74	93	15	1	Trace	—	—	—	4	7	0.5	310	0.06	0.06	0.4	94
220	Cooked, boiled, drained	1 pod	73	95	15	1	Trace	—	—	—	3	7	0.4	310	0.05	0.05	0.4	70
	Potatoes, medium (about 3 per pound raw):																	
221	Baked, peeled after baking	1 potato	99	75	90	3	Trace	—	—	—	21	9	0.7	Trace	0.10	0.04	1.7	20
	Boiled:																	
222	Peeled after boiling	1 potato	136	80	105	3	Trace	—	—	—	23	10	0.8	Trace	0.13	0.05	2.0	22
223	Peeled before boiling	1 potato	122	83	80	2	Trace	—	—	—	18	7	0.6	Trace	0.11	0.04	1.4	20
	French-fried, piece 2 by 1/2 by 1/2 inch:																	
224	Cooked in deep fat	10 pieces	57	45	155	2	7	2	2	4	20	9	0.7	Trace	0.07	0.04	1.8	12
225	Frozen, heated	10 pieces	57	53	125	2	5	1	1	2	19	5	1.0	Trace	0.08	0.01	1.5	12
	Mashed:																	
226	Milk added	1 cup	195	83	125	4	1	—	—	—	25	47	0.8	50	0.16	0.10	2.0	19
227	Milk and butter added	1 cup	195	80	185	4	8	4	3	Trace	24	47	0.8	330	0.16	0.10	1.9	18
228	Potato chips, medium, 2-inch diameter	10 chips	20	2	115	1	8	2	2	4	10	8	0.4	Trace	0.04	0.01	1.0	3
229	Pumpkin, canned	1 cup	228	90	75	2	1	—	—	—	18	57	0.9	14,590	0.07	0.12	1.3	12
230	Radishes, raw, small, without tops	4 radishes	40	94	5	Trace	Trace	—	—	—	1	12	0.4	Trace	0.01	0.01	0.1	10
231	Sauerkraut, canned, solids and liquid	1 cup	235	93	45	2	Trace	—	—	—	9	85	1.2	120	0.07	0.09	0.4	33
	Spinach:																	
232	Cooked	1 cup	180	92	40	5	1	—	—	—	6	167	4.0	14,580	0.13	0.25	1.0	50
233	Canned, drained solids	1 cup	180	91	45	5	1	—	—	—	6	212	4.7	14,400	0.03	0.21	0.6	24
	Squash:																	
	Cooked:																	
234	Summer, diced	1 cup	210	96	30	2	Trace	—	—	—	7	52	0.8	820	0.10	0.16	1.6	21
235	Winter, baked, mashed	1 cup	205	81	130	4	1	—	—	—	32	57	1.6	8,610	0.10	0.27	1.4	27
	Sweetpotatoes:																	
	Cooked, medium, 5 by 2 inches, weight raw about 6 ounces:																	
236	Baked, peeled after baking	1 sweet-potato	110	64	155	2	1	—	—	—	36	44	1.0	8,910	0.10	0.07	0.7	24
237	Boiled, peeled after boiling	1 sweet-potato	147	71	170	2	1	—	—	—	39	47	1.0	11,610	0.13	0.09	0.9	25
238	Candied, 3 1/2 by 2 1/4 inches	1 sweet-potato	175	60	295	2	6	2	3	1	60	65	1.6	11,030	0.10	0.08	0.8	17
239	Canned, vacuum or solid pack	1 cup	218	72	235	4	Trace	—	—	—	54	54	1.7	17,000	0.10	0.10	1.4	30
	Tomatoes:																	
240	Raw, approx. 3-in diam. 2 1/8 in high; wt., 7 oz	1 tomato	200	94	40	2	Trace	—	—	—	9	24	0.9	1,640	0.11	0.07	1.3	742
241	Canned, solids and liquid	1 cup	241	94	50	2	1	—	—	—	10	14	1.2	2,170	0.12	0.07	1.7	41

Fruits and Fruit Products

No.	Food	Measure	Water (%)	Food energy (calories)	Protein (g)	Fat (g)	Saturated fatty acids (g)	Unsaturated oleic (g)	Unsaturated linoleic (g)	Carbohydrate (g)	Calcium (mg)	Iron (mg)	Vitamin A (IU)	Thiamin (mg)	Riboflavin (mg)	Niacin (mg)	Ascorbic acid (mg)
	Tomato catsup:																
242	Cup	1 cup	69	290	6	1	—	—	—	69	60	2.2	3,820	0.25	0.19	4.4	41
243	Tablespoon	1 tbsp.	69	15	Trace	Trace	—	—	—	4	3	0.1	210	0.01	0.01	0.2	2
	Tomato juice, canned:																
244	Cup	1 cup	94	45	2	Trace	—	—	—	10	17	2.2	1,940	0.12	0.07	1.9	39
245	Glass (6 fl oz)	1 glass	94	35	2	Trace	—	—	—	8	13	1.6	1,460	0.09	0.08	1.5	29
246	Turnips, cooked, diced	1 cup	94	35	1	Trace	—	—	—	8	54	0.6	Trace	0.06	0.08	0.5	34
247	Turnips greens, cooked	1 cup	94	30	3	Trace	—	—	—	5	252	1.5	8,270	0.15	0.33	0.7	68
248	Apples, raw (about 3 per lb)[5]	1 apple	85	70	Trace	Trace	—	—	—	18	8	0.4	50	0.04	0.02	0.1	3
249	Apple juice, bottled or canned	1 cup	88	120	Trace	Trace	—	—	—	30	15	1.5	—	0.02	0.05	0.2	2[8]
	Applesauce, canned:																
250	Sweetened	1 cup	76	230	1	Trace	—	—	—	61	10	1.3	100	0.05	0.03	0.1	83
251	Unsweetened or artificially sweetened	1 cup	88	100	1	Trace	—	—	—	26	10	1.2	100	0.05	0.02	0.1	82
	Apricots:																
252	Raw (about 12 per lb)[5]	3 apricots	85	55	1	Trace	—	—	—	14	18	0.5	2,890	0.03	0.04	0.7	10
253	Canned in heavy syrup	1 cup	77	220	2	Trace	—	—	—	57	28	0.8	4,510	0.05	0.06	0.9	10
254	Dried, uncooked (40 halves per cup)	1 cup	25	390	8	1	—	—	—	100	100	8.2	16,350	0.01	0.23	4.9	19
255	Cooked, unsweetened, fruit and liquid	1 cup	76	240	5	1	—	—	—	62	63	5.1	8,550	0.01	0.13	2.8	8
256	Apricot nectar, canned	1 cup	85	140	1	Trace	—	—	—	37	23	0.5	2,380	0.03	0.03	0.5	8[8]
257	Avocados, whole fruit, raw:[5] California (mid- and late-winter; diam. 3 1/8 in)	1 avocado	74	370	5	37	5	17	7	13	22	1.3	630	0.24	0.43	3.5	30
258	Florida (late summer, fall; diam. 3 5/8 in)	1 avocado	78	390	4	33	4	15	7	27	30	1.8	880	0.33	0.61	4.9	43
259	Bananas, raw, medium size[5]	1 banana	76	100	1	Trace	—	—	—	26	10	0.8	230	0.06	0.07	0.8	12
260	Banana flakes	1 cup	3	340	4	1	—	—	—	89	32	0.8	760	0.18	0.24	2.8	7
261	Blackberries, raw	1 cup	84	85	2	1	—	—	—	19	46	1.3	290	0.05	0.06	0.5	30
262	Blueberries, raw	1 cup	83	85	1	1	—	—	—	21	21	1.4	140	0.04	0.08	0.6	20
263	Cantaloups, raw, medium, 5-inch diameter about 1 2/3 pounds[5]	1/2 melon	91	60	1	Trace	—	—	—	14	27	0.8	[9]6,540	0.08	0.06	1.2	63
264	Cherries, canned, red, sour, pitted, water pack	1 cup	88	105	2	Trace	—	—	—	26	37	0.7	1,660	0.07	0.05	0.5	12
265	Cranberry juice cocktail, canned	1 cup	83	165	Trace	Trace	—	—	—	42	13	0.8	Trace	0.03	0.03	0.1	[10]40
266	Cranberry sauce, sweetened, canned, strained	1 cup	62	405	Trace	Trace	—	—	—	104	17	0.6	60	0.03	0.03	0.1	6
267	Dates, pitted, cut	1 cup	22	490	4	1	—	—	—	130	105	5.3	90	0.16	0.17	3.9	0
268	Figs, dried, large, 2 by 1 in	1 fig	23	60	1	Trace	—	—	—	15	26	0.6	20	0.02	0.02	0.1	0
269	Fruit cocktail, canned, in heavy syrup	1 cup	80	195	1	Trace	—	—	—	50	23	1.0	360	0.05	0.03	1.3	5
	Grapefruit:																
270	Raw, medium, 3 3/4-in diam.[5] White	1/2 grapefruit	83	45	1	Trace	—	—	—	12	19	0.5	10	0.05	0.02	0.2	44
271	Pink or red	1/2 grapefruit	89	50	1	Trace	—	—	—	13	20	0.5	540	0.05	0.02	0.2	44
272	Canned, syrup pack	1 cup	81	180	2	Trace	—	—	—	45	33	0.8	30	0.08	0.05	0.5	76

[5]Measure and weight apply to entire vegetable or fruit including parts not usually eaten.

[7]Year-round average. Samples marketed from November through May, average 20 milligrams per 200-gram tomato; from June through October, around 52 milligrams.

[8]This is the amount from the fruit. Additional ascorbic acid may be added by the manufacturer. Refer to the label for this information.

[9]Value for varieties with orange-colored flesh; value for varieties with green flesh would be about 540 I.U.

[10]Value listed is based on products with label stating 30 mg per 6-fl-oz serving.

Table A-1. (Cont.)

#	Food, Approximate Measure, and Weight (in grams)		Water per cent	Food Energy calories	Protein gm	Fat gm	Fatty Acids Saturated (total) gm	Unsaturated Oleic gm	Unsaturated Linoleic gm	Carbohydrate gm	Calcium mg	Iron mg	Vitamin A Value I.U.	Thiamin mg	Riboflavin mg	Niacin mg	Ascorbic Acid mg
		gm															
	Grapefruit juice:																
273	Fresh	1 cup	246	90	95	1	Trace	—	—	—	23	22	0.5	(11)	0.09	0.04	0.4	92
	Canned, white:																
274	Unsweetened	1 cup	247	89	100	1	Trace	—	—	—	24	20	1.0	20	0.07	0.04	0.4	84
275	Sweetened	1 cup	250	86	130	1	Trace	—	—	—	32	20	1.0	20	0.07	0.04	0.4	78
276	Frozen concentrate, unsweetened: Undiluted, can, 6 fluid ounces	1 can	207	62	300	4	1	—	—	—	72	70	0.8	60	0.29	0.12	1.4	286
277	Diluted with 3 parts water, by volume	1 cup	247	89	100	1	Trace	—	—	—	24	25	0.2	20	0.10	0.04	0.5	96
278	Dehydrated crystals	4 oz	113	1	410	6	1	—	—	—	102	100	1.2	80	0.40	0.20	2.0	396
279	Prepared with water (1 pound yields about 1 gallon)	1 cup	247	90	100	1	Trace	—	—	—	24	22	0.2	20	0.10	0.05	0.5	91
	Grapes, raw:[5]																
280	American type (slip skin)	1 cup	153	82	65	1	1	—	—	—	15	15	0.4	100	0.05	0.03	0.2	3
281	European type (adherent skin)	1 cup	160	81	95	1	Trace	—	—	—	25	17	0.6	140	0.07	0.04	0.4	6
	Grapejuice:																
282	Canned or bottled	1 cup	253	83	165	1	Trace	—	—	—	42	28	0.8	—	0.10	0.05	0.5	Trace
	Frozen concentrate, sweetened:																
283	Undiluted, can, 6 fluid ounces	1 can	216	53	395	1	Trace	—	—	—	100	22	0.9	40	0.13	0.22	1.5	(12)
284	Diluted with 3 parts water, by volume	1 cup	250	86	135	1	Trace	—	—	—	33	8	0.3	10	0.05	0.08	0.5	(12)
285	Grapejuice drink, canned	1 cup	250	86	135	Trace	Trace	—	—	—	35	8	0.3	—	0.03	0.03	0.3	(12)
286	Lemons, raw, 2 1/8-in diam., size 165.[5] Used for juice	1 lemon	110	90	20	1	Trace	—	—	—	6	19	0.4	10	0.03	0.01	0.1	39
287	Lemon juice, raw	1 cup	244	91	60	1	Trace	—	—	—	20	17	0.5	50	0.07	0.02	0.2	112
	Lemonade concentrate:																
288	Frozen, 6 fl oz per can	1 can	219	48	430	Trace	Trace	—	—	—	112	9	0.4	40	0.04	0.07	0.7	66
289	Diluted with 4 1/3 parts water, by volume	1 cup	248	88	110	Trace	Trace	—	—	—	28	2	Trace	Trace	Trace	0.02	0.2	17
	Lime juice:																
290	Fresh	1 cup	246	90	65	1	Trace	—	—	—	22	22	0.5	20	0.05	0.02	0.2	79
291	Canned, unsweetened	1 cup	246	90	65	1	Trace	—	—	—	22	22	0.5	20	0.05	0.02	0.2	52
292	Limeade concentrate, frozen: Undiluted, can, 6 fluid ounces	1 can	218	50	410	Trace	Trace	—	—	—	108	11	0.2	Trace	0.02	0.02	0.2	26
293	Diluted with 4 1/3 parts water, by volume	1 cup	247	90	100	Trace	Trace	—	—	—	27	2	Trace	Trace	Trace	Trace	Trace	5
294	Oranges, raw, 2 5/8-in diam., all commercial varieties[5]	1 orange	180	86	65	1	Trace	—	—	—	16	54	0.5	260	0.13	0.05	0.5	66
295	Orange juice, fresh, all varieties	1 cup	248	88	110	2	1	—	—	—	26	27	0.5	500	0.22	0.07	1.0	124
296	Canned, unsweetened	1 cup	249	87	120	2	Trace	—	—	—	28	25	1.0	500	0.17	0.05	0.7	100
297	Frozen concentrate: Undiluted, can, 6 fluid ounces	1 can	213	55	360	5	Trace	—	—	—	87	75	0.9	1,620	0.68	0.11	2.8	360

No.	Food, approximate measure	Measure	Grams	Water (%)	Food energy	Protein (g)	Fat (g)	Fatty acids (sat.)	(oleic)	(linoleic)	Carbohydrate (g)	Calcium (mg)	Iron (mg)	Vitamin A (I.U.)	Thiamin (mg)	Riboflavin (mg)	Niacin (mg)	Ascorbic acid (mg)
298	Diluted with 3 parts water, by volume	1 cup	249	87	120	2	Trace	—	—	—	29	25	0.2	550	0.22	0.02	1.0	120
299	Dehydrated crystals	4 oz	113	1	430	6	2	—	—	—	100	95	1.9	1,900	0.76	0.24	3.3	408
300	Prepared with water (1 pound yields about 1 gallon)	1 cup	248	88	115	2	1	—	—	—	27	25	0.5	500	0.20	0.07	1.0	109
301	Orange-apricot juice drink	1 cup	249	87	125	Trace	Trace	—	—	—	32	12	0.2	1,440	0.05	0.02	0.5	[10]40
	Orange and grapefruit juice: Frozen concentrate:																	
302	Undiluted, can, 6 fluid ounces	1 can	210	59	330	4	1	—	—	—	78	61	0.8	800	0.48	0.06	2.3	302
303	Diluted with 3 parts water, by volume	1 cup	248	88	110	1	Trace	—	—	—	26	20	0.2	270	0.16	0.02	0.8	102
304	Papayas, raw, 1/2-inch cubes	1 cup	182	89	70	1	Trace	—	—	—	18	36	0.5	3,190	0.07	0.08	0.5	102
	Peaches: Raw:																	
305	Whole, medium, 2-inch diameter, about 4 per pound[5]	1 peach	114	89	35	1	Trace	—	—	—	10	9	0.5	[13]1,320	0.02	0.05	1.0	7
306	Sliced	1 cup	168	89	65	1	Trace	—	—	—	16	15	0.8	[13]2,230	0.03	0.08	1.6	12
	Canned, yellow-fleshed, solids and liquid: Syrup pack, heavy:																	
307	Halves or slices	1 cup	257	79	200	1	Trace	—	—	—	52	10	0.8	1,100	0.02	0.06	1.4	7
308	Water pack	1 cup	245	91	75	1	Trace	—	—	—	20	10	0.7	1,100	0.02	0.06	1.4	7
309	Dried, uncooked	1 cup	160	25	420	5	1	—	—	—	109	77	9.6	6,240	0.02	0.31	8.5	28
310	Cooked, unsweetened, 10-12 halves and juice	1 cup	270	77	220	3	1	—	—	—	58	41	5.1	3,290	0.01	0.15	4.2	6
	Frozen:																	
311	Carton, 12 ounces, not thawed	1 carton	340	76	300	1	Trace	—	—	—	77	14	1.7	2,210	0.03	0.14	2.4	[14]135
	Pears:																	
312	Raw, 3 by 2 1/2-inch diameter[5]	1 pear	182	83	100	1	1	—	—	—	25	13	0.5	30	0.04	0.07	0.2	7
	Canned, solids, and liquid: Syrup pack, heavy:																	
313	Halves or slices	1 cup	255	80	195	1	1	—	—	—	50	13	0.5	Trace	0.03	0.05	0.3	4
	Pineapple:																	
314	Raw, diced	1 cup	140	85	75	1	Trace	—	—	—	19	24	0.7	100	0.12	0.04	0.3	24
	Canned, heavy syrup pack, solids and liquids:																	
315	Crushed	1 cup	260	80	195	1	Trace	—	—	—	50	29	0.8	120	0.20	0.06	0.5	17
316	Sliced, slices and juice	2 small or 1 large	122	80	90	Trace	Trace	—	—	—	24	13	0.4	50	0.09	0.03	0.2	8
317	Pineapple juice, canned	1 cup	249	86	135	1	Trace	—	—	—	34	37	0.7	120	0.12	0.04	0.5	[8]22
	Plums, all except prunes:																	
318	Raw, 2-inch diameter, about 2 ounces[5]	1 plum	60	87	25	Trace	Trace	—	—	—	7	7	0.3	140	0.02	0.02	0.3	3
	Canned, syrup pack (Italian prunes):																	
319	Plums (with pits) and juice[5]	1 cup	256	77	205	1	Trace	—	—	—	53	22	2.2	2,970	0.05	0.05	0.9	4

5Measure and weight apply to entire vegetable or fruit including parts not usually eaten.

8This is the amount from the fruit. Additional ascorbic acid may be added by the manufacturer. Refer to the label for this information.

10Value listed is based on product with label stating 30 milligrams per 6-fl-oz serving.

11For white-fleshed varieties value is about 20 I.U. per cup; for red-fleshed varieties, 1,080 I.U. per cup.

12Present only if added by the manufacturer. Refer to the label for this information.

13Based on yellow-fleshed varieties; for white-fleshed varieties value is about 50 I.U. per 114-gm peach and 80 I.U. per cup of sliced peaches.

14This value includes ascorbic acid added by manufacturer.

Table A–1. (Cont.)

	Food, Approximate Measure, and Weight (in grams)	gm	Water per cent	Food Energy calories	Protein gm	Fat gm	Fatty Acids Saturated (total) gm	Unsaturated Oleic gm	Linoleic gm	Carbohydrate gm	Calcium mg	Iron mg	Vitamin A Value I.U.	Thiamin mg	Riboflavin mg	Niacin mg	Ascorbic Acid mg
	Prunes, dried, "softenized," medium:																
320	Uncooked[5] 4 prunes	32	28	70	1	Trace	—	—	—	18	14	1.1	440	0.02	0.04	0.4	1
321	Cooked, unsweetened, 17–18 prunes and 1/3 cup liquid[5] 1 cup	270	66	295	2	1	—	—	—	78	60	4.5	1,860	0.08	0.18	1.7	2
322	Prune juice, canned or bottled 1 cup	256	80	200	1	Trace	—	—	—	49	36	10.5	—	0.03	0.03	1.0	85
	Raisins, seedless:																
323	Packaged, 1/2 oz or 1 1/2 tbsp per pkg. 1 pkg	14	18	40	Trace	Trace	—	—	—	11	9	0.5	Trace	0.02	0.01	0.1	Trace
324	Cup, pressed down 1 cup	165	18	480	4	Trace	—	—	—	128	102	5.8	30	0.18	0.13	0.8	2
	Raspberries, red:																
325	Raw 1 cup	123	84	70	1	1	—	—	—	17	27	1.1	160	0.04	0.11	1.1	31
326	Frozen, 10-ounce carton, not thawed 1 carton	284	74	275	2	1	—	—	—	70	37	1.7	200	0.06	0.17	1.7	59
327	Rhubarb, cooked, sugar added 1 cup	272	63	385	1	Trace	—	—	—	98	212	1.6	220	0.06	0.15	0.7	17
	Strawberries:																
328	Raw, capped 1 cup	149	90	55	1	1	—	—	—	13	31	1.5	90	0.04	0.10	1.0	88
329	Frozen, 10-ounce carton, not thawed 1 carton	284	71	310	1	1	—	—	—	79	40	2.0	90	0.06	0.17	1.5	150
330	Tangerines, raw, medium, 2 3/8-in diam., size 176[5] 1 tangerine	116	87	40	1	Trace	—	—	—	10	34	0.3	360	0.05	0.02	0.1	27
331	Tangerine juice, canned, sweetened 1 cup	249	87	125	1	1	—	—	—	30	45	0.5	1,050	0.15	0.05	0.2	55
332	Watermelon, raw, wedge, 4 by 8 inches (1/16 of 10 by 16-inch melon, about 2 pounds with rind)[5] 1 wedge	925	93	115	2	1	—	—	—	27	30	2.1	2,510	0.13	0.13	0.7	30
	Grain Products																
	Bagel, 3-in diam.:																
333	Egg 1 bagel	55	32	165	6	2	—	1	Trace	28	9	1.2	30	0.14	0.10	1.2	0
334	Water 1 bagel	55	29	165	6	2	—	1	Trace	30	8	1.2	0	0.15	0.11	1.4	0
335	Barley, pearled, light, uncooked 1 cup	200	11	700	16	2	Trace	1	1	158	32	4.0	0	0.24	0.10	6.2	0
336	Biscuits, baking powder from home recipe with enriched flour, 2-in diam. 1 biscuit	28	27	105	2	5	1	2	1	13	34	0.4	Trace	0.06	0.06	0.1	Trace
337	Biscuits, baking powder from mix, 2-in diam. 1 biscuit	28	28	90	2	3	1	2	1	15	19	0.6	Trace	0.08	0.07	0.6	Trace
338	Bran flakes (40% bran), added thiamin and iron 1 cup	35	3	105	4	1	—	—	—	28	25	12.3	0	0.14	0.06	2.2	0
339	Bran flakes with raisins, added thiamin and iron 1 cup	50	7	145	4	1	—	—	—	40	28	13.5	Trace	0.16	0.07	2.7	0
	Breads:																
340	Boston brown bread, slice 3 by 3/4 in 1 slice	48	45	100	3	1	—	—	—	22	43	0.9	0	0.05	0.03	0.6	0
	Cracked-wheat bread:																
341	Loaf, 1 lb 1 loaf	454	35	1,190	40	10	2	5	2	236	399	5.0	Trace	0.53	0.41	5.9	Trace
342	Slice, 18 slices per loaf 1 slice	25	35	65	2	1	—	—	—	13	22	0.3	Trace	0.03	0.02	0.3	Trace

No.	Food	Measure	Weight (g)	Water %	Food energy	Protein	Fat	(sat.)	(oleic)	(linoleic)	Carbohydrate	Calcium	Iron	Vit. A	Thiamin	Riboflavin	Niacin	Ascorbic
	French or Vienna bread:																	
343	Enriched, 1-lb loaf	1 loaf	454	31	1,315	41	14	3	8	2	251	195	10.0	Trace	1.27	1.00	11.3	Trace
344	Unenriched, 1-lb loaf	1 loaf	454	31	1,315	41	14	3	8	2	251	195	3.2	Trace	0.36	0.36	3.6	Trace
	Italian bread:																	
345	Enriched, 1-lb loaf	1 loaf	454	32	1,250	41	4	Trace	1	2	256	77	10.0	0	1.32	0.91	11.8	0
346	Unenriched, 1-lb loaf	1 loaf	454	32	1,250	41	4	Trace	1	2	256	77	3.2	0	0.41	0.27	3.6	0
	Raisin bread:																	
347	Loaf, 1 lb	1 loaf	454	35	1,190	30	13	3	8	2	243	322	5.9	Trace	0.23	0.41	3.2	Trace
348	Slice, 18 slices per loaf	1 slice	25	35	65	2	1	—	—	—	13	18	0.3	Trace	0.01	0.02	0.2	Trace
	Rye bread:																	
	American, light (1/3 rye, 2/3 wheat):																	
349	Loaf, 1 lb	1 loaf	454	36	1,100	41	5	—	—	—	236	340	7.3	0	0.82	0.32	6.4	0
350	Slice, 18 slices per loaf	1 slice	25	36	60	2	Trace	—	—	—	13	19	0.4	0	0.05	0.02	0.4	0
351	Pumpernickel, loaf, 1 lb	1 loaf	454	34	1,115	41	5	—	—	—	241	381	10.9	0	1.04	0.64	5.4	0
	White bread, enriched:[15]																	
	Soft-crumb type:																	
352	Loaf, 1 lb	1 loaf	454	36	1,225	39	15	3	8	2	229	381	11.3	Trace	1.13	0.95	10.9	Trace
353	Slice, 18 slices per loaf	1 slice	25	36	70	2	1	—	—	—	13	21	0.6	Trace	0.06	0.05	0.6	Trace
354	Slice, toasted	1 slice	22	25	70	2	1	—	—	—	13	21	0.6	Trace	0.05	0.05	0.6	Trace
355	Slice, 22 slices per loaf	1 slice	20	36	55	2	1	—	—	—	10	17	0.5	Trace	0.05	0.04	0.5	Trace
356	Slice, toasted	1 slice	17	25	55	2	1	—	—	—	10	17	0.5	Trace	0.05	0.04	0.5	Trace
357	Loaf, 1 1/2 lb	1 loaf	680	36	1,835	59	22	5	12	3	343	571	17.0	Trace	1.70	1.43	16.3	Trace
358	Slice, 24 slices per loaf	1 slice	28	36	75	2	1	—	—	—	14	24	0.7	Trace	0.07	0.06	0.7	Trace
359	Slice, toasted	1 slice	24	25	75	2	1	—	—	—	14	24	0.7	Trace	0.07	0.06	0.7	Trace
360	Slice, 28 slices per loaf	1 slice	24	36	65	2	1	—	—	—	12	20	0.6	Trace	0.06	0.05	0.6	Trace
361	Slice, toasted	1 slice	21	25	65	2	1	—	—	—	12	20	0.6	Trace	0.06	0.05	0.6	Trace
	Firm-crumb type:																	
362	Loaf, 1 lb	1 loaf	454	35	1,245	41	17	4	10	2	228	435	11.3	Trace	1.22	0.91	10.9	Trace
363	Slice, 20 slices per loaf	1 slice	23	35	65	2	1	—	—	—	12	22	0.6	Trace	0.06	0.05	0.6	Trace
364	Slice, toasted	1 slice	20	24	65	2	1	—	—	—	12	22	0.6	Trace	0.06	0.05	0.6	Trace
365	Loaf, 2 lb	1 loaf	907	35	2,495	82	34	8	20	4	455	871	22.7	Trace	2.45	1.81	21.8	Trace
366	Slice, 34 slices per loaf	1 slice	27	35	75	2	1	—	—	—	14	26	0.7	Trace	0.07	0.05	0.6	Trace
367	Slice, toasted	1 slice	23	35	75	2	1	—	—	—	14	26	0.7	Trace	0.07	0.05	0.6	Trace
	Whole-wheat bread, soft-crumb type:																	
368	Loaf, 1 lb	1 loaf	454	36	1,095	41	12	2	6	2	224	381	13.6	Trace	1.36	0.45	12.7	Trace
369	Slice, 16 slices per loaf	1 slice	28	36	65	3	1	—	—	—	14	24	0.8	Trace	0.09	0.03	0.8	Trace
370	Slice, toasted	1 slice	24	24	65	3	1	—	—	—	14	24	0.8	Trace	0.09	0.03	0.8	Trace
	Whole-wheat bread, firm-crumb type:																	
371	Loaf, 1 lb	1 loaf	454	36	1,100	48	14	3	6	3	216	449	13.6	Trace	1.18	0.54	12.7	Trace
372	Slice, 18 slices per loaf	1 slice	25	36	60	3	1	—	—	—	12	25	0.8	Trace	0.06	0.03	0.7	Trace
373	Slice, toasted	1 slice	21	24	60	3	1	—	—	—	12	25	0.8	Trace	0.06	0.03	0.7	Trace
374	Breadcrumbs, dry, grated	1 cup	100	6	390	13	5	1	2	1	73	122	3.6	Trace	0.22	0.22	3.5	Trace
375	Buckwheat flour, light, sifted	1 cup	98	12	340	6	1	—	—	—	78	11	1.0	0	0.08	0.04	0.4	0
376	Bulgur, canned, seasoned	1 cup	135	56	245	8	4	—	—	—	44	27	1.9	0	0.08	0.05	4.1	0
	Cakes made from cake mixes:																	
	Angel food:																	
377	Whole cake	1 cake	635	34	1,645	36	1	—	—	—	377	603	1.9	0	0.03	0.70	0.6	0
378	Piece, 1/12 of 10-in diam. cake	1 piece	53	34	135	3	Trace	—	—	—	32	50	0.2	0	Trace	0.06	0.1	0

[5] Measure and weight apply to entire vegetable or fruit including parts not usually eaten.

[8] This is the amount from the fruit. Additional ascorbic acid may be added by the manufacturer. Refer to the label for this information.

[15] Values for iron, thiamin, riboflavin, and niacin per pound of unenriched white bread would be as follows:

	Iron mg	Thiamin mg	Riboflavin mg	Niacin mg
Soft crumb	3.2	.31	.39	5.0
Firm crumb	3.2	.32	.59	4.1

Table A-1. (Cont.)

| | Food, Approximate Measure, and Weight (in grams) | | Water per cent | Food Energy calories | Pro-tein gm | Fat gm | Fatty Acids | | | Carbo-hy-drate gm | Cal-cium mg | Iron mg | Vita-min A Value I.U. | Thia-min mg | Ribo-flavin mg | Niacin mg | Ascor-bic Acid mg |
		gm					Satu-rated (total) gm	Unsaturated Oleic gm	Unsaturated Lin-oleic gm								
	Cakes made from cake mixes (cont.)																
	Cupcakes, small, 2 1/2 in diam.:																
379	Without icing	1 cupcake	26	90	1	3	1	1	1	14	40	0.1	40	0.01	0.03	0.1	Trace
380	With chocolate icing	1 cupcake	22	130	2	5	2	2	1	21	47	0.3	60	0.01	0.04	0.1	Trace
	Devil's food, 2-layer, with chocolate icing:																
381	Whole cake	1 cake	1,107 / 24	3,755	49	136	54	58	16	645	653	8.9	1,660	0.33	0.89	3.3	1
382	Piece, 1/16 of 9-in diam. cake	1 piece	69 / 24	235	3	9	3	4	1	40	41	0.6	100	0.02	0.06	0.2	Trace
383	Cupcake, small, 2 1/2-in diam	1 cupcake	35 / 24	120	2	4	1	2	Trace	20	21	0.3	50	0.01	0.03	0.1	Trace
	Gingerbread:																
384	Whole cake	1 cake	570 / 37	1,575	18	39	10	19	9	291	513	9.1	Trace	0.17	0.51	4.6	2
385	Piece, 1/9 of 8-in square cake	1 piece	63 / 37	175	2	4	1	2	1	32	57	1.0	Trace	0.02	0.06	0.5	Trace
	White, 2-layer, with chocolate icing:																
386	Whole cake	1 cake	1,140 / 21	4,000	45	122	45	54	17	716	1,129	5.7	680	0.23	0.91	2.3	2
387	Piece, 1/16 of 9-in diam. cake	1 piece	71 / 21	250	3	8	3	3	1	45	70	0.4	40	0.01	0.06	0.1	Trace
	Cakes made from home recipes:[16]																
388	Boston cream pie; piece 1/12 of 8-in diam.	1 piece	69 / 35	210	4	6	2	3	1	34	46	0.3	140	0.02	0.08	0.1	Trace
	Fruitcake, dark, made with enriched flour:																
389	Loaf, 1 lb	1 loaf	454 / 18	1,720	22	69	15	37	13	271	327	11.8	540	0.59	0.64	3.6	2
390	Slice, 1/30 of 8-in loaf	1 slice	15 / 18	55	1	2	Trace	1	Trace	9	11	0.4	20	0.02	0.02	0.1	Trace
	Plain sheet cake:																
	Without icing:																	
391	Whole cake	1 cake	777 / 25	2,830	35	108	30	52	21	434	497	3.1	1,320	0.16	0.70	1.6	2
392	Piece, 1/9 of 9-in square cake	1 piece	86 / 25	315	4	12	3	6	2	48	55	0.3	150	0.02	0.08	0.2	Trace
393	With boiled white icing, piece, 1/9 of 9-in square cake	1 piece	114 / 23	400	4	12	3	6	2	71	56	0.3	150	0.02	0.08	0.2	Trace
	Pound:																
394	Loaf, 8 1/2 by 3 1/2 by 3 in	1 loaf	514 / 17	2,430	29	152	34	68	17	242	108	4.1	1,440	0.15	0.46	1.0	0
395	Slice, 1/2-in thick	1 slice	30 / 17	140	2	9	2	4	1	14	6	0.2	80	0.01	0.03	0.1	0
	Sponge:																
396	Whole cake	1 cake	790 / 32	2,345	60	45	14	20	4	427	237	9.5	3,560	0.40	1.11	1.6	Trace
397	Piece, 1/12 of 10-in diam. cake	1 piece	66 / 32	195	5	4	1	2	Trace	36	20	0.8	300	0.03	0.09	0.1	Trace
	Yellow, 2 layer, without icing:																
398	Whole cake	1 cake	870 / 24	3,160	39	111	31	53	22	506	618	3.5	1,310	0.17	0.70	1.7	2
399	Piece, 1/16 of 9-in diam. cake	1 piece	54 / 24	200	2	7	2	3	1	32	39	0.2	80	0.01	0.04	0.1	Trace
	Yellow, 2-layer, with chocolate icing:																
400	Whole cake	1 cake	1,203 / 21	4,390	51	156	55	69	23	727	818	7.2	1,920	0.24	0.96	2.4	Trace
401	Piece, 1/16 of 9-in diam. cake	1 piece	75 / 21	275	3	10	3	4	1	45	51	0.5	120	0.02	0.06	0.2	Trace
	Cake icings. See Sugars, Sweets																	

No.	Food	Measure	Grams	Water (%)	Food energy (cal)	Protein (g)	Fat (g)	Fatty acids, sat. (g)	Oleic (g)	Linoleic (g)	Carbohydrate (g)	Calcium (mg)	Iron (mg)	Vitamin A (IU)	Thiamin (mg)	Riboflavin (mg)	Niacin (mg)	Ascorbic acid (mg)
	Cookies:																	
402	Brownies with nuts: Made from home recipe with enriched flour	1 brownie	20	10	95	1	6	1	3	1	10	8	0.4	40	0.04	0.02	0.1	Trace
403	Made from mix	1 brownie	20	11	85	1	4	1	2	1	13	9	0.4	20	0.03	0.02	0.1	Trace
404	Chocolate chip: Made from home recipe with enriched flour	1 cookie	10	3	50	1	3	1	1	1	6	4	0.2	10	0.01	0.01	0.1	Trace
405	Commercial	1 cookie	10	3	50	1	2	1	1	Trace	7	4	0.2	10	Trace	Trace	Trace	Trace
406	Fig bars, commercial	1 cookie	14	14	50	1	1	—	—	—	11	11	0.2	20	Trace	0.01	0.1	Trace
407	Sandwich, chocolate or vanilla, commercial	1 cookie	10	2	50	1	2	1	1	Trace	7	2	0.1	0	Trace	Trace	0.1	0
	Corn flakes, added nutrients:																	
408	Plain	1 cup	25	4	100	2	Trace	—	—	—	21	4	0.4	0	0.11	0.02	0.5	0
409	Sugar-covered	1 cup	40	2	155	2	Trace	—	—	—	36	5	0.4	0	0.16	0.02	0.8	0
	Corn (hominy) grits, degermed, cooked:																	
410	Enriched	1 cup	245	87	125	3	Trace	—	—	—	27	2	0.7	[17]150	0.10	0.07	1.0	0
411	Unenriched	1 cup	245	87	125	3	Trace	—	—	—	27	2	0.2	[17]150	0.05	0.02	0.5	0
	Cornmeal:																	
412	Whole-ground, unbolted, dry	1 cup	122	12	435	11	5	1	2	2	90	24	2.9	[17]620	0.46	0.13	2.4	0
413	Bolted (nearly whole-grain) dry	1 cup	122	12	440	11	4	Trace	1	2	91	21	2.2	[17]590	0.37	0.10	2.3	0
	Degermed, enriched:																	
414	Dry form	1 cup	138	12	500	11	2	—	—	—	108	8	4.0	[17]610	0.61	0.36	4.8	0
415	Cooked	1 cup	240	88	120	3	1	—	—	—	26	2	1.0	[17]140	0.14	0.10	1.2	0
	Degermed, unenriched:																	
416	Dry form	1 cup	138	12	500	11	2	—	—	—	108	8	1.5	[17]610	0.19	0.07	1.4	0
417	Cooked	1 cup	240	88	120	3	1	—	—	—	26	2	0.5	[17]140	0.05	0.02	0.2	0
418	Corn muffins, made with enriched degermed cornmeal and enriched flour; muffin 2 3/8-in. diam.	1 muffin	40	33	125	3	4	1	2	Trace	19	42	0.7	[17]120	0.08	0.09	0.6	Trace
419	Corn muffins, made with mix, egg, and milk; muffin 2 3/8-in. diam.	1 muffin	40	30	130	3	4	1	2	1	20	96	0.6	100	0.07	0.08	0.6	Trace
420	Corn, puffed, presweetened, added nutrients	1 cup	30	2	115	1	Trace	—	—	—	27	3	0.5	0	0.13	0.05	0.6	0
421	Corn, shredded, added nutrients	1 cup	25	3	100	2	Trace	—	—	—	22	1	0.6	0	0.11	0.05	0.5	0
	Crackers:																	
422	Graham, 2 1/2-in. square	4 crackers	28	6	110	2	3	1	1	1	21	11	0.4	0	0.01	0.06	0.4	0
423	Saltines	4 crackers	11	4	50	1	1	—	—	—	8	2	0.1	0	Trace	Trace	0.1	0
424	Danish pastry, plain (without fruit or nuts): Packaged ring, 12 ounces	1 ring	340	22	1,435	25	80	24	37	15	155	170	3.1	1,050	0.24	0.51	2.7	Trace
425	Round piece, approx. 4 1/4-in. diam. by 1 in.	1 pastry	65	22	275	5	15	5	7	3	30	33	0.6	200	0.05	0.10	0.5	Trace
426	Ounce	1 oz	28	22	120	2	7	2	3	1	13	14	0.3	90	0.02	0.04	0.2	Trace
427	Doughnuts, cake type	1 doughnut	32	24	125	1	6	1	4	Trace	16	13	[18]0.4	30	[18]0.05	[18]0.05	[18]0.4	Trace
428	Farina, quick-cooking, enriched, cooked	1 cup	245	89	105	3	Trace	—	—	—	22	147	[19]0.7	0	[19]0.12	[19]0.07	[19]1.0	0

[16] Unenriched cake flour used unless otherwise specified.
[17] This value is based on product made from yellow varieties of corn; white varieties contain only a trace.
[18] Based on product made with enriched flour. With unenriched flour, approximate values per doughnut are: iron, 0.2 mg; thiamin, 0.01 mg; riboflavin, 0.03 mg; niacin, 0.2 mg.
[19] Iron, thiamin, riboflavin, and niacin are based on the minimum levels of enrichment specified in standards of identity promulgated under the Federal Food, Drug, and Cosmetic Act.

Table A-1. (Cont.)

Food, Approximate Measure, and Weight (in grams)		gm	Water per cent	Food Energy calories	Protein gm	Fat gm	Saturated (total) gm	Unsaturated Oleic gm	Linoleic gm	Carbohydrate gm	Calcium mg	Iron mg	Vitamin A Value I.U.	Thiamin mg	Riboflavin mg	Niacin mg	Ascorbic Acid mg
Macaroni, cooked: Enriched:																	
429	Cooked, firm stage (undergoes additional cooking in a food mixture) 1 cup	130	64	190	6	1	—	—	—	39	14	191.4	0	190.23	190.14	191.8	0
430	Cooked until tender 1 cup	140	72	155	5	1	—	—	—	32	8	191.3	0	190.20	190.11	191.5	0
	Unenriched:																
431	Cooked, firm stage (undergoes additional cooking in a food mixture) 1 cup	130	64	190	6	1	—	—	—	39	14	0.7	0	0.03	0.03	0.5	0
432	Cooked until tender 1 cup	140	72	155	5	1				32	11	0.6	0	0.01	0.01	0.4	0
433	Macaroni (enriched) and cheese, baked 1 cup	200	58	430	17	22	10	9	2	40	362	1.8	860	0.20	0.40	1.8	Trace
434	Canned 1 cup	240	80	230	9	10	4	3	1	26	199	1.0	260	0.12	0.24	1.0	Trace
435	Muffins, with enriched white flour; muffin, 3-inch diam. 1 muffin	40	38	120	3	4	1	2	1	17	42	0.6	40	0.07	0.09	0.6	Trace
Noodles (egg noodles), cooked:																	
436	Enriched 1 cup	160	70	200	7	2	1	1	Trace	37	16	191.4	110	190.22	190.13	191.9	0
437	Unenriched 1 cup	160	70	200	7	2	1	1	Trace	37	16	1.0	110	0.05	0.03	0.6	0
438	Oats (with or without corn) puffed, added nutrients 1 cup	25	3	100	3	1				19	44	1.2	0	0.24	0.04	0.5	0
439	Oatmeal or rolled oats, cooked 1 cup	240	87	130	5	2			1	23	22	1.4	0	0.19	0.05	0.2	0
Pancakes, 4-inch diam.:																	
440	Wheat, enriched flour (home recipe) 1 cake	27	50	60	2	2	Trace	1	Trace	9	27	0.4	30	0.05	0.06	0.4	Trace
441	Buckwheat (made from mix with egg and milk) 1 cake	27	58	55	2	2	1	1	Trace	6	59	0.4	60	0.03	0.04	0.2	Trace
442	Plain or buttermilk (made from mix with egg and milk) 1 cake	27	51	60	2	2	1	1	Trace	9	58	0.3	70	0.04	0.06	0.2	Trace
Pie (piecrust made with unenriched flour): Sector, 4-in, 1/7 of 9-in-diam. pie:																	
443	Apple (2-crust) 1 sector	135	48	350	3	15	4	7	3	51	11	0.4	40	0.03	0.03	0.5	1
444	Butterscotch (1-crust) 1 sector	130	45	350	6	14	5	6	2	50	98	1.2	340	0.04	0.13	0.3	Trace
445	Cherry (2-crust) 1 sector	135	47	350	4	15	4	7	3	52	19	0.4	590	0.03	0.03	0.7	Trace
446	Custard (1-crust) 1 sector	130	58	285	8	14	5	6	2	30	125	0.8	300	0.07	0.21	0.4	0
447	Lemon meringue (1-crust) 1 sector	120	47	305	4	12	4	6	2	45	17	0.6	200	0.04	0.10	0.2	4
448	Mince (2-crust) 1 sector	135	43	365	3	16	4	8	3	56	38	1.4	Trace	0.09	0.05	0.5	1
449	Pecan (1-crust) 1 sector	118	20	490	6	27	4	16	5	60	55	3.3	190	0.19	0.08	0.4	Trace
450	Pineapple chiffon (1-crust) 1 sector	93	41	265	6	11	3	5	2	36	22	0.8	320	0.04	0.08	0.4	1
451	Pumpkin (1-crust) 1 sector	130	59	275	5	15	5	6	2	32	66	0.7	3,210	0.04	0.13	0.7	Trace
Piecrust, baked shell for pie made with:																	
452	Enriched flour 1 shell	180	15	900	11	60	16	28	12	79	25	3.1	0	0.36	0.25	3.2	0
453	Unenriched flour 1 shell	180	15	900	11	60	16	28	12	79	25	0.9	0	0.05	0.05	0.9	0

338

No.	Food, approximate measure, and weight	Measure	Grams	Water (%)	Food energy (cal.)	Protein (g)	Fat (g)	Saturated fatty acids (g)	Oleic (g)	Linoleic (g)	Carbohydrate (g)	Calcium (mg)	Iron (mg)	Vitamin A (I.U.)	Thiamin (mg)	Riboflavin (mg)	Niacin (mg)	Ascorbic acid (mg)
454	Piecrust mix including stick form: Package, 10 oz, for double crust	1 pkg.	284	9	1,480	20	93	23	46	21	141	131	1.4	0	0.11	0.11	2.0	0
455	Pizza (cheese) 5 1/2-in sector; 1/8 of 14-in diam. pie	1 sector	75	45	185	7	6	2	3	Trace	27	107	0.7	290	0.04	0.12	0.7	4
	Popcorn, popped:																	
456	Plain, large kernel	1 cup	6	4	25	1	Trace	—	—	—	5	1	0.2	—	—	0.01	0.1	0
457	With oil and salt	1 cup	9	3	40	1	2	1	Trace	Trace	5	1	0.2	—	—	0.01	0.2	0
458	Sugar coated	1 cup	35	4	135	2	1	—	—	—	30	2	0.5	—	—	0.02	0.4	0
	Pretzels:																	
459	Dutch, twisted	1 pretzel	16	5	60	2	1	—	—	—	12	4	0.2	0	Trace	Trace	0.1	0
460	Thin, twisted	1 pretzel	6	5	25	1	Trace	—	—	—	5	1	0.1	0	Trace	Trace	Trace	0
461	Sticks, small 2 1/4 inches	10 sticks	3	5	10	Trace	Trace	—	—	—	2	1	Trace	0	Trace	Trace	Trace	0
462	Stick, regular, 3 1/8 inches	5 sticks	3	5	10	Trace	Trace	—	—	—	2	1	Trace	0	Trace	Trace	Trace	0
	Rice, white: Enriched:																	
463	Raw	1 cup	185	12	670	12	1	—	—	—	149	44	[20]5.4	0	[20]0.81	[20]0.06	[20]6.5	0
464	Cooked	1 cup	205	73	225	4	Trace	—	—	—	50	21	[20]1.8	0	[20]0.23	[20]0.02	[20]2.1	0
465	Instant, ready to serve	1 cup	165	73	180	4	Trace	—	—	—	40	5	[20]1.3	0	[20]0.21	[20]—	[20]1.7	0
466	Unenriched, cooked	1 cup	205	73	225	4	Trace	—	—	—	50	21	0.4	0	0.04	0.02	0.8	0
467	Parboiled, cooked	1 cup	175	73	185	4	Trace	—	—	—	41	33	[20]1.4	0	[20]0.19	[20]—	[20]2.1	0
468	Rice, puffed, added nutrients	1 cup	15	4	60	1	Trace	—	—	—	13	3	0.3	0	0.07	0.01	0.7	0
	Rolls, enriched: Cloverleaf or pan:																	
469	Home recipe	1 roll	35	26	120	3	3	1	1	1	20	16	0.7	30	0.09	0.09	0.8	Trace
470	Commercial	1 roll	28	31	85	2	2	Trace	1	Trace	15	21	0.5	Trace	0.08	0.05	0.6	Trace
471	Frankfurter or hamburger	1 roll	40	31	120	3	2	1	1	1	21	30	0.8	Trace	0.11	0.07	0.9	Trace
472	Hard, round or rectangular	1 roll	50	25	155	5	2	Trace	1	Trace	30	24	1.2	Trace	0.13	0.12	1.4	Trace
473	Rye wafers, whole-grain, 1 7/8 by 3 1/2 inches	2 wafers	13	6	45	2	Trace	—	—	—	10	7	0.5	0	0.04	0.03	0.2	0
474	Spaghetti, cooked, tender stage, enriched	1 cup	140	72	155	5	1	—	—	—	32	11	[19]1.3	0	[19]0.20	[19]0.11	[19]1.5	0
	Spaghetti with meat balls, and tomato sauce:																	
475	Home recipe	1 cup	248	70	330	19	12	4	6	1	39	124	3.7	1,590	0.25	0.30	4.0	22
476	Canned	1 cup	250	78	260	12	10	2	3	4	28	53	3.3	1,000	0.15	0.18	2.3	5
	Spaghetti in tomato sauce with cheese:																	
477	Home recipe	1 cup	250	77	260	9	9	2	5	1	37	80	2.3	1,080	0.25	0.18	2.3	13
478	Canned	1 cup	250	80	190	6	2	1	1	1	38	40	2.8	930	0.35	0.28	4.5	10
479	Waffles, with enriched flour, 7-in diam.	1 waffle	75	41	210	7	7	2	4	1	28	85	1.3	250	0.13	0.19	1.0	Trace
480	Waffles, made from mix, enriched, egg and milk added, 7-in diam.	1 waffle	75	42	205	7	8	3	3	1	27	179	1.0	170	0.11	0.17	0.7	Trace
481	Wheat, puffed, added nutrients	1 cup	15	3	55	2	Trace	—	—	—	12	4	0.6	0	0.08	0.03	1.2	0
482	Wheat, shredded, plain	1 biscuit	25	7	90	2	1	—	—	—	20	11	0.9	0	0.06	0.03	1.1	0
483	Wheat flakes, added nutrients	1 cup	30	4	105	3	Trace	—	—	—	24	12	1.3	0	0.19	0.04	1.5	0
	Wheat flours:																	
484	Whole wheat, from hard wheats, stirred	1 cup	120	12	400	16	2	1	1	1	85	49	4.0	0	0.66	0.14	5.2	0

[19] Iron, thiamin, riboflavin, and niacin are based on the minimum levels of enrichment specified in standards of identity promulgated under the Federal Food, Drug, and Cosmetic Act.

[20] Iron, thiamin, and niacin are based on the minimum levels of enrichment specified in standards of identity promulgated under the Federal Food, Drug, and Cosmetic Act. Riboflavin is based on unenriched rice. When the minimum level of enrichment specified in the standards of identity becomes effective the value will be 0.12 mg per cup of parboiled rice and of white rice.

Table A-1. (Cont.)

Food, Approximate Measure, and Weight (in grams)		gm	Water per cent	Food Energy calories	Protein gm	Fat gm	Saturated (total) gm	Oleic gm	Linoleic gm	Carbohydrate gm	Calcium mg	Iron mg	Vitamin A Value I.U.	Thiamin mg	Riboflavin mg	Niacin mg	Ascorbic Acid mg
Wheat flours (cont.)																	
All-purpose or family flour, enriched:																	
485 Sifted	1 cup	115	12	420	12	1	—	—	—	88	18	193.3	0	190.51	190.30	194.0	0
486 Unsifted	1 cup	125	12	455	13	1	—	—	—	95	20	193.6	0	190.55	190.33	194.4	0
487 Self-rising, enriched	1 cup	125	12	440	12	1	—	—	—	93	331	193.6	0	190.55	190.33	194.4	0
488 Cake or pastry flour, sifted	1 cup	96	12	350	7	1	—	—	—	76	16	0.5	0	0.03	0.03	0.7	0
Fats, Oils																	
Butter:																	
Regular, 4 sticks per pound:																	
489 Stick	1/2 cup	113	16	810	1	92	51	30	3	1	23	0	213,750	—	—	—	0
490 Tablespoon (approx. 1/8 stick)	1 tbsp.	14	16	100	Trace	12	6	4	Trace	Trace	3	0	21470	—	—	—	0
491 Pat (1-in sq, 1/3-in high; 90 per lb)	1 pat	5	16	35	Trace	4	2	1	Trace	Trace	1	0	21170	—	—	—	0
Whipped, 6 sticks or 2, 8-oz containers per pound:																	
492 Stick	1/2 cup	76	16	540	1	61	34	20	2	Trace	15	0	212,500	—	—	—	0
493 Tablespoon (approx. 1/8 stick)	1 tbsp.	9	16	65	Trace	8	4	3	Trace	Trace	2	0	21310	—	—	—	0
494 Pat (1 1/4-in sq 1/3-in high; 120 per lb)	1 pat	4	16	25	Trace	3	2	1	Trace	Trace	1	0	21130	—	—	—	0
Fats, cooking:																	
495 Lard	1 cup	205	0	1,850	0	205	78	94	20	0	0	0	0	0	0	0	0
496	1 tbsp.	13	0	115	0	13	5	6	1	0	0	0	0	0	0	0	0
497 Vegetable fats	1 cup	200	0	1,770	0	200	50	100	44	0	0	0	—	0	0	0	0
498	1 tbsp	13	0	110	0	13	3	6	3	0	0	0	—	0	0	0	0
Margarine:																	
Regular, 4 sticks per pound:																	
499 Stick	1/2 cup	113	16	815	1	92	17	46	25	1	23	0	223,750	—	—	—	0
500 Tablespoon (approx. 1/8 stick)	1 tbsp	14	16	100	Trace	12	2	6	3	Trace	3	0	22470	—	—	—	0
501 Pat (1-in sq 1/3-in high; 90 per lb)	1 pat	5	16	35	Trace	4	1	2	1	Trace	1	0	22170	—	—	—	0
Whipped, 6 sticks per pound:																	
502 Stick	1/2 cup	76	16	545	1	61	11	31	17	Trace	15	0	212,500	—	—	—	0
Soft, 2 8-oz tubs per pound:																	
503 Tub	1 tub	227	16	1,635	1	184	34	68	68	1	45	0	227,500	—	—	—	0
504 Tablespoon	1 tbsp	14	16	100	Trace	11	2	4	4	Trace	3	0	22470	—	—	—	0
Oils, salad or cooking:																	
505 Corn	1 cup	220	0	1,945	0	220	22	62	117	0	0	0	—	—	—	—	0
506	1 tbsp	14	0	125	0	14	1	4	7	0	0	0	—	—	—	—	0
507 Cottonseed	1 cup	220	0	1,945	0	220	55	46	110	0	0	0	—	—	—	—	0
508	1 tbsp	14	0	125	0	14	4	3	7	0	0	0	—	—	—	—	0
509 Olive	1 cup	220	0	1,945	0	220	24	167	15	0	0	0	—	—	—	—	0
510	1 tbsp	14	0	125	0	14	2	11	1	0	0	0	—	—	—	—	0
511 Peanut	1 cup	220	0	1,945	0	220	40	103	64	0	0	0	—	—	—	—	0
512	1 tbsp	14	0	125	0	14	3	7	4	0	0	0	—	—	—	—	0

Sugars, Sweets

No.	Food	Measure																
513	Safflower	1 cup	220	0	1,945	0	220	18	37	165	0	0	0	—	0	0	0	0
514		1 tbsp	14	0	125	0	14	1	2	10	0	0	0	—	0	0	0	0
515	Soybean	1 cup	220	0	1,945	0	220	33	44	114	0	0	0	—	0	0	0	0
516		1 tbsp	14	0	125	0	14	2	3	7	0	0	0	—	0	0	0	0
	Salad dressing:																	
517	Blue cheese	1 tbsp	15	32	75	1	8	2	2	4	1	12	Trace	30	Trace	0.02	Trace	Trace
	Commercial, mayonnaise type:																	
518	Regular	1 tbsp	15	41	65	Trace	6	1	1	3	2	2	Trace	30	Trace	Trace	Trace	—
519	Special dietary, low calorie	1 tbsp	16	81	20	Trace	2	Trace	Trace	1	1	3	Trace	40	Trace	Trace	Trace	—
	French:																	
520	Regular	1 tbsp	16	39	65	Trace	6	1	1	3	3	2	0.1	—	—	—	—	—
521	Special dietary, low with artificial sweeteners	1 tbsp	15	95	Trace	Trace	Trace	—	—	—	Trace	2	0.1	—	—	—	—	—
522	Home cooked, boiled	1 tbsp	16	68	25	1	2	1	1	3	2	14	0.1	80	0.01	0.03	Trace	Trace
523	Mayonnaise	1 tbsp	14	15	100	Trace	11	2	2	6	Trace	3	0.1	40	Trace	0.01	Trace	—
524	Thousand island	1 tbsp	16	32	80	Trace	8	1	2	4	3	2	0.1	50	Trace	Trace	Trace	Trace
	Sugars, Sweets																	
	Cake icings:																	
525	Chocolate made with milk and table fat	1 cup	275	14	1,035	9	38	21	14	1	185	165	3.3	580	0.06	0.28	0.6	1
526	Coconut (with boiled icing)	1 cup	166	15	605	3	13	11	1	Trace	124	10	0.8	0	0.02	0.07	0.3	0
527	Creamy fudge from mix with water only	1 cup	245	15	830	7	16	5	8	3	183	96	2.7	Trace	0.05	0.20	0.7	Trace
528	White, boiled	1 cup	94	18	300	1	0	—	—	—	76	2	Trace	0	Trace	0.03	Trace	0
	Candy:																	
529	Carmels, plain or chocolate	1 oz	28	8	115	1	3	2	1	Trace	22	42	0.4	Trace	0.01	0.05	0.1	Trace
530	Chocolate, milk, plain	1 oz	28	1	145	2	9	5	3	Trace	16	65	0.3	80	0.02	0.10	0.1	Trace
531	Chocolate-coated peanuts	1 oz	28	1	160	5	12	3	6	2	11	33	0.4	Trace	0.10	0.05	2.1	Trace
532	Fondant; mints, uncoated; candy corn	1 oz	28	8	105	Trace	1	—	—	—	25	4	0.3	0	Trace	Trace	Trace	0
533	Fudge, plain	1 oz	28	8	115	1	4	2	2	Trace	21	22	0.3	Trace	0.01	0.03	0.1	Trace
534	Gum drops	1 oz	28	12	100	Trace	Trace	—	—	—	25	2	0.1	0	0	Trace	Trace	0
535	Hard	1 oz	28	1	110	0	Trace	—	—	—	28	6	0.5	0	0	0	0	0
536	Marshmallows	1 oz	28	17	90	Trace	Trace	—	—	—	23	5	0.5	0	0	Trace	Trace	Trace
	Chocolate-flavored syrup or topping:																	
537	Thin type	1 fl oz	38	32	90	1	1	Trace	Trace	Trace	24	6	0.6	Trace	0.01	0.03	0.2	0
538	Fudge type	1 fl oz	38	25	125	2	5	3	2	Trace	20	48	0.5	60	0.02	0.08	0.2	Trace
	Chocolate-flavored beverage powder (approx. 4 heaping teaspoons per oz):																	
539	With nonfat dry milk	1 oz	28	2	100	5	1	Trace	Trace	Trace	20	167	0.5	10	0.04	0.21	0.2	1
540	Without nonfat dry milk	1 oz	28	1	100	1	1	Trace	Trace	Trace	25	9	0.6	0	0.01	0.03	0.1	0
541	Honey, strained or extracted	1 tbsp	21	17	65	Trace	0	—	—	—	17	1	0.1	0	Trace	0.01	0.1	Trace
542	Jams and preserves	1 tbsp	20	29	55	Trace	Trace	—	—	—	14	4	0.2	Trace	Trace	0.01	Trace	Trace
543	Jellies	1 tbsp	18	29	50	Trace	Trace	—	—	—	13	4	0.3	Trace	Trace	0.01	Trace	1
	Molasses, cane:																	
544	Light (first extraction)	1 tbsp	20	24	50	—	—	—	—	—	13	33	0.9	—	0.01	0.01	Trace	—
545	Blackstrap (third extraction)	1 tbsp	20	24	45	—	—	—	—	—	11	137	3.2	—	0.02	0.04	0.4	—
	Syrups:																	
546	Sorghum	1 tbsp	21	23	55	—	—	—	—	—	14	35	2.6	—	—	0.02	Trace	—

[19]Iron, thiamin, riboflavin, and niacin are based on the minimum levels of enrichment specified in standards of identity promulgated under the Federal Food, Drug, and Cosmetic Act.

[21]Year-round average.

[22]Based on the average vitamin A content of fortified margarine. Federal specifications for fortified margarine require a minimum of 15,000 I.U. of vitamin A per pound.

341

Table A-1. (Cont.)

Food, Approximate Measure, and Weight		gm	Water per cent	Food Energy calories	Protein gm	Fat gm	Fatty Acids Saturated (total) gm	Unsaturated Oleic gm	Unsaturated Linoleic gm	Carbohydrate gm	Calcium mg	Iron mg	Vitamin A Value I.U.	Thiamin mg	Riboflavin mg	Niacin mg	Ascorbic Acid mg
	Syrups (cont.)																
547	Table blends, chiefly corn, light and dark	1 tbsp	21	24	60	0	0	—	—	—	15	9	0.8	0	0	0	0	0
	Sugars:																
548	Brown, firm packed	1 cup	220	2	820	0	0	—	—	—	212	187	7.5	0	0.02	0.07	0.4	0
	White:																
549	Granulated	1 cup	200	Trace	770	0	0	—	—	—	199	0	0.2	0	0	0	0	0
550		1 tbsp	11	Trace	40	0	0	—	—	—	11	0	Trace	0	0	0	0	0
551	Powdered, stirred before measuring	1 cup	120	Trace	460	0	0	—	—	—	119	0	0.1	0	0	0	0	0
	Miscellaneous Items																
552	Barbecue sauce	1 cup	250	81	230	4	17	2	5	9	20	53	2.0	900	0.03	0.03	0.8	13
	Beverages, alcoholic:																
553	Beer	12 fl oz	360	92	150	1	0	—	—	—	14	18	Trace	—	0.01	0.11	2.2	—
554	Gin, rum, vodka, whiskey: 80 proof	1 1/2 fl oz jigger	42	67	100	—	—	—	—	—	Trace	—	—	—	—	—	—	—
555	86 proof	1 1/2 fl oz jigger	42	64	105	—	—	—	—	—	Trace	—	—	—	—	—	—	—
556	90 proof	1 1/2 fl oz jigger	42	62	110	—	—	—	—	—	Trace	—	—	—	—	—	—	—
557	94 proof	1 1/2 fl oz jigger	42	60	115	—	—	—	—	—	Trace	—	—	—	—	—	—	—
558	100 proof	1 1/2 fl oz jigger	42	58	125	—	—	—	—	—	Trace	—	—	—	—	—	—	—
	Wines:																
559	Dessert	3 1/2 fl oz glass	103	77	140	Trace	0	—	—	—	8	8	—	—	0.01	0.02	0.2	—
560	Table	3 1/2 fl oz glass	102	86	85	Trace	0	—	—	—	4	9	0.4	—	Trace	0.01	0.1	—
	Beverages, carbonated, sweetened, nonalcoholic:																
561	Carbonated water	12 fl oz	366	92	115	0	0	—	—	—	29	—	—	—	—	—	—	0
562	Cola type	12 fl oz	369	90	145	0	0	—	—	—	37	—	—	—	0	0	0	0
563	Fruit-flavored sodas and Tom Collins mixes	12 fl oz	372	88	170	0	0	—	—	—	45	—	—	—	0	0	0	0
564	Ginger ale	12 fl oz	366	92	115	0	0	—	—	—	29	—	—	—	0	0	0	0
565	Root beer	12 fl oz	370	90	150	0	0	—	—	—	39	—	—	—	0	0	0	0
566	Bouillon cubes, approx. 1/2 in	1 cube	4	4	5	1	Trace	—	—	—	Trace	—	—	—	—	—	—	—
	Chocolate:																
567	Bitter or baking	1 oz	28	2	145	3	15	8	6	Trace	8	22	1.9	20	0.01	0.07	0.4	0
568	Semisweet, small pieces	1 cup	170	1	860	7	61	34	22	1	97	51	4.4	30	0.02	0.14	0.9	0
	Gelatin:																
569	Plain, dry powder in envelope	1 envelope	7	13	25	6	Trace	—	—	—	0	—	—	—	—	—	—	—
570	Dessert powder, 3-oz package	1 pkg	85	2	315	8	0	—	—	—	75	—	—	—	—	—	—	—
571	Gelatin dessert, prepared with water	1 cup	240	84	140	4	0	—	—	—	34	—	—	—	—	—	—	—

No.	Food, approximate measure	Measure	Grams	Water (%)	Food energy (cal)	Protein (g)	Fat (g)	Saturated (g)	Oleic (g)	Linoleic (g)	Carbohydrate (g)	Calcium (mg)	Iron (mg)	Vitamin A (IU)	Thiamin (mg)	Riboflavin (mg)	Niacin (mg)	Ascorbic acid (mg)
572	Olives, pickled: Green	4 medium or 3 extra large or 2 giant	16	78	15	Trace	2	Trace	2	Trace	Trace	8	0.2	40	—	—	—	—
573	Ripe: Mission	3 small or 2 large	10	73	15	Trace	2	Trace	2	Trace	Trace	9	0.1	10	Trace	Trace	Trace	—
	Pickles, cucumber:																	
574	Dill, medium, whole, 3 3/4 in long, 1 1/4 in diam.	1 pickle	65	93	10	1	Trace	—	—	—	1	17	0.7	70	Trace	0.01	Trace	4
575	Fresh, sliced, 1 1/2 in diam., 1/4 in thick	2 slices	15	79	10	Trace	Trace	—	—	—	3	5	0.3	20	Trace	Trace	Trace	1
576	Sweet, gherkin, small, whole, approx. 2 1/2 in long, 3/4 in diam.	1 pickle	15	61	20	Trace	Trace	—	—	—	6	2	0.2	10	Trace	Trace	Trace	1
577	Relish, finely chopped, sweet	1 tbsp	15	63	20	Trace	Trace	—	—	—	5	3	0.1	—	—	—	—	—
	Popcorn. See Grain Products																	
578	Popsicle, 3-fl oz size	1 popsicle	95	80	70	0	0	0	0	0	18	0	Trace	0	0	0	0	0
	Pudding, home recipe with starch base:																	
579	Chocolate	1 cup	260	66	385	8	12	7	4	Trace	67	250	1.3	390	0.05	0.36	0.3	1
580	Vanilla (blanc mange)	1 cup	255	76	285	9	10	5	3	Trace	41	298	Trace	410	0.08	0.41	0.3	2
581	Pudding mix, dry form, 4-oz package	1 pkg	113	2	410	3	2	1	1	Trace	103	23	1.8	Trace	0.02	0.08	0.5	0
582	Sherbet	1 cup	193	67	260	2	2	—	—	—	59	31	Trace	120	0.02	0.06	Trace	4
	Soups: Canned, condensed, ready-to-serve: Prepared with an equal volume of milk:																	
583	Cream of chicken	1 cup	245	85	180	7	10	3	3	3	15	172	0.5	610	0.05	0.27	0.7	2
584	Cream of mushroom	1 cup	245	83	215	7	14	4	4	5	16	191	0.5	250	0.05	0.34	0.7	1
585	Tomato	1 cup	250	84	175	7	7	3	2	1	23	168	0.8	1,200	0.10	0.25	1.3	15
	Prepared with an equal volume of water:																	
586	Bean with pork	1 cup	250	84	170	8	6	1	2	2	22	63	2.3	650	0.13	0.08	1.0	3
587	Beef broth, bouillon consommé	1 cup	240	96	30	5	0	—	—	—	3	Trace	0.5	Trace	Trace	0.02	1.2	—
588	Beef noodle	1 cup	240	93	70	4	3	1	1	1	7	7	1.0	50	0.05	0.07	1.0	Trace
589	Clam chowder, Manhattan type (with tomatoes, without milk)	1 cup	245	92	80	2	3	—	—	—	12	34	1.0	880	0.02	0.02	1.0	—
590	Cream of chicken	1 cup	240	92	95	3	6	1	2	3	8	24	0.5	410	0.02	0.05	0.5	Trace
591	Cream of mushroom	1 cup	240	90	135	2	10	1	3	5	10	41	0.5	70	0.02	0.12	0.7	Trace
592	Minestrone	1 cup	245	90	105	5	3	—	2	Trace	14	37	1.0	2,350	0.07	0.05	1.0	—
593	Split pea	1 cup	245	85	145	9	3	1	1	1	21	29	1.5	440	0.25	0.15	1.5	1
594	Tomato	1 cup	245	90	90	2	2	Trace	—	—	16	15	0.7	1,000	0.05	0.05	1.2	12
595	Vegetable beef	1 cup	245	92	80	5	2	—	—	—	10	12	0.7	2,700	0.05	0.05	1.0	—
596	Vegetarian	1 cup	245	92	80	2	2	—	—	—	13	20	1.0	2,940	0.05	0.05	1.0	—
	Dehydrated, dry form:																	
597	Chicken noodle (2-oz package)	1 pkg	57	6	220	8	6	2	3	1	33	34	1.4	190	0.30	0.15	2.4	3
598	Onion mix (1 1/2-oz package)	1 pkg	43	3	150	6	5	1	2	1	23	42	0.6	30	0.05	0.03	0.3	6
599	Tomato vegetable with noodles (2 1/2-oz pkg)	1 pkg	71	4	245	6	6	2	3	1	45	33	1.4	1,700	0.21	0.13	1.8	18
	Frozen, condensed: Clam chowder, New England type (with milk, without tomatoes):																	
600	Prepared with equal volume of milk	1 cup	245	83	210	9	12	—	—	—	16	240	1.0	250	0.07	0.29	0.5	Trace

Table A-1. (Cont.)

	Food, Approximate Measure, and Weight (in grams)		gm	Water per cent	Food Energy calories	Pro-tein gm	Fat gm	Fatty Acids			Carbo-hy-drate gm	Cal-cium mg	Iron mg	Vita-min A Value I.U.	Thia-min mg	Ribo-flavin mg	Niacin mg	Ascor-bic Acid mg
								Satu-rated (total) gm	Unsaturated									
									Oleic gm	Lin-oleic gm								
	Soups, frozen (cont.)																	
	Clam chowder, New England type																	
601	Prepared with equal volume of water	1 cup	240	89	130	4	8	—	—	—	11	91	1.0	50	0.05	0.10	0.5	—
	Cream of potato:																	
602	Prepared with equal volume of milk	1 cup	245	83	185	8	10	5	3	Trace	18	208	1.0	590	0.10	0.27	0.5	Trace
603	Prepared with equal volume of water	1 cup	240	90	105	3	5	3	2	Trace	12	58	1.0	410	0.05	0.05	0.5	—
	Cream of shrimp:																	
604	Prepared with equal volume of milk	1 cup	245	82	245	9	16	—	—	—	15	189	0.5	290	0.07	0.27	0.5	Trace
605	Prepared with equal volume of water	1 cup	240	88	160	5	12	—	—	—	8	38	0.5	120	0.05	0.05	0.5	—
	Oyster stew:																	
606	Prepared with equal volume of milk	1 cup	240	83	200	10	12	—	—	—	14	305	1.4	410	0.12	0.41	0.5	Trace
607	Prepared with equal volume of water	1 cup	240	90	120	6	8	—	—	—	8	158	1.4	240	0.07	0.19	0.5	—
608	Tapioca, dry, quick cooking	1 cup	152	13	535	1	Trace	—	—	—	131	15	0.6	0	0	0	0	0
	Tapioca desserts:																	
609	Apple	1 cup	250	70	295	1	Trace	—	—	—	74	8	0.5	30	Trace	Trace	Trace	Trace
610	Cream pudding	1 cup	165	72	220	8	8	4	3	Trace	28	173	0.7	480	0.07	0.30	0.2	2
611	Tartar sauce	1 tbsp	14	34	75	Trace	8	1	1	4	1	3	0.1	30	Trace	Trace	Trace	Trace
612	Vinegar	1 tbsp	15	94	Trace	Trace	0	—	—	—	1	1	0.1	—	—	—	—	—
613	White sauce, medium	1 cup	250	73	405	10	31	10	10	1	22	288	0.5	1,150	0.10	0.43	0.5	2
	Yeast:																	
614	Bakers', dry, active	1 pkg	7	5	20	3	Trace	—	—	—	3	3	1.1	Trace	0.16	0.38	2.6	Trace
615	Brewers', dry	1 tbsp	8	5	25	3	Trace	—	—	—	3	17	1.4	Trace	1.25	0.34	3.0	Trace
	Yogurt. See Milk, Cheese, Cream, Imitation Cream																	

Exchange List	Measure	Carbohydrate gm	Protein gm	Fat gm	Energy kcal
Milk, list 1					
nonfat	1 cup	12	8	tr	80
1 per cent fat	1 cup	12	8	2.5	105
2 per cent fat	1 cup	12	8	5	125
whole	1 cup	12	8	10	170
Vegetables, list 2	½ cup	5	2		25
Fruits, list 3	varies	10			40
Breads, cereals, and starchy vegetables, list 4	varies	15	2		70
prepared foods	varies	15	2	5–10	115–160
Meat, list 5					
lean	1 ounce		7	3	55
medium fat	1 ounce		7	5.5	80
high fat	1 ounce		7	8	100
Fat, list 6	1 teaspoon			5	45

* The data for this table and the *exchange lists* in this book are based on materials in *Exchange Lists for Meal Planning* prepared by committees of the American Diabetes Association, Inc., and The American Dietetic Association in cooperation with The National Institute of Arthritis, Metabolism and Digestive Diseases and the National Heart and Lung Institute, National Institutes of Health, Public Health Service, U.S. Department of Health, Education, and Welfare.

LIST 1—MILK

MILK, NONFAT, FORTIFIED. USE ONLY THIS LIST FOR DIETS RESTRICTED IN SATURATED FAT.

	Amount to Use
Skim or nonfat milk	1 cup
Powdered (nonfat dry)	⅓ cup
Canned, evaporated, skim	½ cup
Buttermilk, made from skim milk	1 cup
Yogurt, made from skimmed milk, plain unflavored	1 cup

MILK, LOW-FAT, FORTIFIED

1 per cent fat, fortified (omit ½ fat exchange)	1 cup
2 per cent fat, fortified (omit 1 fat exchange)	1 cup
Yogurt, made from 2 per cent fortified, plain, unflavored (omit 1 fat exchange)	1 cup

Milk, Whole (omit two fat exchanges)

Whole milk	1 cup
Canned evaporated whole	½ cup
Buttermilk made from whole milk	1 cup
Yogurt made from whole milk (plain unflavored)	1 cup

List 2—Vegetables

One-Half Cup Equals One Exchange

Asparagus	Greens:
Bean Sprouts	Mustard
Beets	Spinach
Broccoli	Turnip
Brussels Sprouts	Mushrooms
Cabbage	Okra
Carrots	Onions
Cauliflower	Rhubarb
Celery	Rutabaga
Cucumbers	Sauerkraut
Eggplant	String Beans, green or yellow
Green Pepper	Summer Squash
Greens:	Tomatoes
Beet	Tomato Juice
Chards	Turnips
Collards	Vegetable Juice Cocktail
Dandelion	Zucchini
Kale	

The following raw vegetables may be used as desired:

Chicory	Lettuce
Chinese Cabbage	Parsley
Endive	Radishes
Escarole	Watercress

Starchy Vegetables are found in the Bread Exchange List.

List 3—Fruit Exchanges

	Amount to Use		*Amount to Use*
Apple	1 small	Blueberries	½ cup
Apple Juice	⅓ cup	Raspberries	½ cup
Applesauce (unsweetened)	½ cup	Strawberries	¾ cup
Apricots, fresh	2 medium	Cherries	10 large
Apricots, dried	4 halves	Cider	⅓ cup
Banana	½ small	Dates	2
Berries		Figs, fresh	1
Blackberries	½ cup	Figs, dried	1

346

	Amount to Use		Amount to Use
Grapefruit	½	Papaya	¾ cup
Grapefruit Juice	½ cup	Peach	1 medium
Grapes	12	Pear	1 small
Grape Juice	¼ cup	Persimmon, native	1 medium
Mango	½ small	Pineapple	½ cup
Melon		Pineapple Juice	⅓ cup
Cantaloupe	¼ small	Plums	2 medium
Honeydew	⅛ medium	Prunes	2 medium
Watermelon	1 cup	Prune Juice	¼ cup
Nectarine	1 small	Raisins	2 tablespoons
Orange	1 small	Tangerine	1 medium
Orange Juice	½ cup		

Cranberries may be used as desired if no sugar is added.

LIST 4—BREAD, CEREAL, AND STARCHY VEGETABLE EXCHANGES

	Amount to Use		Amount to Use
Bread		Cornmeal (dry)	2 tablespoons
White (including French and Italian)	1 slice	Flour	2½ tablespoons
Whole Wheat	1 slice	Wheat Germ	¼ cup
Rye or Pumpernickel	1 slice	Crackers	
Raisin	1 slice	Arrowroot	3
Bagel, small	½	Graham, 2½" sq.	2
English Muffin, small	½	Matzoth, 4" × 6"	½
Plain Roll, bread	1	Oyster	20
Frankfurter Roll	½	Pretzels, 3⅛" long × ⅛" dia.	25
Hamburger Bun	½	Rye Wafers, 2" × 3½"	3
Dried Bread Crumbs	3 tablespoons	Saltines	6
Tortilla, 6"	1	Soda, 2½" sq.	4
Cereal		Dried Beans, Peas and Lentils	
Bran Flakes	½ cup	Beans, Peas, Lentils (dried and cooked)	½ cup
Other ready-to-eat unsweetened Cereal	¾ cup	Baked Beans, no pork (canned)	¼ cup
Puffed Cereal (unfrosted)	1 cup	Starchy Vegetables	
Cereal (cooked)	½ cup	Corn	⅓ cup
Grits (cooked)	½ cup	Corn on Cob	1 small
Rice or Barley (cooked)	½ cup		

	Amount to Use		Amount to Use
Pasta (cooked)	½ cup	Lima Beans	½ cup
Spaghetti, Noodles,		Parsnips	⅔ cup
Macaroni		Peas, Green (canned	½ cup
Popcorn (popped,		or frozen)	
no fat added)	3 cups	Potato, White	1 small
Potato (mashed)	½ cup	Muffin, plain small	1
Pumpkin	¾ cup	(omit 1 Fat Exchange)	
Winter Squash, Acorn		Potatoes, French Fried,	
or Butternut	½ cup	length 2" to 3½"	8
Yam or Sweet Potato	¼ cup	(omit 1 Fat Exchange)	
Prepared Foods		Potato or Corn Chips	15
Biscuit 2" dia.	1	(omit 2 Fat Exchanges)	
(omit 1 Fat Exchange)		Pancake, 4" × ½"	1
Corn Bread, 2" × 2" × 1"	1	(omit 1 Fat Exchange)	
(omit 1 Fat Exchange)		Waffle, 5" × ½"	1
Corn Muffin, 2" dia.	1	(omit 1 Fat Exchange)	
(omit 1 Fat Exchange)			
Crackers, round butter type	5		
(omit 1 Fat Exchange)			

List 5 Meat and Protein-Rich Exchanges

Lean Meat, Protein-Rich Exchanges. Use only this list for diets low in saturated fat and cholesterol.

	Amount to Use
Beef: Baby Beef (very lean), Chipped Beef, Chuck, Flank Steak, Tenderloin, Plate Ribs, Plate Skirt Steak, Round (bottom, top), All cuts Rump, Spare Ribs, Tripe	1 ounce
Lamb: Leg, Rib, Sirloin, Loin (roast and chops), Shank, Shoulder	1 ounce
Pork: Leg (Whole Rump, Center Shank), Ham, Smoked (center slices)	1 ounce
Veal: Leg, Loin, Rib, Shank, Shoulder, Cutlets	1 ounce
Poultry: Meat without skin of Chicken, Turkey, Cornish Hen, Guinea Hen, Pheasant	1 ounce
Fish: Any fresh or frozen	1 ounce
Canned Salmon, Tuna, Mackerel, Crab and Lobster,	¼ cup
Clams, Oysters, Scallops, Shrimp,	5 or 1 ounce
Sardines, drained	3
Cheeses containing less than 5% butterfat	1 ounce
Cottage Cheese, Dry and 2% butterfat	¼ cup
Dried Beans and Peas (omit 1 Bread Exchange)	½ cup

MEDIUM FAT MEAT AND PROTEIN-RICH EXCHANGES. OMIT ½ FAT EXCHANGE FOR EACH
MEAT EXCHANGE USED FROM THIS LIST.

	Amount to Use
Beef: Ground (15% fat), Corned Beef (canned), Rib Eye, Round (ground commercial)	1 ounce
Pork: Loin (all cuts Tenderloin), Shoulder Arm (picnic), Shoulder Blade, Boston Butt, Canadian Bacon, Boiled Ham	1 ounce
Liver, Heart, Kidney and Sweetbreads (these are high in cholesterol)	1 ounce
Cottage Cheese, creamed	¼ cup
Cheese: Mozzarella, Ricotta, Farmer's cheese, Neufchatel, Parmesan	1 ounce 3 tablespoons
Egg (high in cholesterol)	1
Peanut Butter (omit 2 additional Fat Exchanges)	2 tablespoons

HIGH FAT MEAT AND PROTEIN-RICH EXCHANGES. OMIT 1 FAT EXCHANGE FOR EACH
MEAT EXCHANGE USED FROM THIS LIST

	Amount to Use
Beef: Brisket, Corned Beef (Brisket), Ground Beef (more than 20% fat), Hamburger (commercial), Chuck (ground commercial), Roasts (Rib), Steaks (Club and Rib)	1 ounce
Lamb: Breast	1 ounce
Pork: Spare Ribs, Loin (Back Ribs), Pork (ground), Country style Ham, Deviled Ham	1 ounce
Veal: Breast	1 ounce
Poultry: Capon, Duck (domestic), Goose	1 ounce
Cheese: Cheddar Types	1 ounce
Cold Cuts	4½" x ⅛" slice
Frankfurter	1 small

List 6—Fat Exchanges

For a diet low in saturated fat and higher in polyunsaturated fat select only from this list.

	Amount to Use
Margarine, soft, tub, or stick (made with corn, cottonseed, safflower, soy, or sunflower oil)	1 teaspoon
Avocado, 4 in. diam.	⅛
Nuts	
Almonds *	10 whole
Peanuts *	
Spanish	20 whole
Virginia	10 whole
Pecans *	2 large, whole
Walnuts	6 small
Other nuts	6 small
Oil: corn, cottonseed, safflower, soy, sunflower	1 teaspoon
Oil: olive or peanut *	1 teaspoon
Olives *	5 small
Salad dressings, if made with corn, cottonseed, safflower, soy, or sunflower oil	
French dressing	1 tablespoon
Italian dressing	1 tablespoon
Mayonnaise	1 teaspoon
Salad dressing, mayonnaise type	2 teaspoons

    * Fat content is primarily monounsaturated.

The following fat exchanges may be used only on diets not restricted in saturated fat.	
Margarine, regular stick	1 teaspoon
Butter	1 teaspoon
Bacon fat	1 teaspoon
Bacon, crisp	1 strip
Cream, light	2 tablespoons
Cream, sour	2 tablespoons
Cream, heavy	1 tablespoon
Cream cheese	1 tablespoon
Lard	1 teaspoon
Salad dressings (permitted on restricted diets only if made with allowed oils)	
French dressing	1 tablespoon
Italian dressing	1 tablespoon
Mayonnaise	1 teaspoon
Salad dressing, mayonnaise type	2 teaspoons
Salt pork	¾ in. cube

TABLE A–3 SUGGESTED WEIGHTS FOR HEIGHTS FOR MEN AND WOMEN *

| Height (without shoes) | | Weight (without clothing) | | | | | |
| | | Low | | Medium | | High | |
cm	in.	kg	lb	kg	lb	kg	lb
				Men			
160	63	54	118	59	129	64	141
163	64	55	122	60	133	66	145
165	65	57	126	62	137	68	149
167	66	59	130	65	142	70	155
170	67	61	134	67	147	73	161
173	68	63	139	69	151	75	166
175	69	65	143	70	155	77	170
178	70	67	147	72	159	80	174
180	71	68	150	74	163	81	178
183	72	70	154	76	167	83	183
185	73	72	158	77	171	85	188
188	74	74	162	80	175	87	192
191	75	75	165	81	178	89	195
				Women			
152	60	45	100	50	109	54	118
155	61	47	104	51	112	55	121
157	62	49	107	52	115	57	125
160	63	50	110	54	118	58	128
163	64	51	113	55	122	60	132
165	65	53	116	57	125	61	135
167	66	55	120	59	129	63	139
170	67	56	123	60	132	65	142
173	68	57	126	62	136	66	146
175	69	59	130	64	140	69	151
178	70	60	133	65	144	71	156
180	71	62	137	67	148	73	161
183	72	64	141	69	152	75	166

* Data for heights in inches and weights in pounds taken from: M. L. Hathaway, and E. D. Foard, *Heights and Weights of Adults in the United States.* Home Economics Research Report No. 10, U.S. Department of Agriculture, Washington, D.C., Table 80, p. 111.

Conversions to centimeters and kilograms were rounded off to the nearest whole number.

TABLE A-4 RECOMMENDED DAILY NUTRIENT INTAKES—CANADA, REVISED 1974

(Committee for Revision of the Canadian Dietary Standard, Bureau of Nutritional Sciences, Health and Welfare, Ottawa, Canada

Age (years)	Sex	Weight (kg)	Height (cm)	Energy [a] (kcal)	Protein (gm)	Thiamin (mg)	Niacin [e] (mg)	Riboflavin (mg)	Vitamin B_6 [f] (mg)	Folate [g] (mcg)	Vitamin B_{12} (mcg)	Ascorbic Acid (mg)
								Water-Soluble Vitamins				
0–6 mos.	both	6		kg × 117	kg × 2.2 (2.0) [d]	0.3	5	0.4	0.3	40	0.3	20 [h]
7–11 mos.	both	9		kg × 108	kg × 1.4	0.5	6	0.6	0.4	60	0.3	20
1–3	both	13	90	1400	22	0.7	9	0.8	0.8	100	0.9	20
4–6	both	19	110	1800	27	0.9	12	1.1	1.3	100	1.5	20
7–9	M	27	129	2200	33	1.1	14	1.3	1.6	100	1.5	30
	F	27	128	2000	33	1.0	13	1.2	1.4	100	1.5	30
10–12	M	36	144	2500	41	1.2	17	1.5	1.8	100	3.0	30
	F	38	145	2300	40	1.1	15	1.4	1.5	100	3.0	30
13–15	M	51	162	2800	52	1.4	19	1.7	2.0	200	3.0	30
	F	49	159	2200	43	1.1	15	1.4	1.5	200	3.0	30
16–18	M	64	172	3200	54	1.6	21	2.0	2.0	200	3.0	30
	F	54	161	2100	43	1.1	14	1.3	1.5	200	3.0	30
19–35	M	70	176	3000	56	1.5	20	1.8	2.0	200	3.0	30
	F	56	161	2100	41	1.1	14	1.3	1.5	200	3.0	30
36–50	M	70	176	2700	56	1.4	18	1.7	2.0	200	3.0	30
	F	56	161	1900	41	1.0	13	1.2	1.5	200	3.0	30
51+	M	70	176	2300 [b]	56	1.4	18	1.7	2.0	200	3.0	30
	F	56	161	1800 [b]	41	1.0	13	1.2	1.5	200	3.0	30
Pregnant				+300 [c]	+20	+0.2	+2	+0.3	+0.5	+50	+1.0	+20
Lactating				+500	+24	+0.4	+7	+0.6	+0.6	+50	+0.5	+30

a Recommendations assume characteristic activity pattern for each age group.
b Recommended energy allowance for age 66+ years reduced to 2000 for men and 1500 for women.
c Increased energy allowance recommended during second and third trimesters. An increase of 100 kcal per day is recommended during the first trimester.
d Recommended protein allowance of 2.2 gm per kg body weight for infants age 0–2 mos., and 2.0 gm per kg body weight for those age 3–5 mos. Protein recommendation for infants, 0–11 mos., assumes consumption of breast milk or protein of equivalent quality.
e Approximately 1 mg of niacin is derived from each 60 mg of dietary tryptophan.
f Recommendations are based on the estimated average daily protein intake of Canadians.
g Recommendations given in terms of free folate.
h Considerably higher levels may be prudent for infants during the first week of life to guard against neonatal tyrosinemia.

Fat-Soluble Vitamins | | | *Minerals* | | | | | |

Vitamin A [1] (mcg RE)	Vitamin D [j] (mcg cholecalciferol)	Vitamin E (mg α-tocopherol)	Calcium (mg)	Phosphorus (mg)	Magnesium (mg)	Iodine (mcg)	Iron (mg)	Zinc (mg)	Age (years)
400	10	3	500[l]	250[l]	50[l]	35[l]	7[l]	4[l]	0– 6 mos.
400	10	3	500	400	50	50	7	5	7–11 mos.
400	10	4	500	500	75	70	8	5	1– 3
500	2.5[k]	5	500	500	100	90	9	6	4– 6
700	2.5[k]	6	700	700	150	110	10	7	7– 9 M
700	2.5[k]	6	700	700	150	100	10	7	7– 9 F
800	2.5[k]	7	900	900	175	130	11	8	10–12 M
1000	2.5[k]	7	1000	1000	200	120	11	9	10–12 F
1000	2.6[k]	9	1200	1200	250	140	13	10	13–15 M
800	2.5[k]	7	800	800	250	110	14	10	13–15 F
1000	2.5[k]	10	1000	1000	300	160	14	11	16–18 M
800	2.5[k]	6	700	700	250	110	14	12	16–18 F
1000	2.5[k]	9	800	800	300	150	10	11	19–35 M
800	2.5[k]	6	700	700	250	110	14	10	19–35 F
1000	2.5[k]	8	800	800	300	140	10	9	36–50 M
800	2.5[k]	6	700	700	250	100	14	10	36–50 F
1000	2.5[k]	8	800	800	300	140	10	9	51 + M
800	2.5[k]	6	700	700	250	100	9	10	51 + F
+100	+2.5[k]	+1	+500	+500	+25	+15	+1 m	+3	Pregnant
+400	+2.5[k]	+2	+500	+500	+75	+25	+1 m	+7	Lactating

¹ One mcg retinol equivalent (1 mcg RE) corresponds to a biological activity in humans equal to 1 mcg retinol (3.33 IU) and 6 mcg β-carotene (10 IU).

ʲ One mcg cholecalciferol is equivalent to 40 IU vitamin D activity.

ᵏ Most older children and adults receive enough vitamin D from irradiation but 2.5 mcg daily is recommended. This recommended allowance increases to 5.0 mcg daily for pregnant and lactating women and for those who are confined indoors or otherwise deprived of sunlight for extended periods.

ˡ The intake of breast-fed infants may be less than the recommendation but is considered to be adequate.

ᵐ A recommended total intake of 15 mg daily during pregnancy and lactation assumes the presence of adequate stores of iron. If stores are suspected of being inadequate, additional iron as a supplement is recommended.

TABLE A–5 APPROXIMATE CONVERSIONS TO AND FROM METRIC MEASURES

If Measure Is in	Multiply by	To Find
Length		
inches	2.5	centimeters
feet	30	centimeters
centimeters	0.4	inches
meters	3.3	feet
Weight		
ounces	28	grams
pounds	0.45	kilograms
grams	0.035	ounces
kilograms	2.2	pounds
Volume		
teaspoons	5	milliliters
tablespoons	15	milliliters
fluid ounces	30	milliliters
cups	0.24	liters
pints	0.47	liters
quarts	0.95	liters
milliliters	0.03	fluid ounces
liters	2.1	pints
liters	1.06	quarts
Temperature		
Fahrenheit	subtract 32; then multiply by $\frac{5}{9}$	Celsius
Celsius	$\frac{9}{5}$; then add 32	Fahrenheit

TABLE A–6   SOME EXAMPLES OF DRUG AND FOOD/NUTRIENT INTERACTIONS

Drugs	Possible Effects on Nutrition *
Anticonvulsants	
phenytoin	Anorexia; nausea; vomiting; deficiency of folacin and vitamins D and K; osteomalacia
Antidepressants	
MAO inhibitors	React with tyramine in foods (aged cheese, yogurt, herring, banana, chocolate, wine, and others): headache, severe hypertension; diarrhea
Antimicrobials	Sore mouth; nausea; vomiting; diarrhea
neomycin	Sterilizes gastrointestinal tract; reduces synthesis of folacin, vitamin K; lowers absorption of Ca, Na, K, Fe, carotene, vitamin B_{12}
tetracycline	Binds mineral elements
para-aminosalicylic acid	Lowers absorption of folacin, vitamin B_{12}, iron
Antipyretics	
aspirin	Nausea; vomiting; epigastric distress; gastric ulceration
indomethacin	Anorexia; abdominal pain; peptic ulceration; bleeding
Antituberculars	
isoniazid	Dry mouth; epigastric distress; increased excretion of vitamin B_6
Cardiovascular Agents	
digitalis	Nausea; vomiting
anti-hypertensives chlorothiazide furosemide methyldopa reserpine	Fluid and electrolyte imbalance; hypokalemia; hyperglycemia; hyperuricemia; gastrointestinal upset
hypocholesteremic cholestyramine	Nausea; constipation or diarrhea; binds bile acids; lowers absorption fat-soluble vitamins, folacin, vitamin B_{12}
clofibrate	Unpleasant taste sensation; nausea; diarrhea; anemia; lowered absorption of glucose, iron, vitamins A and B_{12}
Chemotherapeutic Agents	Nausea; vomiting; altered taste sensation; sore mouth; esophagitis; gastrointestinal bleeding; diarrhea
aminopterin 5-fluorouracil	Reduced absorption of folacin, vitamin B_{12}
methotrexate	Reduced absorption of folacin, vitamin B_{12}; elevated prothrombin

355

TABLE A–6   *(Continued)*

Drugs	*Possible Effects on Nutrition**
Hormones	
ACTH	Gastric inflammation; fluid imbalance
contraceptives (oral)	Lowered serum levels of ascorbic acid, folacin, vitamin B_6, and riboflavin
prednisone	Gastric ulceration; anemia; decreased glucose tolerance
Laxatives	Chronic use of any reduces absorption of all nutrients; protein-losing enteropathy
mineral oil	Reduced absorption of fat-soluble vitamins
milk of magnesia	Draws water into the gut; reduced absorption
Uricosuric Agents	
colchicine	Nausea; vomiting; diarrhea; high doses reduce nutrient absorption
probenecid	Gastrointestinal irritation
Other drugs	
ferrous sulfate	Nausea; vomiting
griseofulvin	Altered sense of taste
potassium chloride	Bitter after taste; nausea; vomiting

* Adverse reactions between drugs and food/nutrient utilization occur with (1) long term use, and (2) abuse of drugs, for example, laxatives. The effects are more pronounced when the nutritional status is poor and when the diet is of marginal quality.

TABLE A–7 PROPRIETARY FORMULAS FOR ORAL OR TUBE FEEDINGS

Name of Product	Composition per 1000 ml †				Osmolality** mOsm/Kg water	Description of Product ††
	Energy kcal	Protein gm	Fat gm	Carbo-hydrate gm		
Blenderized Feedings						Typical ingredients: purées of meat, fruit, vegetables; nonfat dry milk, vegetable oil, added carbohydrate, minerals, vitamins.
Carnacal (Hospital Diet) *	1008	40	40	122	575	
Compleat-B (bottles) (Doyle)	1068	43	43	128	405	Generally well tolerated
Formula 2 (Cutter)	1000	38	40	123		
Magnacal-B (Hospital Diet)	1509	50	73	163	725	
Milk-base Formulas						Typical ingredients: nonfat dry or concentrated skim milk, corn syrup solids, vegetable oil, calcium and sodium caseinate, minerals, vitamins .
Formula 1 (Gerber)	1000	50	33	125		
Meritene Liquid (Doyle)	1000	60	33	115		
Nutri-1000 (Syntex)	1060	40	55	101	500	
Suppurt-M (Hospital Diet)	1000	30	40	130	475	
Sustacal (Mead Johnson)	1000	60	23	138	625	

TABLE A-7 (Continued)

Name of Product	Energy kcal	Composition per 1000 ml†				Osmolality** mOsm/Kg water	Description of Product ††
		Protein gm	Fat gm	Carbo-hydrate gm			
Lactose-free—blenderized							
Vegecal (Hospital Diet)	1080	36	40	144		525	All vegetable blend: soy protein
Vitaneed (Hospital Diet)	1020	35	40	130		435	Meat, fruit, vegetable blend
Lactose-free							
Ensure (Ross)	1060	37	37	145			Typical ingredients: soy protein, calcium and sodium caseinate, corn syrup solids, vegetable oil, minerals, vitamins
Ensure Osmolite (Ross)	1060	37	38	143		300	Includes medium chain triglycerides
Isocal (Mead Johnson)	1057	34	44	130		350	
Nutri-1000 LF (Syntex)	1060						
Renu (Hospital Diet)	1012	33	40	130		345	
Low-residue and Elemental Diets							
Flexical (Mead Johnson)	1000	22	34	155		835	Hydrolyzed casein, amino acids, medium-chain triglycerides, soy oil, corn syrup solids, vitamins, minerals
Precision LR Diet (Doyle)	1110	26	2	248		525	Egg white solids, maltodextrin, sucrose, minerals, vitamins

Product						Ingredients
Precision High Nitrogen Diet (Doyle)	1050	44	1	216	557	
Precision Isotonic Diet (Doyle)	1000	30	31	150	300	Glucose oligosaccharides, egg white solids, sucrose, soy oil, vitamins, minerals
Vital (Ross)	1000	42	10	185	450	Glucose oligo- and polysaccharides, hydrolyzed proteins (soy, whey, meat), sucrose, corn starch, sunflower oil . . . free amino acids
Vivonex Standard (Eaton)	1000	20	1	226		Purified amino acids, linoleic acid, glucose, oligosaccharides
Vivinex High Nitrogen (Eaton)	1000	42	1	210		

* Consult manufacturers for information on ingredients, nutritive values and uses: Cutter Medical, Division of Cutter Laboratories, Inc., Berkeley, CA 94710; The Doyle Pharmaceutical Company, Minneapolis, MN 55416; Eaton Laboratories, Division of Morton-Norwich Products, Inc., Norwich, N.Y. 13815; Gerber Products Company, Fremont, Mich 49412; Hospital Diet Products Corporation, Buena Park, CA 90621; Mead Johnson Laboratories, Evansville, Ind. 47721; Syntex Laboratories, Inc., Palo Alto, CA 94304

† Values are given for standard dilutions of the product. All formulas listed furnish minerals and vitamins to meet or exceed the Recommended Dietary Allowances and/or U.S. Recommended Dietary Allowances when ingested at appropriate energy levels.

** The osmotic pressure of blood plasma is about 300 mOsm per kilogram. Feedings with an osmolality similar to that of blood reduces the likelihood of gastrointestinal discomfort.

Appendix B

GLOSSARY

FOREWORD TO THE STUDENT

The first step in the study of any subject is gaining an understanding of the vocabulary. Every student should have a standard dictionary and should form the habit of using it whenever he comes across a word he does not know.

This glossary includes words frequently used in medicine and nutrition and that are not, for the most part, defined fully in the text. Many terms directly related to nutrition are defined in the text, and the student should refer to the chapters in which these terms are discussed. Consult the index for page references to such terms.

absorption. In physiology, the uptake of nutrients by the walls of the small intestine for transfer to the circulation.

acetone bodies. Intermediate products in the oxidation of fatty acids; acetone, aceto-acetic acid, and beta-hydroxy-butric acid.

acidosis. Abnormal accumulation of acids in the body, or loss of base.

ACTH (adrenocorticotropic hormone). A hormone produced by the pituitary gland that controls the action of the adrenal cortex; sodium metabolism, for example.

acute. Sudden, severe symptoms of short duration.

adipose. Fatty tissue; body stores of fat.

adrenal. Organ near the kidney that secretes several hormones.

amylase (amylopsin). An enzyme in saliva or pancreatic juice that digests starch.

anemia. A decrease in the number of red blood cells or hemoglobin or both.

anion. Chemical substance that carries a negative electrical charge.

anorexia. Loss of appetite.

360

antibiotic. A substance that checks the growth of microorganisms.

antibody. A protein substance produced within the body that destroys bacteria.

antioxidant. A substance that prevents oxidation; often added to foods to prevent rancidity.

anuria. Absence of urinary output.

ascites. Accumulation of fluid in the abdominal cavity.

atherosclerosis. Thickening of inside wall of arteries by fat-cholesterol containing deposits.

avitaminosis. Deficiency or lack of vitamins in the diet, or failure to absorb them; specific symptoms result from each vitamin deficiency.

bile. Secretion of the liver that aids in fat digestion and absorption.

blanch. To preheat in boiling water or steam; used to inactivate enzymes before freezing food, or to remove the skins of fruits.

bland. Mild in flavor.

braise. To cook food in a tightly covered pan with a small amount of liquid.

buffer. A substance that lessens the change in pH that otherwise would occur with the addition of acids or alkalies.

calcification. Hardening of tissue by deposits of calcium salts; bone, for example.

calculi. Hard substances formed in the body; kidney stones.

caliper. An instrument for measuring the thickness of an object; used in medicine to measure thickness of fat layers.

calorimeter. An instrument for measuring heat change. A bomb calorimeter measures calories in food; a respiration calorimeter measures oxygen and carbon dioxide exchange of an individual.

carboxylase. An enzyme necessary for the metabolism of glucose; thiamin is a component.

catalyst. A substance that speeds up a chemical reaction.

cation. Chemical substance that carries a positive electrical charge.

cecum. The large blind pouch in which the large intestine begins.

cellular. Pertaining to the function of cells that make up the tissues.

chlorophyll. The green coloring matter in plants that is responsible for the process of photosynthesis.

cholecystokinin. A hormone secreted in the wall of the duodenum when fat is present; causes contraction of the gallbladder and flow of bile.

chronic. Of long duration; opposed to acute.

chyme. The liquid food mass that has been digested in the stomach and is ready for passage through the duodenum.

coagulation. Change from a fluid to a semisolid or solid state; curd; clot.

coenzyme. A substance such as a vitamin that is a part of an enzyme.

colitis. Inflammation of the colon.

colon. The large intestine, beginning at the cecum.

coma. Unconsciousness; may result from accumulation of acids as in diabetes mellitus.

congenital. Present at birth.

consistency. Refers to the texture of a diet; liquid, soft, low-fiber, etc.

convulsion. Involuntary contraction of the muscles; may occur in eclampsia, uremic poisoning, and many other conditions.

cortisone. A hormone of the adrenal gland.

cretin. An individual who has inadequate physical and mental development because of insufficient thyroid secretion.

cultural. In study of food habits, refers to social, religious, national habits of a group of people.

decompensation, heart. Failure of the heart to adequately pump blood through the circulation.

dehydration. Abnormal loss of water from the body. Also, removal of water from food.

delirium. Mental disturbance characterized by physical restlessness, excitement, confusion, and delusions.

denaturation. The change of the physical state of a substance; for example, the coagulation of a protein.

dentine. The major calcified portion of the tooth; covered by enamel over the crown, and by cementum on the root portion of the tooth.

dermatitis. Inflammation of the skin.

dextrose. A single sugar; also called glucose.

dietetic food. A food prepared for specific uses in modified diets; for example, low-sodium, or packed without sugar.

distention. The state of stretching or enlarging; often refers to the accumulation of gases in the intestinal tract and the resultant feeling of fullness.

diuretic. Any substance that increases the volume of the urine.

DNA (deoxyribonucleic acid). A protein substance in the nucleus that carries genetic information.

duodenum. The first part of the small intestine beginning at the pylorus.

dysentery. An inflammation of the colon; often caused by bacterial or parasitic infection.

edema. Accumulation of fluid in the body.

electrolyte. Chemical substance in body fluids that can carry an electrical charge, for example, sodium (Na^+) or chlorine (Cl^-).

embryo. Early stage of development of the fetus.

emulsification. The breaking up of large particles into much smaller particles and suspending them in another liquid; for example, bile breaks up fat into minute droplets for digestion.

endemic. Refers to a disease being prevalent in a particular area.

endocrine. Any of the ductless glands such as the thyroid, adrenal, pituitary that secrete hormones into the blood circulation.

endosperm. The starchy portion of the cereal grain.

enzyme. A substance formed by living cells that speeds up chemical reactions: a living catalyst.

epithelium. Outer layer of the skin; includes the linings of the hollow organs, the respiratory, gastrointestinal, and genitourinary tracts.

erepsin. A group of protein-splitting enzymes secreted by the small intestine.

esophageal varices. Varicose veins of the esophagus.

extracellular. Around the cells.

extractive, meat. Nonprotein, nitrogen-containing, water-soluble substances in meat.

fallout. The radioactive dust that settles following explosion of a nuclear bomb.
feces. Excretion from the bowels.
fetus. Unborn young, especially in the later stages of development.
fibrinogen. A protein in blood necessary for clotting.
flatulence. Gas in the intestinal tract.

gastrectomy. Operation for removal of part or all of the stomach.
gastritis. Inflammation of the stomach.
genetic. Dealing with heredity.
genitourinary. Pertaining to the organs of reproduction and the urinary tract.
geriatrics. Branch of medicine concerned with diseases of older people.
gluten. Protein substance in cereal grains, especially wheat, that gives elastic quality to doughs.
glycerol. The organic compound to which fatty acids are attached to form a fat.
gristle. The tough connective-tissue fibers of meat.

hemicellulose. A complex, indigestible carbohydrate found in cell walls of plants.
hemoglobin. Red pigment in blood cells that carries oxygen.
hemorrhage. Loss of blood.
hepatic. Refers to the liver.
herbs. Group of plants having odors and flavors useful in the seasoning of foods; for example, sage, marjoram, thyme, and many others.
hormone. Chemical substance produced by a gland of the body and transported by the blood for activity in other tissues; thyroxine, insulin, and others.
hydrolysis. The splitting of a substance into simpler compounds by the addition of water.
hyper-. A prefix meaning increased, or greater than normal.
hyperalimentation. Intravenous feedings of solutions that are more concentrated than substances in blood.
hyperglycemia. Increased level of glucose in the blood.
hyperlipidemia. Elevation of one or more fatty components of blood, such as triglycerides, cholesterol, or lipoproteins.
hypertension. High blood pressure.
hypervitaminosis. Excess of vitamin storage in the body; for example, from an overdosage of vitamin A or D.
hypo-. A prefix meaning below normal.
hypochromic. Less color than normal; for example, hypochromic anemia.
hypothyroidism. Inadequate secretion of thyroid gland.

ileum. Lower part of the small intestine.
insulin. Hormone secreted by the islands of Langerhans in the pancreas; changes blood glucose to glycogen, increases uptake of glucose by the cell, and facilitates the formation of fat.
intracellular. Within the cell.
intravenous. Within the veins.
irradiation. Expose to rays such as ultraviolet rays, x-rays.

jejunum. Middle part of the small intestine, beginning at the duodenum and extending to the ileum.

ketosis. Condition resulting from the accumulation of ketones (acetone bodies) as a result of incomplete oxidation of fatty acids.

labile. Easily destroyed.

lactase. Enzyme produced by the small intestine; splits lactose to glucose and galactose.

lacteal. A small lymphatic vessel that takes up fatty substances from the intestinal wall.

legumes. Class of plant foods including beans, lentils, peas, peanuts.

lignin. Indigestible carbohydrate found in the cell wall of plants.

lipase. Enzyme produced by the pancreas that digests fats.

macrocyte. Giant red blood cell.

malabsorption. Failure to absorb the various nutrients from the intestinal tract; occurs in celiac disease, sprue, dysentery, diarrhea, and others.

maltase. Enzyme that splits maltose to two molecules of glucose.

marbled. Referring to meat, fine streaks of fat appearing throughout the lean portion of meat.

marinate. To soak meat, fish, or salad ingredients in a seasoned mixture such as wine, vinegar, French dressing.

median. The middle point; half of the values in a series of measurements will be above and half below this point.

micro-. Prefix meaning small; for example, *microcyte* is a very small cell; *microorganisms* include bacteria, yeasts, molds.

myo-. Refers to muscle; *myocardium* is the heart muscle; *myoglobin* is the iron-containing pigment in muscle.

nausea. Sick at the stomach with tendency to vomit.

nephritis. Inflammation of the kidney.

nyctalopia. Night blindness.

osmosis. Passage of fluid through membranes from weaker to stronger solution.

ossification. Hardening of the bone.

oxidase. A class of enzymes that brings about oxidation of products in metabolism.

oxidation. Combination of a substance with oxygen; an increase in the positive valence of an atom through the loss of electrons.

parathyroid. Gland located near the thyroid that secretes hormone for control of calcium metabolism.

parenteral. Outside the gastrointestinal tract; for example, injection into vein, under the skin.

pasta. Spaghetti, macaroni, noodles, and the like made from durum wheat flour.

pathogenic. Disease-producing.

pectin. A complex indigestible carbohydrate that has the capacity to hold water; found in many fruits such as apples.

pepsin. Enzyme secreted by the stomach for digestion of proteins.

peptidases. Class of enzymes that split peptides to amino acids.

peptones. Intermediate products in protein digestion.

peristalsis. Waves of contraction of muscle fibers in the intestinal tract that cause food to move through the tract.

photosynthesis. The process by which plants synthesize carbohydrates from carbon dioxide and water in the presence of light.

placenta. Organ attached to the wall of the uterus through which the fetus receives nourishment.

plasma. Fluid portion of the blood.

poly-. Prefix meaning much or many.

polydipsia. Excessive thirst.

polyneuritis. Inflammation of the nerves as in thiamin deficiency.

polypeptide. Groups of amino acids; intermediate stage in protein digestion.

polyphagia. Excessive appetite.

polyuria. Excessive amount of urine.

protease. Group of enzymes that digest proteins.

ptyalin. Starch-splitting enzyme in the saliva; also known as amylase.

purée. The pulp obtained by pressing food through a sieve to remove the fiber.

purines. Nitrogen-containing substances of a nonprotein nature occurring especially in meats; metabolized to uric acid.

pylorus. Circular opening of the stomach into the duodenum.

rancid. Having a disagreeable flavor or odor; usually affects foods high in fat content.

rectum. The lower part of the large intestine extending to the anal canal.

regimen. Dietary program.

rehabilitation. Restoration of health and efficiency as much as possible by physical, dietary, or other therapy.

renal. Referring to the kidney.

rennin. Enzyme secreted by the stomach that brings about coagulation of milk.

retina. The layer of the eye that receives the image and is connected to the brain by the optic nerve.

secretin. Hormone produced by the duodenum; stimulates pancreatic activity.

sedentary. Occupied in quiet activities; sitting, for example.

serum. Clear liquid that separates from clotted blood.

sphincter. A muscle surrounding and closing an opening; for example, pyloric sphincter.

spore. Reproductive part of a microorganism; very resistant to heat.

stabilizer. A substance added to food to help maintain quality over a period of time.

steapsin. Enzyme in the small intestine that digests fat; also called lipase.

steatorrhea. Excessive amount of fat in the feces.

subcutaneous. Beneath the skin.

sucrase. Enzyme produced by the small intestine that splits sucrose to glucose and fructose.

supplementary. Additional.

syndrome. A number of symptoms occurring together that are typical of a certain disease; for example, malabsorption syndrome.

synthesis. Formation of complex substances from simpler substances.

tenderizer. An enzyme preparation that partially breaks down meat fibers, thereby making the meat more tender.

thrombosis. Formation of clot in blood vessel, as in heart (coronary thrombosis) or brain (cerebral thrombosis).

toxemia. Condition in which the blood contains poisonous substances; for example, excess of nitrogenous wastes.

toxin. Poisonous product produced by cells; for example, botulin.

trauma. Injury.

trypsin. Protein-splitting enzyme produced by the pancreas.

ultraviolet rays. Light rays of shorter wave length than visible rays.

urea. The chief nitrogenous waste product in the urine.

uremia. Elevation of nitrogenous constituents in blood because of failure of kidney to remove them; renal failure.

uric acid. Nitrogenous product resulting from the breakdown of purines.

uterus. The womb.

vascular. Refers to the blood and lymph vessels in the body.

villus. Tiny fingerlike projection on the mucous lining of the small intestine; supplied with blood and lymph vessels.

viosterol. Activated ergosterol; vitamin D.

visual purple. Organic compound in retina of the eye that is changed to yellow by light; vitamin A is required for its synthesis.

INDEX

Information provided in tables is indicated by the letter *t* following page numbers; illustrations are indicated by numbers that appear in **bold-face** type.